Oxford Guide to Surviving as a CBT Therapist

Oxford Guides in Cognitive Behavioural Therapy

Oxford Guide to Low Intensity CBT Interventions
Bennett-Levy, Richards, Farrand, Christensen, Griffiths, Kavanagh, Klein, Lau, Proudfoot, Ritterband, Williams, and White

Oxford Guide to Surviving as a CBT Therapist
Mueller, Kennerley, McManus, and Westbrook

Oxford Guide to Metaphors in CBT
Stott, Mansell, Salkovskis, Lavender, and Cartwright-Hatton

Also published by Oxford University Press

The Oxford Guide to Behavioural Experiments in Cognitive Therapy
Bennett-Levy, Butler, Fennell, Hackmann, Mueller, and Westbrook

Oxford Guide to Surviving as a CBT Therapist

Edited by

Martina Mueller

Helen Kennerley

Freda McManus

David Westbrook

OXFORD
UNIVERSITY PRESS

OXFORD
UNIVERSITY PRESS

Great Clarendon Street, Oxford OX2 6DP

Oxford University Press is a department of the University of Oxford.
It furthers the University's objective of excellence in research, scholarship,
and education by publishing worldwide in

Oxford New York

Athens Auckland Bangkok Bogotá Buenos Aires Cape-Town
Chennai Dar es Salaam Delhi Florence Hong Kong Istanbul Karachi
Kolkata Kuala Lumpur Madrid Melbourne Mexico City Mumbai Nairobi
Paris São Paulo Shanghai Singapore Taipei Tokyo Toronto Warsaw

with associated companies in Berlin Ibadan

Oxford is a registered trade mark of Oxford University Press
in the UK and in certain other countries

Published in the United States
by Oxford University Press Inc., New York

First published 2010

British Library Cataloguing in Publication Data

Data available

Library of Congress Cataloging in Publication Data

Data available

Typeset in Minion by Glyph International, Bangalore, India
Printed in Great Britain
on acid-free paper by
Clays Ltd, St Ives Plc

ISBN 978–0–19–956130–8

10 9 8 7 6 5 4 3 2 1

Acknowledgements

We would like to express our gratitude to our colleagues, supervisees and those who came before us, whose ideas and skills we so fruitfully build on in our clinical practice. Above all we would like to thank our patients for their openness and willingness to change, and for teaching us the art of being a CBT therapist.

Preface

In the Oxford Cognitive Therapy Centre we meet, teach and supervise many CBT therapists. They tell us how content they are with their work, but we also hear about the difficulties they experience: the concerns of those who are newly trained and lacking confidence in their ability to apply their skills and knowledge outside a protected training milieu; the stresses of those working in isolation and therefore finding it difficult to widen their scope or bounce ideas off other CBT therapists; the particular problems of those who are faced with a therapy dilemma but who have no local expertise to guide them. Not infrequently, we have found ourselves relating to some of the difficulties—just how do you get practical advice on setting up group therapy? How do we marry theory with ethical practice? How does one maintain CBT integrity when combining it with the business of private practice? Which are the most important components to include if you only have six sessions?

One of the editors (MM) had the idea that we could draw on a wealth of knowledge amongst OCTC staff and associates that could form the basis of a 'How to...' book: a practical guide to dealing with some of the common challenges that arise in the working lives of CBT therapist. We all felt that this was a good idea and in 2008 several of us met for a mellow brainstorming exercise in front of a roaring fire. We were fortunate at that time in being joined by Melanie Fennell and Jon Wheatley whose contributions helped to shape this text. Very quickly our ideas fell into three categories: those concerning general clinical issues (such as common clinical dilemmas and ethical practice); those which addressed the challenges of working in specific settings or with specific patient groups (such as working within an IAPT low intensity setting or within an in-patient unit) and finally, those which considered continuing professional development, such as how we might develop as CBT therapists, supervisors, trainers and researchers.

When we began to shape ideas for the book we were very aware that we were doing so at a time when the UK government had announced that it would be committing a large amount of new funding to the NHS 'Improving Access to Psychological Therapies' (IAPT) programme, which aimed to train and employ thousands of new therapists, mostly doing CBT. We felt that this large group of newly, and often rapidly, trained therapists would particularly benefit from a practical guide to surviving the rigours of being a CBT therapist in practice, and we took this into account in including chapters on low intensity (LI) practice as well as practice in primary care and specialist settings.

When we sounded out our colleagues, we were thrilled by their enthusiasm and we have been very impressed by, and grateful for, their generosity in giving their time and careful consideration to writing what we feel are highly relevant chapters. We want to stress that the compilation of the book has been a group effort and reflects the hard work and expertise of a very wide range of contributors. The process of writing this book has been relatively harmonious and there has been great accord on the relevance of our choice of chapters.

However, there was one heated debate which, as far as we know, continues to fuel discussions—and that was the word we should use to describe the recipients of CBT: 'patient' or 'client'? Many passionate e-mails were exchanged and many of the authors felt strongly about this issue. Those who preferred the term 'patient' argued that this denotes someone for whom we care and do what is necessary to best help that person, whereas a 'client' is someone with whom we have a contractual relationship and for whom we do what is needed to fulfil the contract but no more. Authors who preferred the term 'client' thought that 'patient' was too medicalized a term, associated with a power imbalance and conveying passivity, while 'client' conveyed autonomy and the right to expect certain standards. In the end the vote for 'patient' was greater, partly because the evidence seems to be that that term is preferred by 'patients', and so we have stuck with that. We appreciate that not all readers will feel entirely comfortable with our choice but, to echo Wittgenstein, the meaning we ultimately ascribe to the term reflects how it is used. We feel that it has consistently been used to reflect a caring and respectful working relationship.

Prefaces usually say something about 'how to use the book' and in this case we would say that it depends on where you are in your career development, your particular interests, and what the demands of your current role are. You might dip into one or two chapters because you need a succinct overview of how you might move to private practice or how you can develop your supervision knowledge and skills, or you might feel that it would be useful to you to focus on a particular section: for example if you are just starting out in your career and want to review your options more widely you might focus on section 2 in particular. Our aim in writing this book was that you should use it how best suits you, and we hope that the material contained in it is of use to you in your career as a CBT therapist.

Martina Mueller, Helen Kennerley,
Freda McManus & David Westbrook

Contents

Contributors

James Bennett-Levy
Associate Professor at the
Northern Rivers University,
Department of Rural Mental Health,
Sydney University and Southern
Cross University,
Australia

Nicky Boughton
Associate Clinical Director for
Eating Disorders,
Cotswold House Specialist Eating
Disorders Service,
Oxfordshire and Buckinghamshire
Mental Health NHS Foundation Trust,
Oxford, UK

Sue Clohessy
Clinical Tutor, Oxford Doctoral
Course in Clinical Psychology,
Oxfordshire and Buckinghamshire
Mental Health NHS Foundation Trust,
Oxford and Consultant Clinical
Psychologist,
Berkshire Traumatic Stress Service,
Berkshire NHS Foundation Trust,
Traumatic Stress Service,
Reading, UK

Helen Close
Consultant Clinical Psychologist,
Psychological Services,
Oxfordshire and Buckinghamshire
Mental Health NHS Foundation
Trust,
Oxford, UK

Alison J. Croft
Consultant Clinical Psychologist,
Oxford Cognitive Therapy Centre and
Psychological Services,
Oxfordshire and Buckinghamshire
Mental Health NHS Foundation Trust,
Oxford, UK

June Dent
Consultant Clinical Psychologist,
Oxfordshire and Buckinghamshire
Mental Health NHS Foundation Trust,
Oxford, UK

Melanie Fennell
Consultant Clinical Psychologist and
Co-Director of the Oxford Course in
Advanced Cognitive Therapy Studies,
Oxford Cognitive Therapy Centre,
Oxfordshire and Buckinghamshire
Mental Health NHS Foundation Trust,
Oxford, UK;
Co-Director of the MSC in
Mindfulness-Based Cognitive Therapy,
Oxford University Department of
Psychiatry,
Warneford Hospital,
Oxford, UK

Ann Hackmann
Consultant Clinical Psychologist,
Oxford University Department of
Psychiatry and Oxford Cognitive
Therapy Centre,
Oxfordshire and Buckinghamshire
Mental Health NHS Foundation Trust,
Oxford, UK

Louise Hankinson
Clinical Psychologist,
Clinical Health Psychology,
Berkshire Healthcare NHS
Foundation Trust,
Oxford, UK

Patsy Holly
Consultant Clinical Psychologist,
Thames Valley Forensic Mental
Health Service,
Oxfordshire and Buckinghamshire
Mental Health NHS Foundation Trust,
Oxford, UK

Tony Hope
Professor of Medical Ethics,
The Ethox Centre, University of
Oxford; and
Honorary Consultant Psychiatrist

Helen Jenkins
Clinical Psychologist and Clinical Tutor,
Oxford Doctoral Course in
Clinical Psychology,
Oxfordshire and Buckinghamshire
Mental Health NHS Foundation Trust,
Oxford, UK

Helen Kennerley
Consultant Clinical Psychologist,
Oxford Cognitive Therapy Centre
and Psychological Services,
Oxfordshire and Buckinghamshire
Mental Health NHS Foundation
Trust,
Oxford, UK

David Kingdon
Professor of Mental Health Care
Delivery,
University of Southampton,
Southampton, UK

Joan Kirk
Clinical Psychologist in Private
Practice

Claudia Koch
Principal Clinical Psychologist,
Prison Mental Health In-Reach Team,
Oxfordshire and Buckinghamshire
Mental Health NHS Foundation Trust,
Oxford, UK

Freda McManus
Clinical Research Fellow,
Department of Psychiatry,
University of Oxford, and
Course Director,
Oxford Diploma in Cognitive Therapy,
Oxford Cognitive Therapy Centre,
Oxfordshire and Buckinghamshire
Mental Health NHS Foundation Trust,
Oxford, UK

Rebecca Mitchell
Consultant Clinical Psychologist,
Psychological Services,
Oxfordshire and Buckinghamshire
Mental Health NHS Foundation Trust,
Oxford, UK

Harriet Montgomery
Consultant Clinical Psychologist,
Psychological Services,
Oxfordshire and Buckinghamshire
Mental Health NHS Foundation Trust,
Oxford, UK

Martina Mueller
Consultant Clinical Psychologist
Oxford Cognitive Therapy Centre
and Psychological Services,
Oxfordshire and Buckinghamshire
Mental Health NHS Foundation Trust,
Oxford, UK

Farooq Naeem
Research Fellow,
Southampton University,
Southampton, UK

Peter Phiri
Research Fellow,
Southampton University,
Southampton, UK

Shanaya Rathod
Consultant Psychiatrist,
Mid Hampshire and Eastleigh
NHS Trust,
Winchester, UK

Dave Richards
Professor of Mental Health
Services Research,
School of Psychology,
University of Exeter,
Exeter, UK

Jill Roberts
Clinical Nurse Specialist,
Cotswold House Specialist Eating
Disorders Service, Oxfordshire and
Buckinghamshire Mental Health
NHS Foundation Trust,
Oxford, UK

Kate Rosen
Clinical Psychologist in Private
Practice

Joanne Ryder
Consultant Clinical Psychologist,
Oxford Cognitive Therapy Centre
and Psychological Services,
Oxfordshire and Buckinghamshire
Mental Health NHS Foundation
Trust,
Oxford, UK

Heather Salt
Consultant Clinical Psychologist,
Department Psychological Medicine,
Oxfordshire and Buckinghamshire
Mental Health NHS Foundation Trust,
Oxford and IAPT Course Director
(PWP),
University of Reading,
Reading, UK

Diana Sanders
Counselling Psychologist,
Department of Psychological
Medicine,
Oxfordshire and Buckinghamshire
Mental Health NHS Foundation Trust,
Oxford, UK

Anne Stewart
Consultant Child and Adolescent
Psychiatrist,
Oxford City CAMHS,
Oxfordshire and Buckinghamshire
Mental Health NHS Foundation Trust,
Oxford, and
Honorary Senior Clinical Lecturer,
University of Oxford,
Oxford, UK

Ailsa Stuart
Clinical Psychologist,
Psychological Services,
Oxfordshire and Buckinghamshire
Mental Health NHS Foundation Trust,
Oxford, UK

Christina Surawy
Clinical Psychologist,
Department Psychological Medicine,
Oxfordshire and Buckinghamshire
Mental Health NHS Foundation Trust,
Oxford, UK

David Westbrook
Director of Oxford Cognitive
Therapy Centre,
Oxfordshire and Buckinghamshire
Mental Health NHS Foundation Trust,
Oxford, UK

Daniel Zahl
Clinical Psychologist,
Buckinghamshire PCT, High Wycombe,
and Department of Infectious Diseases,
Oxford Radcliffe Trust,
Oxford, UK

Chapter 1

Common problems in therapy

David Westbrook, Martina Mueller, Helen Kennerley, and Freda McManus

Introduction

Anyone who has practised cognitive behavioural therapy (CBT) with more than a few patients knows that it is not as easy as it sometimes seems in books or videos. The smooth courses of CBT described there can seem a long way from the messy, difficult, and sometimes frustrating courses of therapy that are normal daily experience for many of us. This is perhaps particularly striking when we move from the more protected existence of a trainee to a post-qualification job, with its increased responsibilities and heavier caseload, often at the same time as supervision is reduced. Some patients do not make the best use of therapy, therapists sometimes feel at sea, and some courses of CBT do not end satisfactorily. The aim of this chapter is therefore to set the scene for the rest of this book by addressing life as a clinician 'in the real world'. The rest of the book will then go on to consider more specialized aspects of developing as a CBT therapist and applying your skills in a range of settings.

We are concerned here with the everyday problems that may, for example, make it difficult to engage patients in treatment, dilute the effectiveness of CBT, or make it hard to end treatment well. We are not aiming to teach you basic CBT strategies—there are many texts that do that very well—nor even to reproduce the work of more advanced books. Our aim is to consider some of the common clinical problems that may arise for therapists and patients who are doing *any* kind of CBT with *any* kind of patient or problem.

What factors affect the outcome of therapy?

A course of CBT is shaped by both therapist and patient, by their interactions with each other, and by the therapy model (which tells us what patient and therapist are expected to do, how they are to achieve their goals, and so on). Both therapist and patient also live and work within their own contexts *outside* the therapy sessions, and these contexts can also affect therapy. Your patient might live in adverse circumstances, or the service in which you work might impose seemingly impossible restrictions on therapy. Some of these contextual factors are easily noticeable, for example, when a patient tells you that she has had a significant bereavement in the past week. Others can sneak up on the unwary: for example, you might not notice that the quality of therapy is compromised by your always seeing a patient last thing on a Friday afternoon, when you are both too tired to apply yourselves well.

Figure 1.1 summarizes this picture of the interacting factors that may determine the outcome of therapy.

So if we are thinking about where difficulties may arise, we need to consider any or all of these factors as potential sources of difficulty.

The therapy model

- The characteristics of the therapy, its demands and expectations, its theoretical models, and its understanding of the nature of psychological problems and appropriate treatment strategies.
- The interaction between either patient or therapist and the therapy model: what they make of it, how they approach it, and so on.

The therapist

- The therapist's personal characteristics (personality, style, knowledge and skills, attitudes and beliefs, etc.)
- The therapist's contexts (organizational factors, service constraints and demands, personal situation, family, social, and cultural setting, etc.)

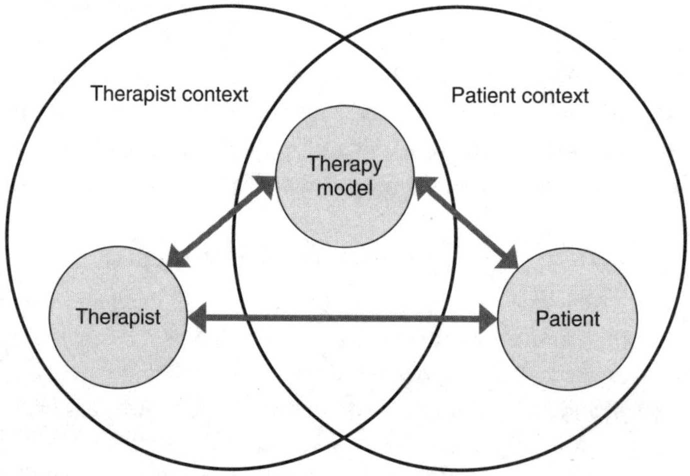

Fig. 1.1 Factors affecting therapy.

The patient

- The patient's personal characteristics (personality, problems, previous therapeutic history, attitudes and beliefs, etc.)
- The patient's contexts (work situation, family, social, and cultural setting, etc.)

Therapist-patient interaction

- Processes by which the interactions between therapist and patient characteristics may become unhelpful.

This chapter will examine some of the common problems in these different areas and provide some guidance on how to manage them, as well as pointing you towards other chapters in this book that expand on some of these topics.

The golden rule: *use* the CBT model...

Before moving on to consider particular common problems, let us begin with some general guidance that can be summed up by a simple motto:

> In cognitive therapy, you should doubt everything...except cognitive therapy!

This motto is a reminder that you should always be skeptical, and look for evidence to support or contradict your or your patient's hypotheses; but also that when you run into problems with the model, you should not drop it too rapidly, but rather *use* cognitive therapy to understand what is going on and find possible solutions (*cf.* Schulte's work described below).

Use the formulation

So when you run into difficulties the golden rules are:

1. Understand the patient's (and/or your own) thoughts, feelings, and behaviours; and then
2. Consider how you can work with these so as to improve the therapy.

And of course the way to encapsulate that understanding is through a CBT *formulation* that tells you what thoughts and behaviours are affecting this problem in therapy, and what processes are preventing the problems from being resolved (see Westbrook *et al.*, 2007, Chapter 4 on formulation; also Chapter 9 of the present volume, on systemic formulations).

Any exploration of treatment problems therefore begins with your assessment and formulation: either the original formulation, which may already enable you to understand what is going on; or, if it does not, then a new or modified formulation that will extend your understanding. This might be a 'mini-formulation' of the specific obstacle, or a total reformulation of your patient's difficulties. In either case, when you become aware of an impediment to therapy, do just what we recommend to patients: stand back and try to conceptualize what's going on, taking account of the areas that we have noted in Fig. 1.1, and which are described further in following sections (and, of course, make use of your clinical supervision to help you reflect on the problems).

Use collaboration

Another key feature of CBT to use when there are problems is its open and collaborative approach. In other words, *talk* to your patient about any difficulties and use *both* the heads in the room to look for solutions.

> *Lindsey had been referred for CBT for recurrent depression and low self-esteem. By the time she entered treatment her mood had improved significantly, but Lindsey's self-esteem remained low. She found it difficult to make day-to-day choices, felt anxious about making even small decisions (especially in relation to her boyfriend), and struggled to do anything pleasant for herself. She and her therapist constructed a formulation based on Fennell's model of low self-esteem and proceeded to work on key maintaining cycles. After 8 sessions, despite Lindsey's very active participation in treatment, nothing seemed to be changing. Problems seemed to vanish on closer inspection, or impossible obstacles arose from nowhere. Concerned about the lack of progress, the therapist began to dread the sessions.*
>
> *The therapist took his concern to supervision and decided to schedule a review session with Lindsey. Lindsey said that she found the sessions valuable but that progress was perhaps slower than expected, and they agreed to revise the formulation to include a greater focus on the interpersonal aspects of Lindsey's difficulties. The sessions continued with this slight change of direction, but still nothing changed and the therapist still felt guilty and at sea. Then, during the 10th session, Lindsay noticed a (switched off) digital voice recorder on her therapist's desk. She became anxious and distressed, and requested that the recorder be removed from the office. This struck the therapist as an unusual request, so he tried to find out what might be causing Lindsey's reaction. However she became uncharacteristically opaque, and answered questions in monosyllables.*
>
> *The therapist decided to change his approach and reflected on Lindsey's changed demeanour. Slowly she was able to reveal that she had "this thing" that she didn't like to talk about and which caused her a great deal of anxiety. It gradually became clear that she had long standing OCD, with concerns about harm to important others. Her worry was that she might say something upsetting which might then come to their attention, and that this in turn might lead them to harm themselves, accidentally or deliberately.*
>
> *By expressing his concerns about therapy, Lindsey's therapist was able to pave the way towards a more meaningful re-formulation and a more manageable treatment approach. He was able to reinforce the importance of her honest input, which in turn helped tackle her belief that she was not capable. Without addressing the*

lack of progress directly with Lindsay, it is likely that her OCD issues would not have come to light and thus it would not have been possible to make progress in CBT as it was these difficulties that were exacerbating her low self-esteem.

Use structure

It is easy to get lost and meander when things do not go smoothly in therapy. Make sure that you keep your sessions under review, regularly taking stock of your agenda, therapy goals, and treatment protocol.

Lindsey's therapist realized that he had "coasted" for a couple of sessions after she had first revealed that she was not making progress. In his attempt to be supportive, and in order to buy himself some time to work out what was going on, he had allowed the sessions to turn into supportive counselling rather than CBT. With hindsight, he realized that it would have been more productive to stick firmly but compassionately with homework tasks that were then properly reviewed. This would have quickly shed light on unhelpful safety behaviours, would have helped them to construct more realistic assignments, and would have informed the re-formulation more rapidly.

Use the empirical approach

The last aspect of the general CBT approach that can be usefully applied to obstacles in therapy is to adopt an empirical style. In other words, follow the general CBT preference for the gathering and careful consideration of *evidence*, rather than sticking blindly to some theoretical preconception. If you or your patient thinks that some particular factor is interfering with therapy, don't get into endless sterile discussions—or even worse, arguments!—about how to tackle the problem; instead, try things out through behavioural experiments and *see* what works best to remove the obstacles.

Following the re-formulation described above, Lindsey agreed to a number of in-session experiments to test the nature of her fears and to find out whether harm does come to others simply by mentioning them in conversation.

Once Lindsey appreciated that she could give honest feedback during the development of homework, she and her therapist devised tasks that she was more inclined to try out. Her longstanding worries meant that she still felt reluctant, but at least she now expressed this. She and her therapist highlighted the "no-lose" status of behavioural experiments—that either she would be able to complete the experiment and thus learn something important that was relevant to her difficulties, or she wouldn't be able to complete the experiment but would learn more about what made it difficult for her in such situations. This view gave her licence to "have a go" even if she was not confident of success. She began to make progress both with her original goals and with the therapy-interfering beliefs that were identified when her difficulties were re-formulated.

The role of CBT as a therapy model

Let us now turn to some of the specific areas for common difficulties identified in Fig. 1.1. This section will consider the role of CBT as a therapy model, and how that may interact with particular therapists or patients.

Characteristics and demands of CBT

CBT nowadays is a very broad church, and we have neither the space nor the expertise to examine the characteristics of every type of therapy that might be included under that heading. Therefore, like most other chapters in this book, we will focus on what is probably currently 'mainstream' CBT in the United Kingdom, based on the 'Beckian' model first developed by Beck (1976). This approach to therapy has several characteristics that may be important to consider when you run into problems:

- It rests on a *collaborative* relationship between patient and therapist, in which both work together to solve problems.
- It is usually relatively *short term* (typically 5–20 sessions).
- It assumes that the patient has—or can easily learn to get—*access to thoughts and emotions.*
- It is *structured*, for example, in setting agendas, working towards clear goals, incorporating standard session elements, etc.
- It expects patients to be able—with appropriate help—to *confront* their fears and *tolerate* negative emotions.
- *Behaviour change* is often a central part of the process.
- It uses *homework* as an essential element of treatment.

Assessing 'suitability' for CBT

It follows from the preceding list of qualities that problems may arise in therapy to the extent that patients or therapists do *not* fit with these assumptions, and it may therefore be important to consider them in assessment. One approach to such assessment is the Suitability for Short-term Cognitive Therapy scale (SSCT; Safran and Segal, 1990). Based on an interview with the patient, the therapist rates 10 factors as follows:

1 Accessibility of automatic thoughts
2 Awareness and differentiation of emotions
3 Acceptance of personal responsibility for change
4 Compatibility with the cognitive rationale (acceptance of links between thoughts and feelings, role of homework, etc.)
5 Alliance potential 1 (*in-session evidence* of ability to develop therapeutic relationship)

6 Alliance potential 2 (*out-of-session* evidence of ability to develop relationships, i.e. in patient's 'real life' in the world outside the therapy room)

7 (Lack of) Chronicity of problems

8 (Lack of) Security operations (i.e. unhelpful strategies to reduce anxiety or maintain self-esteem)

9 Focality (ability to work with a specific problem focus)

10 Client optimism regarding therapy[1]

For more details and scoring criteria, see Safran and Segal (1990) and Safran *et al.* (1993).

The SSCT is scored in such a way that high scores indicate greater likelihood of response, and there is some evidence that scores on the SSCT correlate with the outcome of therapy (Safran *et al.*, 1993; Myhr *et al.*, 2007). However, it is important to be clear that this is a statistical association, and definitely *not* strong enough to be a clear guide to selection in an individual case. The status of the evidence is like the evidence that men are on average taller than women. That is of course true, but we would not expect to make accurate judgements about gender if we picked a height—say 5 feet 10 inches—and classed everyone less than that as a woman and everyone taller than that as a man: such a decision procedure would lead to many errors! Similarly there is no simple cut-off score on the SSCT below which we can say with confidence that an individual will *not* respond to CBT. Indeed, Safran and Segal themselves have said that such decisions ultimately must rest on the therapist's clinical judgement. The SSCT may help to structure and inform such judgements, but it is not a simple answer that can *substitute* for judgement.

The same problem affects any simple procedure for classifying patients as 'suitable' or not, and therefore many clinicians believe that the best way of determining suitability in any individual case is to 'suck it and see': in other words, to have a trial period of therapy and see how it works out in practice. Figure 1.2 shows a procedural diagram of how such a process might work.

Although this kind of process is widely used, there are potential problems. Therapists often find it difficult to say 'This isn't working' (for fear of upsetting patients; because there is no reasonable alternative treatment available; because it makes them feel incompetent; or for many other reasons). Therefore, the obvious danger is that what is supposed to be a careful decision-making procedure actually ends up as an endless loop round the central part of Fig. 1.2, with the therapist constantly thinking that 'just a bit more' treatment will do the trick … with the end result that 5–20 sessions becomes 50–200! How can you minimize such problems?

[1] This item seems to have been dropped in the version of the SSCT described in Safran *et al.* (1993).

- Be clear and consistent with your patients in conveying the message that this *is* a trial of therapy, not an open-ended commitment: 'We will keep things under review to see if CBT is helpful for you. If at any time we feel that it isn't, then we can consider other options…'
- Set clear goals that are operationalized, so that both you and the patient can tell whether they have been achieved or not (of course these should not be too ambitious for a short trial).
- When it is necessary to say 'This isn't working', do it in a way that minimizes negative messages as far as possible. For instance, not 'You (the patient) have failed' but 'CBT might not be quite right for you, maybe we should think about alternatives…'; 'Maybe you would be better off with… (some alternative approach)'; or 'It seems like the time is not right for you at the moment, but maybe you could try again at some future time…'. Of course, such explanations should only be used if they are founded on truth.

There may also be occasions when you decided to persist even though there *isn't* any good reason to believe that another few sessions will do the trick. For example, you might persist with a patient who is suicidal, even though your CBT is not likely to result in anything like full recovery, because it seems the suicide risk would be increased by stopping; or you (together with your manager/supervisor) might decide that it is worth giving a longer-than-usual trial

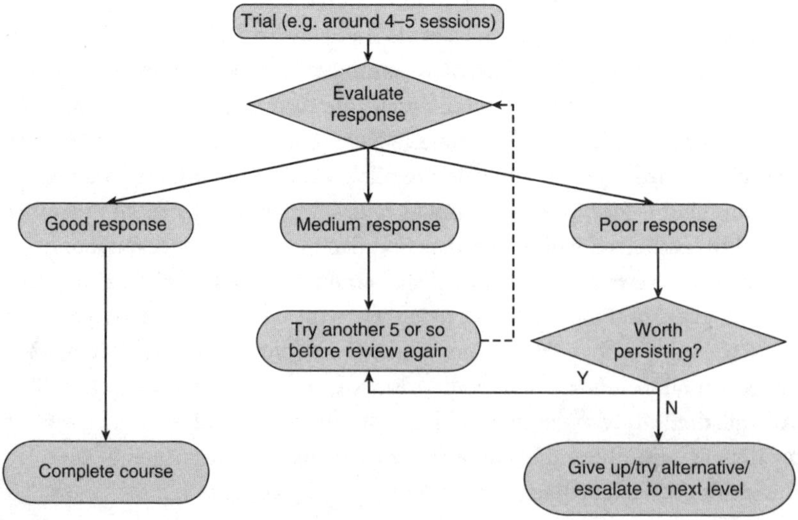

Fig. 1.2 Possible procedure for a trial of therapy.

of treatment to someone with a history of treatment resistance, in order to make sure that all reasonable options have been exhausted.

Difficulties in applying the model

Of course we would all like to work with patients who respond positively to CBT and are comfortable with all the features outlined above, but real-life patients are often not like that. So what happens if your patient does not fit with one or more of the above characteristics of CBT? Let us consider some of these possible problems.

Difficulties in collaboration

A common problem in collaboration comes from patients who adopt a very passive attitude, conveying the message that it is up to you to fix their problems. The golden rule tells us that the first step is to identify possible factors contributing to this attitude. For example:

- Is your patient feeling very defeated and hopeless, so that he cannot imagine being able to make a difference to the problems himself?
- Has your patient come from a hierarchical or authoritarian background that leads her to believe that it is the expert's job to tell her what to do?
- Has your patient had previous experiences of medical or psychiatric care that was delivered in such a 'top-down' manner, and therefore understandably assumes that you will follow the same model?

Identifying the thoughts and emotions contributing to passivity may enable you to explore and modify them using standard CBT methods for testing beliefs.

A particularly difficult version of this problem is the patient who seems to be saying 'Solve my problems but don't make me change'. In other words, I want things to *be* different, but I don't want to have to *do* anything different. Possible thoughts or beliefs leading to this attitude include hopelessness, as above, or possibly fear—fear either of what is necessary to overcome the problem (e.g. difficult behavioural experiments, reflecting on traumatic memories, or experiencing strong emotion); or fear of what may follow if the problem is tackled (e.g. my family won't like it, or my employers will demand more of me). A good analogy to help patients think about this is to think about how one might tackle being overweight. Most patients can see that (barring surgical or similar methods) no doctor will be able to help them to lose weight without *their* changing—either the amount they eat or the amount of energy they use. Nevertheless, a weight loss clinic may be able to help them find the best way to change their behaviour, to problem-solve difficulties, and to support them through the process—and a CBT therapist can take a similar role.

A common attribution that therapists make when a patient does not seem to be fully contributing to therapy is that he/she is 'not motivated'. This can sometimes be no more than an easy excuse that lets us off the hook: 'The failure is not mine, it's because the patient is not motivated…' Nevertheless there are of course differences in the degree of commitment that patients show to therapy. Many factors may contribute to this, but a simple rule of thumb is that 'motivation' for a particular therapy or therapeutic procedure depends on the patient's:

- *Understanding* why the procedure might be useful;
- *Believing* that you and they are capable of doing it; and
- *Evaluating* the balance of costs and benefits of the procedure as having more pros than cons.

Thus, 'poor motivation' may come from a lack of understanding of the relevance of a strategy, a lack of belief in their own or your capacity to implement it, or seeing the costs as outweighing the benefits. Look at these factors with your patient and see whether any of these perceptions may be distorted or inaccurate (but also be prepared to acknowledge that for some patients the balance will come out *against* taking part in therapy, at least at this time).

At the opposite extreme is the patient who is unable to accept any input from you as therapist, but who feels she has to control every part of therapy herself. Let her! Or at least, let her try it out as an experiment, so long as you can agree how to evaluate the effect of doing that. This can be a classic 'no lose' strategy: either she is right and she makes better progress this way; or she has some evidence that may help her to adopt a different approach which will in turn lead to better progress.

From the beginning of his course of CBT, Bill was reluctant to discuss tasks he might do between sessions. He had no objection to the idea of homework in principle, but thought that he needed to "mull things over for a bit" after each session before deciding what sort of task would be most helpful or important for him, rather than plan them in session with his therapist. Bill's therapist outlined her concerns about this strategy: "Homework really matters"; "The more specific and tailored it is the more useful it is likely to be"; "Two heads might be better than one in deciding what might be useful and doable"; and so on. But Bill, in a calm but definite manner, remained firm: "Yeah, but I'm going to try it my way, and see how far I get". And that is what he did, perhaps not in a textbook order or in quite the careful, controlled, "no lose" way that his therapist might have liked, but his homework was always useful, always linked to issues that had been addressed in session—and usually recorded on colourful bits of scrap paper!

Difficulties in short-term therapy

In principle, CBT is adaptable to longer-term work as well as the classic short-term CBT of 5–20 sessions. For example, in schema-focused therapy for personality disorders, treatment may consist of 3 years of twice-weekly sessions (Giesen-Bloo *et al.*, 2006). But what can you do if you are working in a context where therapy is fairly strictly limited to 10 or 20 sessions, but you are still trying to help people with multiple complex problems because there is nowhere else for them to go? Some thoughts:

- Remember that in many areas there is actually little clear evidence that very long treatments do much better than shorter ones, so it is not *necessarily* the case that longer treatment is better (Howard *et al.*, 1986; Baldwin *et al.*, 2009).
- Pick one specific focus for therapy that your formulation suggests might have an effect on other problems, and work with that (e.g. just tackle the post-traumatic stress disorder [PTSD] or the obsessive-compulsive disorder [OCD] or the eating disorder…). In many cases, there are 'ripple' effects from treating one problem that lead on to improvements in other problems (but you may need to help your patient appreciate *how* she might generalize, rather than just leaving it up to her to work it out).
- Remember that it may be better for you and your patient to think of therapy as *teaching skills* rather than *curing problems*. In other words, therapy does not always have to solve all your patient's problems. It may be as good or better to help them to learn the psychological skills they need to tackle their problems for themselves, so they can then use those skills to make progress over a much longer time period than just a course of therapy.
- Work in collaboration with others who can continue where you leave off. For example, a community mental health team, a specialist eating disorder service, or a general practitioner might provide ongoing support during your intervention, and also help your patient maintain progress after you have discharged her.

Difficulties in accessing thoughts or emotions

Some patients may find it difficult to report thoughts or, more rarely, emotions in the way that the CBT approach asks them to do. Possible approaches to this include:

- Sometimes negative thoughts are not accessible because the patient has become so adept at avoidance or other safety behaviours that he/she no longer experiences the thoughts. In such cases, it may be useful to do behavioural experiments, not so much as a directly therapeutic strategy but rather as an assessment strategy: if the patient can stop or reduce the safety behaviours, then the negative thoughts may become more prominent.

- Sometimes there are no *clear* negative thoughts, in words or images: instead it may be more productive to ask your patient about the *meaning* of the event or situation: 'What did this seem to be saying about you (or the world, or other people, or the future)?'; 'What was it about this situation that bothered you?'; 'What was the worst thing about it?'
- Or you might ask about the *opposite* of the problem: 'What would have to be different for you to feel OK about this?'; 'What would have to change about the situation (or yourself), for this not to be a problem for you?'
- Some patients find it difficult or impossible to describe, or even directly experience, emotional states (a problem known as *alexithymia*). This often arises from experiences which have led the person to see emotion as dangerous or destructive, and hence to avoid expressing or even experiencing emotion. As always it is important to formulate the factors causing or maintaining this avoidance and see what you can do to modify them. The avoidance is often based on a 'slippery slope' belief: that allowing one small bit of negative emotion will result in collapsing and being completely unable to cope. A graduated approach to identifying emotions and allowing experience of them, first in sessions and then elsewhere, may lead to some reduction in this belief.

  Alicia was experiencing severe PTSD following an assault. Before the assault she had always seen herself as a strong person who was able to cope with life. Her subsequent PTSD symptoms made her see herself as one of the "weak" people whom she had previously looked down on for not keeping their emotional reactions under control. Alicia's need to be in control of her emotions was very difficult in CBT for PTSD, as it meant that she was not willing to do the re-living component. She feared that her emotional reactions would be uncontainable and that she would be permanently "broken" if she let her emotions spiral out of control in this way. Several behavioural experiments to test out the consequences of letting herself get upset were required before she was able to engage in the more emotional tasks of therapy.

Difficulties with structure

Some patients have difficulty with the relatively high degree of structure and focus in CBT. We ask people to set agendas, focus on particular topics agreed for the agenda, put their efforts into changing specific problems, and so on. Some patients may find this degree of structure difficult simply because of their own natural approach: they just have a more discursive style and experience structure as constricting. For such patients it may be best to be flexible, within reason, to accommodate their preferences. However, it is also important to be aware that some patients may find it hard to focus on specific topics because of their psychological problems. Perhaps they find it extremely aversive to look at their negative thoughts or beliefs, or social anxiety makes them nervous about allowing any silence during an interaction. In such cases, their difficulty with the structure of CBT may be a problem that needs tackling if therapy is to be as effective as possible. As always, follow the golden rules of discussing with your patient and formulating the problem, in order to choose the best course of action.

After six sessions with Patrick his therapist was becoming concerned that they didn't seem to be making progress with his OCD after the initial formulation. The sessions were entirely taken up with Patrick's trying to tell her every detail of his perceived "sins", and seeking reassurance that she didn't think he was a bad person and that he hadn't inadvertently caused harm to his family. No time was left for focused CBT.

Addressing this reassurance-seeking directly meant that the therapist was able to get Patrick to agree to more structure for their sessions. He agreed (a) to spend no more than 10 minutes reviewing the week; and (b) that when he sought reassurance, instead of giving it, the therapist would help Patrick either to devise a behavioural experiment to test whether he had caused anyone harm, or to complete a thought record to evaluate whether his actions meant he was a bad person. They also added "Seeking reassurance from authority figures" as a maintenance cycle in the formulation. Then when it occurred in sessions they were able to identify it, note it as something that maintained the problem rather than solved it, and move on.

Difficulties in facing difficult situations

All of us who do CBT are sometimes amazed and humbled by the courage with which our patients face up to situations which are immensely painful, or which seem to them to involve terrible risks. But no one can be brave all the time, and sometimes your patient may find it difficult or impossible to face up to some difficult situations. Common factors that may be part of the formulation for such problems include:

- When avoidance has been someone's main coping strategy for difficult situations for a long time.
- Particularly strong fearful beliefs, for example, patients with OCD who have little doubt that the disasters they fear for themselves or their family will really happen.
- 'Head versus heart'—when people say for example, 'I know (some disaster) is not really likely to happen but when I'm in the situation it *feels* as if it is'.
- Hopelessness, when your patient feels it is pointless to go through the difficulties, because they are bound to fail anyway.
- 'If I don't try then I can't fail'—which is usually driven by a strong fear of looking foolish or being criticized if they fail to complete a task.

In many such cases it may be useful to look for a more limited initial goal; it is surprising how often pulling back to a slightly less ambitious target will result in success, and boost confidence in a way that then allows your patient to face up to something more difficult.

Although Aseem's ultimate goal was to be able to give presentations at work, he felt too anxious to be able to approach this at all in his CBT for social phobia. He and his therapist had tried to devise behavioural experiments that involved giving a talk to an audience, without success. Aseem was expressing hopelessness about therapy, so his therapist attempted to scale back the task to something that Aseem might be more able to manage.

They began with his practising standing reading from a book in an entirely empty room; then progressed to reading aloud with the therapist in the room; then moved on to his watching a video of this experiment. The video gave him more confidence that his anxiety symptoms were not as obvious as he had feared and he was soon able to move on to giving a short talk in front of the therapist. By working gradually and reviewing the videos along the way, Aseem was eventually able to give talks to the therapist's colleagues and finally in his own place of work.

Alternatively of course, work with specific problematic beliefs that are getting in the way, to see if there are ways to help your patient reconsider them, and therefore be more able to tackle the area of difficulty. See the section on patient characteristics below for further discussion of some of these problems.

Difficulties with homework

We all know that homework plays a central role in CBT, for several reasons:

- There is evidence of a positive link between homework and outcome in CBT (e.g. Kazantzis *et al.*, 2000; Schmidt and Woolaway-Bickel, 2000).
- It helps to engage patients in the collaborative approach.
- It helps patients to transfer learning from the therapy room to 'real life' in the outside world, and thus helps us to make best use of limited session time.

Homework obviously needs collaboration between you and your patient and also often involves facing difficulties, so some of the factors outlined above may apply here as well. Other factors may be more specific to homework:

- Patients may genuinely forget, or misunderstand, what they are supposed to do and how they are supposed to do it. Avoiding such problems is all about preparation. Did you discuss the homework collaboratively? Did you make sure your patient understood what was to be done and why it would be useful? Did you anticipate any practical problems? Did you ensure that your patient had, and was able to use, any diaries, record forms, rating scales, etc.? Did you check how demanding it was likely to be? Did you—or preferably, your patient—write down exactly what was to be done, when and how? If the answer to any of these questions is 'No', then you know what to try first!

- Of course if your patient *keeps on* 'forgetting', or running into other problems, despite reasonable attempts at reminders and problem-solving, then you may need to look more carefully at the formulation and identify possible blocking beliefs.
- It is a cliché—but no less true for that—that some patients do not like the word *homework*, because it brings back unpleasant memories of demanding but pointless tasks from schooldays. Therefore, it may be helpful to find different words for the concept: *self-help exercises*, or *therapy tasks*, or anything else that feels better for your patient.

The nature of the problem

Perhaps the most common difficulty in applying the CBT model is when patients do not easily fit into the established protocols for treating specific disorders. There are two frequent reasons for this:

- *The patient has multiple problems ('co-morbidity').*
  One should note that this pattern is, if anything, the rule rather than the exception. In clinical practice, a high proportion of patients have problems that do not fit neatly into one diagnostic category. In such cases it can be hard to know how to proceed. Should you follow the treatment model for problem 1, followed by the model for problem 2, followed by…? And if so, in what order? Or try to tackle them all at once? If so, how?

  There are two possible approaches here. First, it may be worth seeing whether the problems can reasonably be understood as linked together in some way, perhaps by a common feature such as 'fear of failure'. If so, then an intervention targeted at that common feature may be an economical way of tackling the problem. Such a formulation may also be helpful in unifying different parts of therapy: in the above example, whatever you're working on in any particular session, it can be related back to the central idea of 'fear of failure'.

  Alternatively, it may be better to see whether your formulation suggests that one of the problems appears to be of more central importance, so that you might reasonably suppose that improvement in that problem might have an effect on other problems as well. If so, tackle that problem according to the protocol. Craske *et al.* (2007) provide some interesting evidence that for patients with panic disorder plus at least one co-morbid disorder, CBT focused just on the panic actually had better outcomes for *both* disorders than did CBT that tried to tackle the co-morbid disorder(s) as well.

- *The patient has a problem for which there is no established treatment.* In such cases it is clearly impossible to follow a protocol! However, remember that the generic CBT model can be applied to pretty much any psychological problem (and has been), so it may be possible to proceed by formulating the problem(s) from first principle. Ask yourself how you might use basic CBT ideas to make sense of the problem(s) in a way that is credible and offers some useful guide to treatment. There are many common maintenance processes that operate across different disorders, and you may be able to formulate using these (see Westbrook *et al.*, 2007, Chapter 4, for some examples of such common processes; also see Harvey *et al.*, 2004, for a fascinating exploration of a 'transdiagnostic' approach to CBT).

  In considering this question, take care not to cause yourself difficulty by confusing diagnosis, or problem label, with the possible aetiology of that problem. Therapists sometimes say things like 'This patient has been referred with childhood trauma and there is no treatment protocol for that'. Even if that is true, the childhood trauma is not a disorder in itself, but rather part of the aetiology of what may be a clear presenting disorder, such as depression, or PTSD, or another anxiety disorder—all of which *do* have research-based treatment protocols.

With a creative use of basic CBT principles, it should be possible to arrive at a formulation and hence derive a reasonable treatment plan for almost any type of problem.

Therapists and their contexts

Therapist 'adherence'

In this section, we will highlight some of the problems that can arise when as therapists we know what we *ought* to be doing for a particular kind of problem, and yet we don't do it. Why not? Many factors may contribute to this, but to start with we will highlight two recent papers with some provocative ideas about these questions.

Schulte and Eifert (2002) describe an interesting approach to the problem of applying proven psychological therapy methods, such as CBT, to individual cases. They put forward what they call a 'dual model' of therapy. The fundamental idea of this model is that there are two tasks that therapists have to carry out in successful therapy:

1 Applying effective (research-backed) treatment protocols ('*method-related strategies*')
2 Helping patients maintain behaviours that are essential prerequisites for the application of those treatment techniques ('*process-related strategies*'). The patient behaviours that are the focus of this second task are termed '*basic behaviours*' and comprise, for example:
   - Seeking treatment (vs. dropping out)
   - Cooperation (high vs. low)
   - Self-disclosure (vs. withdrawal)
   - Exploring and testing out new patterns of behaviour (vs. refusal)
   - (No) resistance as an active form of non-cooperation.

One of the findings from Schulte and colleagues' research programme is that therapists tend to switch from a focus on Task 1 (i.e. treatment protocols) to a focus on Task 2 (process-related strategies) too early and too frequently, and that this has a detrimental effect on outcome (Schulte and Eifert, *op. cit.*). The implication of this is that when the treatment model seems to be running into problems, we should not abandon it for more process-oriented strategies too quickly, but instead work hard at implementing known effective treatment strategies. A switch of focus to process-related strategies will of course sometimes be necessary—but maybe not as often and not as early as we tend to think.

Waller (2009) also tackles head-on the problem of what he calls 'therapist drift', or the ways in which therapists contribute to ineffective therapy. He suggests that several factors may be involved in producing such drift, including therapist beliefs, emotions, and behaviours (see next section). He also identifies situations where we may be at high risk of drifting, such as when we constantly shift focus through a succession of crises; or when we feel an excessive need to protect our patients. His paper makes invaluable reading for any CBT therapist, and some of the same issues are discussed below.

Therapist beliefs and attitudes

It is assumed in the CBT approach that the theory's ideas about the influence of thoughts and beliefs apply as much to therapists as they do to patients. It is therefore obvious that our own beliefs may sometimes get in the way of our attempts to provide the best possible therapy for our patients. In this section we will look at some common problematic therapist beliefs.

I must not upset my patients

As CBT therapists, we try to be open with patients about therapy often being hard work and sometimes distressing. Patients may need to tolerate increased anxiety while testing out anxious predictions, or to push themselves to engage in activities when they do not feel like it, in the hope that this will have an effect on improving mood. Of course our aim is always to help patients improve in the longer term, but we may find it difficult to adopt the supportive but firm stance that is sometimes necessary for effective CBT. For example, there is evidence that clinicians relatively rarely implement the reliving or exposure components of CBT for PTSD, in spite of the evidence supporting its efficacy (Becker *et al.*, 2004). Similarly, therapists are often reluctant to adopt the strict kind of exposure and response prevention that seems to be most effective in treating OCD (Abramowitz, 1996), because it is clearly difficult and distressing for patients.

There is a limit to *how much* distress it is reasonable to contemplate, and any potentially distressing procedures need to be agreed collaboratively with your patient. But sometimes it may become apparent to you or your supervisor that it is not the patient's beliefs that are getting in the way of a demanding procedure, but your own. If you have this kind of belief, it may be helpful to think through the implications, alone or with your supervisor. Do you think it is actually right to give patients less than optimal therapy, because it causes some temporary but not excessive distress? Would you say the same of a medical procedure, for example, that doctors should not do surgery unless it was *completely* painless? If *you* were a patient with one of these conditions, which would you prefer: a therapist who was supportive but encouraged you to stick with it, or a therapist who allowed you off the hook too easily? Similarly, in supervision, you may have felt that it would be more helpful in improving your therapy skills if your supervisor was a bit more critical and put you on the spot more. In all these case the easier, pain-free option is not necessarily the best option.

There can come a point for any intervention when it is causing too much distress for it to be either ethical or productive to continue—we must always pay attention to that possibility, and respect our patients' wishes—but we may not do patients any favours by being *so* supportive and sensitive that we give up, and allow them to give up, too soon (see Chapter 4).

The research evidence doesn't apply to my practice

Another possible problem is when therapists too easily abandon evidence-based interventions and choose to employ some new or fashionable approach instead of those that have strong evidence. For example, at the time of writing there is limited evidence to support using mindfulness-based cognitive therapy with a currently depressed patient who had not yet had an adequate trial of either anti-depressant medication or conventional CBT; similarly the evidence for using schema-focused cognitive therapy is currently rather limited, and such approaches certainly cannot be said to be superior to conventional CBT for *all* problems.

This is not to say that there is no room for innovation! Clearly if everyone only ever did what had already been shown to be effective, we would end up with a static field in which no progress was ever made. But when you deviate from the treatment approach for which there is greatest evidence of efficacy, you should always be asking yourself whether this is actually justified by the literature, or by some aspect of the patient's presentation, rather than just a product of your own personal preference (or indeed a reflection of your own beliefs or assumptions—sometimes one of the factors driving therapists towards these 'non-standard' approaches is the kind of belief described just above; that is, an alternative approach may feel better because it avoids the more 'difficult' aspects of CBT that cause a temporary increase in distress).

If there is some good reason to be using a 'non-standard' approach then be clear what it is, discuss it in supervision, and consider how you will evaluate its effects, so that you and others can tell whether it is useful or not.

It's the therapist what gets the blame...

A common therapist distortion, akin to 'filtering out the positive' in depression, is the attitude that if anything goes wrong in therapy or the patient does not get better, then that is my fault; although if things go well and the patient *does* get better, then obviously that had nothing to do with me and was just luck or coincidence.

Like any such belief, this is not helpful in the long run because it involves taking either too much or too little responsibility. Therapy is a classic example of a service that is 'co-produced': that is, the ultimate form and content (and effect) of therapy are not simply decided by the professional, nor by the patient, but are *co-produced* out of the interaction between both parties, and therefore responsibility for what happens must also be shared by both parties. If you claim some responsibility for *poor* outcomes, you must also take some responsibility for *good* ones!

I have to help everyone *or* I cannot help anyone

As therapists we may sometimes slip into perfectionism (I ought to be able to help everyone) or its mirror image, hopelessness (I have no skills to help anyone). As with the previous belief, we need to find a reasonable and moderate approach to our work. There is no one in the real world who can help *every* patient (not least because, as noted above, there are two people in the room, not just one, so as therapists we cannot have complete control over what happens). On the other hand if you are getting through your training, or have already qualified, then it is unlikely that you are truly unable to help *anyone*! Most people in our professions have had thoughts that they are faking it and that 'other people will soon find out that actually I cannot do this, they made a mistake in accepting me, all my patients get better without my help…' and so on. We all have those thoughts sometimes, but that does not make them true!

These ideas are probably partly driven by the fact that therapy is hidden most of the time: no one except you and your patient actually observes what goes on. Therefore, this is yet another area where supportive supervision, coupled with the courage to expose yourself to scrutiny, may be invaluable. Record sessions, play them to your supervisor, and get some realistic feedback … and hopefully some disconfirmation of your fears.

Therapist contexts

Contextual factors that influence the way the therapist delivers CBT include the work environment, contracts and other service requirements, the resources available (from supervision and training to access to multidisciplinary teams and other specialist services), work load, and personal concerns and difficulties. We look at four contextual factors that we feel merit more discussion.

Service constraints on treatment

Many services nowadays work under tight constraints: they may have fairly strict limits on the number of sessions any patient can receive; they may have demanding requirements for the rate of patient contacts for clinicians; they are constrained by national targets for waiting times; and they have rules for paperwork that can seem as if they value recording your work more highly than actually doing the work. All of these requirements may understandably make your job feel demanding and pressured.

There are no simple answers to these problems—all we can do is try our best to make sure these demands do not adversely affect the quality of the service we give to patients. Other chapters in this book have relevant advice, including Chapters 3 and 7. Guidelines might include:

- Recognizing that brief and focused therapy can be just as valuable as supposedly more 'in depth' work, and is actually the best option for many patients (see Chapters 6 and 7).

- Making sure that you have good supervision in which you can share and problem-solve any such frustrations.
- Being creative in thinking about how to meet service demands, for example, by modifying the classic (but not research-based) '1 hour a week' approach to therapy. What about groups (see Chapter 8), or shorter individual sessions, or 'advice clinics' (Lovell *et al.*, 2003), or leaving more time between sessions and putting a greater emphasis on between-session assignments…? There is plenty of scope for innovation that may be effective for your patients and interesting for you.
- It is obvious, but still worth remembering, that working within strict time limits means that you need to make the best possible use of the time available. Therapy needs to be tightly focused and efficient, and to be efficient you need to make sure that you prepare well for each session.

Availability of supervision

Clinical supervision is generally seen as being crucial for the safe and effective practice of any psychotherapy. CBT is no exception, and a certain amount of supervision is a requirement for BABCP (British Association for Behavioural and Cognitive Psychotherapies) accreditation as a CBT therapist. However sometimes it can be hard to find supervision, for several reasons: perhaps there are no other CBT therapists close to you; perhaps you are expected to supervise everyone else, but no one is available to supervise you; perhaps there is some difficulty with potential supervisors. It is important to find some way around this, and remember that one-to-one, face-to-face supervision is not the only way of doing it. Considerable benefit can also come out of peer group supervision, or supervision via the phone or the Internet: there is nearly always *some* way of overcoming the problem. See Westbrook *et al.* (2007, Chapter 19) for further thoughts about using supervision, and Chapter 16 of this book about becoming a supervisor.

Type of service

The fact that different kinds of service have different approaches is not necessarily a problem in itself. A primary care service with a 6-session limit for mild-moderate common mental health problems is different to a tertiary service working with particularly severe and complex problems. They each have their own ways of working and they each have their own challenges. Problems are likely to arise, however, when there is a 'one size fits all' approach: for example, when the primary care service is trying to treat people for multiple, complex, and long-standing problems within its 6-session limit. It is important for us as therapists, and our managers, to recognize the limits of any particular approach and not try to apply it in areas where it will not work. By all means innovate (as noted above), but be careful to evaluate such innovations so that you know what works and what does not.

Other demands from outside work

We all know, even if we do not often speak about it, that therapists are neither super-heroes nor saints. We do not sail through life unaffected by external problems, and we are not always happy and focused. Like everyone else, we have worries, relationship problems, financial stress, and so on. Although we do our best to leave those concerns at the door of the therapy room, we cannot always succeed in doing that completely. So perhaps the first rule is to recognize that you are human, and that sometimes you will be working at less than 100% efficiency. The second rule is to know when you are *so* badly affected that you need to do something about it: talk to a partner or friend, talk to your supervisor, take a holiday, or whatever may be appropriate. See Chapter 3 for other advice on looking after yourself.

Patients and their contexts

There are some patient behaviours that you will probably recognize as warning signs of possible problems in therapy. For example:

- Not turning up to, or frequently cancelling, appointments.
- Not appearing to engage with the formulation or the therapeutic approach.
- Regularly not doing homework.
- Persistently finding it difficult to talk about important thoughts, feelings, or behaviours.
- 'Going through the motions', that is, only being engaged at an intellectual rather than an emotional and behavioural level.
- Consistently finding it hard to face feared thoughts, emotions, or situations.

This section will examine some of the factors involving patients and their contexts that may contribute to such problems, with some guidelines on how you might tackle them. As always, the first approach is to follow the golden rules outlined at the beginning of this chapter: understand the problems through a formulation, then work with the factors identified, using a collaborative and empirical approach.

Patient characteristics

So what factors might you need to consider in formulating (or reformulating) problems that arise during therapy?

Patients with highly avoidant coping style

All of us sometimes find it difficult to face anxiety-provoking situations, but some patients find it particularly hard and have a long history of coping with difficulties primarily by trying to avoid them. This can obviously cause problems in implementing some of the behaviour change that CBT requires. Approaches that may be useful in formulating and working with such avoidance include the following:

- Make sure you convey to the patients that you understand their desire to avoid and that it is indeed difficult to face up to things they have always avoided (partly because the avoidance itself means that they have no real experience on which to base their expectations of what will happen).
- Help them think through the pros and cons of avoidance. It is understandable that it feels better in the short run to avoid, but what are the long-term costs, to them, their family and friends, or to other people? Is it possible that it might be worth some short-term pain in order to avoid the long-term misery that often follows from frequent avoidance?
- Identify whether the avoidance is driven by particularly extreme or unrealistic negative appraisals. A common approach is to help your patient to think through 'What is the worst that could really happen here?' Often people have never actually identified clearly what might happen and, when they do, they sometimes discover that it is less awful than their fantasy about it.
- Adjust behavioural experiments to tackle smaller steps and/or use therapist-assisted experiments: brainstorm anything that might make it even a little bit easier for your patient to get over this 'hump in the road'.

Patients who find it difficult to disclose clear information

Talking about their thoughts and feelings to a stranger is not easy for most people, but some find it harder than average. This poses a problem because without reasonable knowledge of your patient's thoughts and feelings, obviously you have little to work with. There are several common factors that might fit into your formulation of such difficulties:

- Some patients have greater concerns about confidentiality: they fear that other people will get access to private information and perhaps use it in some way, or perhaps just disapprove of them. Discuss confidentiality with your patients—and its limits (e.g. that you might have to break confidentiality if you had reason to suspect serious potential harm to the patient or others). There is sometimes room for negotiation, for example, about exactly how much information is recorded in reports or letters to referrers or other third parties: there may be information that you need to know but which is not vital for others to know.

- Some patients have greater fears of negative evaluation, leading them to conceal information that they think will lead you to disapprove, or think they are stupid, or whatever. As always, identifying and formulating your patient's specific worries is vital. Sometimes there are specific fears, such as that telling you about their obsessional thoughts concerning harming people will lead to your informing the authorities or getting social services to take their children away.

The first step is understanding what the block is. People can often talk about *why* they can't tell you something, even when they can't tell you exactly what the 'something' is. You may then be able to work with those fears so as to reduce them and lead on to greater disclosure. Of course a vital component here is a good, trusting therapeutic relationship, in which your patient feels safe. It may be sensible to consider with your supervisor whether you need to do more to build up your patient's trust.

If you have some rough idea about the general kind of thought your patient is struggling with, then a specific strategy is to discuss some common *possible* thoughts of that kind with your patient: 'I wonder if you've ever had thoughts or feelings like…' There is an obvious danger here of putting words into your patient's mouth, so it is important to be very clear that these are only examples and that it is perfectly OK if their response is 'No, nothing like that!' But it can be very helpful for patients to have such evidence that you are familiar with the kind of thoughts or feelings that concern them, and that you will therefore not be shocked by them.

Patients who find it hard to move from 'head' to 'heart'

You will almost certainly have had some experience of patients who express ideas along the lines of 'I can see that in principle my thoughts/beliefs may be exaggerated or unhelpful, but when I get into difficult situations it still *feels* as if they are true'. For many people this is a temporary phenomenon, but others get 'stuck' in this position. In such cases, it is worth trying one or more of the following strategies:

- In terms of verbal/cognitive strategies, look for 'Yes, but…' thoughts. This often indicates that there are negative thoughts or beliefs that have not been tackled, or which only arise when the patient is actually in a difficult situation. For example, a patient who panics might genuinely believe while sitting in your office that this is due to anxiety and not a heart attack; but when he is having a panic outside in the real world, he may think 'Yes, but...sensations this strong *must* be due to some physical problem'. Identify such thoughts and work with them as any others.

- Explore carefully to see whether there are unnoticed safety behaviours that may be blocking belief change. For example, the above patient might be able to test out his fears in sessions because he is thinking 'It's a hospital, there will be doctors to save me if I do have a heart attack'; but he may be unable to do the same thing elsewhere because of the lack of such reassuring facilities.

  If you can identify such safety behaviours, look for ways to test out dropping them in behavioural experiments (see next point).
- Such 'head versus heart' dilemmas are one of the main target areas for behavioural experiments (Bennett-Levy *et al.*, 2004). Behavioural experiments can often consolidate new learning at a 'gut level' in a way that verbal testing never can. So work with your patient to look for ways to test out thoughts and beliefs through action in the real world outside the therapy session: 'What could we *do* to test out these old ideas (or these new ideas)?'
- Consider using imagery rescripting to transform negative images or to construct a new positive image (Holmes *et al.*, 2007).
- As noted above, such head/heart splits are a frequent temporary experience in therapy, so it may be that the split will reduce simply with more time and more repetition. Strong beliefs do not usually disappear or change in one flash of insight! Change far more commonly happens in small, incremental steps, which demand repetition; so be prepared for that, and prepare your patients for it as well.

Patients whose problems are driven by fixed beliefs

We can work at the level of negative automatic thoughts (NATs) most of the time but when therapy grinds to a halt or therapy-interfering behaviours are apparent, it may become necessary to check out what is driving the NATs. It is then useful to ask whether there are more fixed beliefs that make sense of the patient's enduring emotional state and/or behaviour, and which may be stopping progress. You can find guidance in identifying these more fundamental cognitions in basic and specialist CBT texts (e.g. Beck *et al.*, 2004; Westbrook *et al.*, 2007). The key is recognizing that you are stuck, and that it is appropriate to explore more deeply.

Despite being able to challenge his NATs and repeatedly carrying out behavioural experiments, Ned's fear of leaving home and being far from a hospital remained intact. Further exploration revealed this was because he had had, since childhood, a firmly fixed belief that he would one day have a heart attack just as his father had. Despite his coping experiences in therapy he retained a nagging, "Yes but... I am still bound to die just like my dad" This explained his head–heart gap, his fear of relinquishing safety-seeking behaviours, the lack of progress in sessions, and his frequent cancellations.

There will be times when your formulation needs to incorporate deeper level cognitions. This can then provide a rationale for an approach which addresses core beliefs or schemata (Beck *et al.*, 2004). In Ned's case it was this which eventually shifted the conviction in his belief and he was able to overcome his fears.

Patients who have poor memory

Sometimes people may fail to make the best use of therapy partly because of memory problems: they may simply have a poor memory, or their memory may be adversely affected by their mood state, by drug or alcohol abuse, by psychological trauma, or by sleep deprivation or ageing.

Frances was severely depressed and her therapist felt as though they were always taking one step forward only to slip back two steps the following week. In discussion with Frances, her therapist realized that she had underestimated how profoundly Frances' memory was affected by her mood state, and that her poor memory contributed to the lack of momentum in the therapy, the apparent lack of engagement in the work, and her struggling to recall or reflect on recent events.

If you think that poor memory is disadvantaging your patient then:

- Focus even more than usual on using Socratic methods to *elicit* information in the first place, as information gained in this way will usually then be retained better by your patient.
- Make sure you use memory aids such as therapy notebooks and recordings of sessions.
- Use repetition, in the form of regular summaries given to and elicited from the patient.
- Make sure that you encourage your patient to reflect and process new information gathered through therapy, considering the personal implications and how they might take it forward. Such reflection will enhance the retention of learning.

Patients who have very biased information processing

It is a key idea in CBT that information processing can be biased, and it is probably routine for you to help patients rein in exaggerated and distorted thinking. However, some patients have particularly *extreme* styles of processing, so we need to be prepared for more challenging scenarios. For example:

- The highly anxious person who dissociates into a state of de-realization or de-personalization.

Greg just didn't engage. He attended sessions and he did homework but he remained somehow detached from the therapy and made little progress in overcoming his social anxiety. His therapist began to interrupt sessions at times when Greg seemed particularly disengaged and asked him what was happening. He revealed that he had "spaced out" for a moment and it became apparent that this happened frequently both within the sessions and outside. It became clear that high emotions triggered Greg's "spacing out", and this explained several perplexing aspects of therapy: his frequent passivity, his difficulties in being specific and remembering events clearly, and his struggle to talk about emotions. It also explained his struggle to shift his affect and close the "head-heart" gap.

- The traumatized patient who experiences flashbacks.
- The patient with borderline personality disorder who has extremely dichotomous (all-or-nothing) thinking.
- The patient suffering from psychosis who has exaggerated paranoid or catastrophic ideas.

As always, the first step is to *formulate* the impact of extreme thinking on emotions and behaviours. Next, introduce methods of addressing these maintaining cycles:

- Teach 'decentring' to help your patients get a more objective, detached view of their information processing style and therefore reduce its emotional consequences.
- Use continuum techniques to combat dichotomous thinking (see Beck *et al.*, 2004).
- Teach grounding skills to help in the management of depersonalization and feelings of unreality (Kennerley, 1996; Kennerley, 2000).
- Teach specific techniques to help your patient manage intrusive images (Hackmann and Holmes, 2004; Holmes *et al.*, 2007).

It may also be helpful to become more familiar with the fundamental mechanisms of information processing: a good resource is Williams *et al.* (1997).

Patients who misuse alcohol, street drugs, or prescribed medication

It is important to bear in mind that your patient's use of various types of drug may play a part in limiting the impact of therapy. For example, there is some evidence that benzodiazepines (e.g. Valium) may significantly reduce the impact of CBT for anxiety disorders, especially when taken 'when needed', as opposed to on a regular regime (Westra and Stewart, 1998). Alcohol or other drugs may also interfere with therapy, although the evidence of a severe negative impact from alcohol dependence is not as clear as one might think (McEvoy and Shand, 2008). Nevertheless, it is obvious that if a patient is still using substances regularly then it may be difficult either for them to access thoughts and emotions effectively, or to retain evidence gathered from verbal or behavioural testing of thoughts. Self-harming, such as cutting or burning, can also have a similar 'addictive' pattern, with attempts to resist the behaviour provoking a strong sense of craving.

Such problems can account for some engagement and adherence problems. For example, a person with an addiction might be ambivalent about trying to give up their addictive behaviour; the neurochemical changes experienced during or after drug use or self-harming can interfere with engagement in therapy and attendance at sessions; engagement in illegal activities can lead to the patient's withholding key information; and failure to control such behaviour can contribute to a sense of lost momentum. Amongst the approaches which can help are the following:

- As with any potentially dangerous behaviour, clearly it is important to assess risk and have a plan to deal with any increase in risk.
- Motivational interviewing can help engage a patient who is ambivalent about therapy (Miller and Rollnick, 2002).
- Specialist CBT may be useful to understand and challenge the specific belief systems that support such problem behaviours (Beck *et al.*, 1993; Kennerley, 2004).
- Negotiating less damaging responses (e.g. non-injurious cathartic or soothing behaviours, or controlled drinking) can also play a key part in managing harmful activities (Kennerley, 2004).

Patient contexts

A patient's circumstances can either enhance or diminish the effectiveness of treatment. Although many of our patients live within a context that supports their therapy, others do not. Some will go home to dysfunctional families; some will have to deal with financial difficulties that cause chronic stress; others are under impossible pressure at work. In these situations, you might feel like a firefighter rather than a proper cognitive therapist, always trying to put out the latest flare-up sparked by external stresses. In this section, we shall look at some of the most common contextual factors that affect patients.

Psychosocial support and wider systemic factors

CBT makes many demands on patients. They are asked to face their fears, trust the therapist enough to be open about problems, and try out new ways of seeing and doing things—and they also have to find the time and money to attend regular sessions. Patients will obviously find it easier to cope with these demands when they are adequately supported by their social network. The quality of social support can therefore help or hinder progress in treatment, as well as affecting the maintenance of treatment gains. Your assessment and formulation therefore needs to address questions about these areas:

- How well supported is the patient by family and/or friends in doing CBT?
- How does the patient perceive the available support? What if anything would the patient like to be different?
- Are relatives and friends who are trying to be supportive nevertheless inadvertently acting in ways likely to be maintaining the problem (see more on this below)?
- What impact, both positive and negative, might change in the presenting problem(s) have on the social network and the support available?

Sometimes you may be able to establish clear answers to these questions right from the start of therapy, but at other times the full picture will only emerge gradually.

Even if the patient is well supported, maintaining that support will be helped by ensuring that relatives and friends have access to good quality information about the treatment you are offering. Discuss with your patient what information he/she might want to share about his/her experience of treatment, and what he/she can do to make it easier for others to help and support the process of therapy. You may be able to recommend a self-help or information book for his/her relatives to read.

Of course, social networks can also be problematic in a range of ways, which we consider in more detail below.

Inadequate social support

Some patients may never have had much social support, while in other cases the disorder itself may have contributed to the erosion of social support over time (King *et al.*, 2006). There are several options you might like to try to increase the level of support:

- Reactivate support networks that have withered. For example, encourage your patients to get back in touch with existing networks, help them to problem-solve any obstacles, and use behavioural rehearsal and experiments to deal with those obstacles.
- Consider the possibility of building temporary *new* support networks, perhaps provided by the NHS (National Health Service) or voluntary services. You could request the help of a support worker or make a referral to a befriending service until the patient recovers sufficiently to begin to develop natural support networks.
- Provide additional support yourself, outside regular sessions, by offering telephone or email contact at specified times or intervals during the week.

This can be particularly useful at key stages in treatment when it might be difficult to keep the therapeutic momentum going, for example, to support your patient in keeping his/her activity schedule going, or reviewing the progress of a particular behavioural experiment.

- Consider possible ways in which your patient might consciously or unconsciously be rejecting available help, for example, through thoughts like 'I'm fine now and don't need any help', or through being hostile to people who offer help. Could he/she experiment with alternative strategies?

The support network is hostile to treatment

Sometimes social networks are actively *hostile* to therapy. Family or friends may believe it is the wrong treatment, or even that it is potentially harmful. For example, the wife of a patient with chronic and severe PTSD was concerned that CBT would open old wounds and overwhelm her husband, thus putting him at risk of self-harm or suicide.

Conjoint sessions are usually the most helpful way to address such fears with the wider network. It can be useful to schedule conjoint review sessions from time to time, and to agree on a shared plan of action should the relative or friend become concerned about the course of treatment.

The support network has unrealistic expectations of treatment

Unrealistic expectations of treatment outcome or the speed of recovery can be a burden for patients and therapists alike. They can cause us to try to run before we can walk, lead to dismissing small achievements, and create hopelessness in the face of obstacles. If they are constantly expecting more, then the support network is less likely to value whatever progress the patient has made, and thus less likely to be encouraging. Try to help your patients arrive at realistic expectations (e.g. this will take time, and is likely to be 'two steps forward and one step back'), and support them in conveying such expectations to other people.

The support network inadvertently maintains aspects of the problem

Most of the time, family and friends are not *intentionally* unhelpful: they are usually doing what they believe to be in the best interest of their loved one. Nevertheless it is quite common that they do things that are *in fact* unhelpful. Common examples of such maintaining processes to look out for are:

- Providing repeated reassurance.
- Enabling or encouraging avoidance.

- Joining in with safety behaviours (e.g. helping a health-anxious patient check for symptoms, or helping an obsessional patient's rituals).
- Sharing and reinforcing unhelpful beliefs (e.g. the friends of a patient with an eating disorder openly admiring underweight celebrities and swapping dieting tips).

When such processes are identified, it is important to formulate them (see Chapter 9 on systemic formulation) and then address them, first with the patient and then, if your patient feels he/she needs support in changing these patterns, with his/her family or friends as well. It may be helpful to invite others to join part of an early session, to help you gain a detailed picture and to share ideas about how to work together productively.

Apart from unhelpful involvement, the other side of the coin is that patients' social networks may be able to play a useful role in helping them test the validity of their negative thinking, in supporting and encouraging the dropping of safety behaviours, or in conducting behavioural experiments. The role of others in treatment might be relatively limited—perhaps helping with the practicalities of freeing time to attend the session by being available to look after the children—or quite extensive, as, for example tackling family involvement in obsessional rituals. See Chapter 9 for more on a systemic approach to CBT.

Real-life adversity

The relationship between adversity, psychological morbidity, and treatment outcome is complex and not fully understood. Stressful events, economic disadvantage, and the lack of individual resources tend to be accompanied by a lack of community services and support. Furthermore, stressful events are more likely to occur in the context of disadvantaged living conditions. The effect is to make stress multiplicative, rather than merely additive, and thus it becomes much harder for patients to stay on top of problems and maintain helpful coping. Growing up in disadvantaged communities may encourage the development of beliefs, attitudes, and coping styles which make people vulnerable to psychological difficulties, and engender a pervasive sense of hopelessness that makes the possibility of change seem unattainable.

Possible approaches to this kind of problem include:

- Acknowledge the reality. Remember—and remind your patient—that CBT is not about thinking positively but about thinking *realistically*. If there are real-life problems then you need to consider how much the patient's thoughts or beliefs are contributing to the problems versus how much they are problems *anyone* would have to much the same degree in that situation.

- Conceptualize the impact of adverse circumstances on the problem and work with your patient in a more problem-solving mode to see what if anything can be done to change or ameliorate those circumstances.
- Be realistic about taking smaller steps both in and out of sessions, and try to help your patient maintain regular attendance at sessions.

Also see Moorey (1996) for an insightful approach to working with 'realistic' negative thoughts in adverse life circumstances.

When life gets in the way of treatment

The death of a parent, acute illness, the loss of a job...we all experience significant life events from time to time, and of course this can happen to patients during the course of treatment. Some life events can be contained by the patient, and perhaps even become an opportunity to practice coping and integrate new learning. At other times, therapists and patients face a significant dilemma: should we carry on as usual, or do we need to consider other options? You may need to consider various possibilities:

- Continuing treatment, perhaps after reviewing aims and goals, or using a session to problem-solve how they can best cope with the recent event.
- Taking a break from treatment for a defined period, or until some event has passed (e.g. until a court case has been decided).
- Ending treatment for the time being, and picking it up again when the patient is more ready.

In such circumstances, you need to discuss and agree the best way forward with your patient, taking account of factors such as:

- How far through the course of treatment you are (e.g. if you have only just started, it may be more sensible to stop and pick it up again later).
- How long the difficult events or situations are likely to last (if relatively brief then a break in treatment may be easier).
- To what extent current or planned treatment strategies might actually help your patient cope with the crisis, and should therefore be continued.
- Whether the therapeutic relationship is likely to be badly affected by a break in treatment.

If there is to be a break, try to maintain treatment gains by working on a temporary blueprint that highlights the most important lessons from your work so far. As with any blueprint, this should cover:

- How did the problem develop?
- What keeps the problem going?

- What has been helpful in treatment so far?
- What are the most unhelpful thoughts and beliefs I have so far identified?
- What might be reasonable alternatives?
- What have I learned that might help me manage this current crisis?
- What pitfalls might there be and how might I cope with these?
- What do I need to do to maintain the progress I have made so far?
- What supportive resources are still available to me?

Therapist-patient interaction

Those factors that relate specifically to the patient, therapy, and context have been addressed above. We will end this chapter with a consideration of some of the problems that can arise not from patient or therapist in isolation, but from the *interaction* between patient and therapist characteristics.

Most therapists feel that they work better with certain patients or 'types' of patients—indeed, this is one factor that often affects our choice of specialty. However, most of us still have occasional patients who appear 'suitable' but who fail to benefit from CBT. The interaction between patient and therapist may be a cause of some of those failures.

Shireen sought CBT for health anxiety and obsessional checking. Shireen was a senior doctor at a local hospital, with a strong academic profile. When, after a year of regular sessions, the first therapist concluded that she wasn't benefitting from treatment, she decided the problem was her lack of experience in treating health anxiety and OCD, and organized a handover to a therapist with specialist skills in those disorders. However, further CBT with this second therapist had equally limited impact.

There was no obvious explanation for Shireen's failure to benefit from CBT: she was intelligent and psychologically minded; seemed well-motivated; the issues she wanted help with were of a kind for which there is considerable evidence for the efficacy of CBT; and both therapists were experienced and accredited CBT practitioners, with one of them having many years' experience of successfully treating similar patients.

The therapists had the opportunity to reflect together on how they might understand this treatment failure. One common theme was that they had both found it very difficult to implement specific treatment procedures. Instead, the sessions were eaten up by academic debate about the differences between different therapeutic procedures, and what the likely impact of any specific therapeutic manoeuvre might be. This made the therapists less willing to take therapeutic risks, and thus less active in pushing for behavioural change. In addition, they both felt somewhat intimidated by the patient, and in dealing with the health anxiety, they felt that they had to defer to the patient's greater medical knowledge. This resulted in the

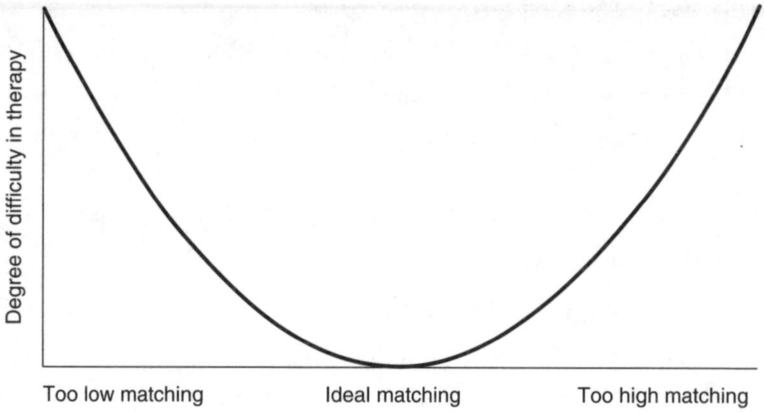

Fig. 1.3 How patient-therapist matching may affect therapy.

therapists feeling inhibited by a fear of negative evaluation of their clinical skills and feeling that their suggestions were "trumped" by the "expert" patient, and thus they found it more difficult to be as active and directive as they normally would be.

Problems with the interaction between patients and therapists can arise from 'matching' between patient and therapist that goes too far in either direction. In other words, they may match too well (e.g. over-empathizing and sharing assumptions); or they may not match well enough (e.g. there is a lack of empathy, clashing value systems, dislike between the parties, etc.)

Given that there is evidence that the therapeutic alliance affects outcome in any therapy (Castonguay *et al.*, 2006), and that the alliance is a product of the interaction between you and your patient, it is likely that this matching between you and your patient will have an impact on the therapy. See Fig. 1.3 for an illustration of how the degree of matching may affect the course of therapy.

Let us look further at these problems.

Too low matching

A lack of matching can lead to a lack of empathy, disliking each other, or the therapist lacking credibility in the patient's eyes. For example, when you and your patient have very different value systems, or opposing assumptions, it may be difficult for you to show the warmth and empathy that is the necessary grounding for effective CBT interventions. That in turn may make it difficult for them to feel supported in doing behavioural experiments, or they may find it difficult to be open about their beliefs and feelings. Similarly, if you are not perceived by your patient as belonging to a group whose opinion they value, this can undermine the effects of any therapeutic feedback from the therapist (e.g. 'It might be OK for a wimp like you to express emotions or show signs of anxiety in public, but it is totally unacceptable for people like me'). Additionally, the greater the difference between the therapist's world and the patient's, the harder both parties will have to work to develop a shared understanding of the problem.

Difficulties with a poor match between therapist and patient can arise when the therapist reminds the patient of a previous negative experience, or vice versa. For example, it may cause problems if you have the same name as, or physically resemble, someone who abused the patient. This has the potential to be a healing experience if it can be overcome (e.g. 'Not all men with beards called John will take advantage of me') but clearly also has the potential to have a detrimental effect on therapy. On the other side of this coin, your patient may activate memories of one of your own previous negative experience, which may contaminate your behaviour during therapy.

A therapist whose childhood was disrupted by her father's frequent affairs struggled to empathize with a patient who was trying to decide whether to stay with his wife or leave her for his mistress. The therapist, who had empathized with her own mother's distress at her father's affairs, found it hard to disentangle this from her patient's need to come to a satisfactory choice between the two women in his life. This was particularly salient as the patient felt that one of the factors preventing him from making the decision was his assumption about having to "follow the rules/do the right thing" and to "look after others' needs first". Understandably, he wanted help in learning to prioritize his own needs. However, the therapist struggled to keep this as the therapeutic priority and felt that her behaviour in therapy was contaminated by empathizing more with his wife's position than with her patient's.

Although therapists are entitled to their own opinions about the way in which life should be lived, this therapist was concerned that her beliefs about his situation, and her emotional reaction to it, compromised her ability to help her patient evaluate his beliefs and options in an unbiased way.

Clearly no therapist can hope to suit every patient ideally, but you should be alert for mismatches that are bad enough to affect treatment. Supervision is crucial in helping you to identify and address any unhelpful patient-therapist interactions. Early warning signs may be your having particularly strong emotional reactions to the patient (positive or negative), or noticing deviations from your normal practice, even if only in the pace of treatment. If there does seem to be a problem of mismatch then supervision may help you to diminish any negative effects, for example, by seeking a better understanding and formulation for your patient. In extreme cases, it may be necessary to consider referral to a different therapist.

Too high matching

A high degree of sharing of beliefs may help you to empathize with and understand the patient's difficulties. However, if the match is too close you may not be able to see the patient's situation objectively and may empathize *so* much that your ability to intervene effectively is compromised—instead of Socratically questioning unhelpful beliefs, you may end up saying, in effect, 'You're right'!

Many of the dysfunctional assumptions targeted in CBT are widely held by the general population, including therapists (e.g. 'I should do well at everything' or 'I must be nice to everyone all the time'). What differentiates those who come for treatment is not so much the pure *content* of their beliefs but the degree of conviction and rigidity with which they are held. Hence, it is likely that patients and therapists will sometimes share beliefs that are relevant to the patient's treatment, and this may cause problems. For example, an unassertive therapist who has a high need to please others may not have sufficient assertiveness skills to teach patients, and may struggle to help the patient find an alternative perspective. Or a very slender therapist who is clearly concerned about appearance may lack credibility when trying to convince patients with eating disorders not to evaluate themselves in terms of their shape and weight. Of course, this can also work in a helpful way—a perfectionist therapist may know only too well the pitfalls of rigidly adhering to such beliefs, and furthermore may have useful experiences of experimenting with lower standards in pursuit of a more enjoyable life…

As well as sharing beliefs or assumptions, there may be significant overlap in *experiences* between patients and therapists. For example, reliving in PTSD will be difficult if your own matching experiences make it particularly aversive, and the result may be allowing the patient to avoid exposure to the trauma. Therapists may cope with such 'weak spots' by avoiding taking on patients whose traumas are likely to activate their own beliefs (assuming that it is possible to predict in advance who these will be…), and that may work well, so long as there are others in the service who can see the 'avoided' patients.

Possible clues that such identification is occurring include having particularly strong emotional reactions to the patient ('I just feel so sorry for him'), or finding yourself deviating from your standard treatment. For example, if you would normally have begun reliving by the third session and yet it is session seven and you still haven't managed to do any, then you may need to stop and think why; or if you normally use behavioural experiments and yet find with a particular patient that you haven't got around to them yet, then again you may need to think about what has stopped you. These would be important issues to discuss in supervision and may even necessitate some re-evaluation of your belief system.

Conclusion

In this chapter, we have highlighted some common clinical issues that you might encounter, along with some suggestions for managing them. Some of the chapters in the rest of this book will highlight specific challenges in more detail. In combination with the fundamental CBT skills of formulating difficulties,problem-solving, and helping people test their cognitions, we hope that these guidelines will help you move forward in your CBT practice and career.

Key points

- The course of CBT does not always run smoothly. In attempting to understand any difficulties your first port of call should be the CBT model and the formulation of the patient's problems.
- The process and outcome of treatment are shaped by both therapist and patient, and their interactions with each other, with the CBT model, and with their individual living and working situations.
- Not everyone is equally suited to CBT, but there is scope for creativity in developing effective goals and methods for a wide variety of patients.
- When you run into problems, use CBT flexibly to try to understand what is happening and to try out strategies that might improve things.
- Watch out for your own attitudes and beliefs that might cause you to drift away from effective treatment protocols.
- The context in which you and your patients live and work matters. If it gets in the way of good CBT try out ways to improve things for either of you.

Further reading

Beck, J.S. (2005). *Cognitive Therapy for Challenging Problems: What to do When the Basics Don't Work.* New York, NY: Guilford Press.

Butler, G., Fennell, M. and Hackmann, A. (2008). *Cognitive-behavioural Therapy for Anxiety Disorders: Mastering Clinical Challenges.* New York, NY: Guilford Press.

Gilbert, P. and Leahy, R. (eds.). (2007). *The Therapeutic Relationship in the Cognitive Behavioural Psychotherapies.* London: Routledge.

Kuyken, W., Padesky, C. and Dudley, R. (2009). *Collaborative Case Conceptualization: Working Effectively With Clients in Cognitive-behavioral Therapy.* New York, NY: Guilford Press.

Tarrier, N. (2006). *Case Formulation in Cognitive Behaviour Therapy.* London: Routledge.

References

Abramowitz, J. (1996). Variants of exposure and response prevention in the treatment of obsessive-compulsive disorder: a meta-analysis. *Behavior Therapy*, **27**, 583–600.

Baldwin, S., Berkeljon, A., Atkins, D., Olsen, J. and Nielsen, S. (2009). Rates of change in naturalistic psychotherapy: contrasting dose–effect and good-enough level models of change. *Journal of Consulting and Clinical Psychology*, **77**, 203–211.

Beck. A.T, Wright, F.D, Newman, C.F., and Liese, B.S. (1993). *Cognitive therapy of substance abuse.* New York, NY: Guilford Press.

Beck, A.T., Freeman, A., Davis, D.D. and associates (2004). *Cognitive Therapy of Personality Disorders.* Second edition. New York, NY: Guilford Press.

Beck, J.S. (2005). *Cognitive Therapy for Challenging Problems: What to do When the Basics Don't Work.* New York, NY: Guilford Press.

Becker, C.B., Zayfert, C. and Anderson, E. (2004). A survey of psychologists' attitudes towards and utilization of exposure therapy for PTSD. *Behaviour Research and Therapy*, **42**, 277–292.

Bennett-Levy, J., Butler, G., Fennell, M., Hackmann, A., Mueller, M. and Westbrook, D. (eds.) (2004). *The Oxford Guide to Behavioural Experiments in Cognitive Therapy.* Oxford: Oxford University Press.

Castonguay, C.G., Constantiona, M.J. and Grosse Holtforth, M.G. (2006). The Working Alliance: where are we and where should we go? *Psychotherapy: Theory, Research, Practice, Training*, **43**, 198–205.

Craske, M.G., Farchione, T.J., Allen, N.B., Barrios, V., Stoyanova, M. and Rose, R. (2007). Cognitive behavioural therapy for panic disorder and comorbidity: more of the same or less of more? *Behaviour Research and Therapy*, **45**, 1095–1109.

Giesen-Bloo, J., van Dyck, R., Spinhoven, P., van Tilburg, W., Dirksen, C., van Asselt, T., Kremers, I., Nadort, M. and Arntz, A. (2006). Outpatient psychotherapy for borderline personality disorder: randomized trial of schema-focused therapy vs transference-focused psychotherapy. *Archives of General Psychiatry*, **63**, 649–658.

Hackmann, A. and Holmes, E.A. (2004). Reflecting on imagery: a clinical perspective and overview of the special issue of *Memory* on mental imagery and memory in psychopathology. *Memory*, **12**, 389–402.

Harvey, A., Watkins, E., Mansell, W. and Shafran, R. (2004). *Cognitive Behavioural Processes Across Psychological Disorders: A Transdiagnostic Approach to Research and Treatment.* Oxford: Oxford University Press.

Holmes, E.A., Arntz, A. and Smucker, M.R. (2007). Imagery rescripting in cognitive behaviour therapy: images, treatment techniques and outcomes. *Journal of Behavior Therapy and Experimental Psychiatry*, **38**, 297–305.

Howard, K.I., Kopta, S.M., Krause, M.S. and Orlinsky, D.E. (1986). The dose-effect relationship in psychotherapy. *American Psychologist*, **41**, 159–164.

Kazantzis, N., Deane, F. and Ronan, K. (2000). Homework assignments in cognitive and behavioural therapy: a meta-analysis. *Clinical Psychology Science and Practice*, **7**, 189–202.

Kennerley, H. (1996). Cognitive therapy of dissociative symptoms associated with trauma. *British Journal of Clinical Psychology*, **35**, 325–340.

Kennerley, H. (2000). *Overcoming Childhood Trauma.* London: Constable-Robinson.

Kennerley, H. (2004). Self-injurious behaviour, in Bennett-Levy, J., Butler, G., Fennell, M., Hackmann, A., Mueller, M. and Westbrook, D. (eds.), *The Oxford Guide to Behavioural Experiments in Cognitive Therapy*. Oxford: Oxford University Press.

King, D., Taft, C., King, L., Hammond, C. and Stone, E. (2006). Directionality of the association between social support and posttraumatic stress disorder: a longitudinal investigation. *Journal of Applied Social Psychology*, **36**, 2980–2992.

Lovell, K., Richards, D. and Bower, P. (2003). Improving access to primary mental health care: uncontrolled evaluation of a pilot self-help clinic. *British Journal of General Practice*, **53**, 133–135.

McEvoy, P.M. and Shand, F. (2008). The effect of comorbid substance use disorders on treatment outcome for anxiety disorders. *Journal of Anxiety Disorders*, **22**, 1087–1098.

Miller, W.R. and Rollnick, S. (2002). *Motivational Interviewing: Preparing People for Change.* Second edition. New York, NY: Guilford Press.

Moorey, S. (1996). When bad things happen to rational people: cognitive therapy in adverse life situations, in Salkovskis, P. (ed.), *Frontiers of Cognitive Therapy*. New York, NY: Guilford Press.

Myhr, G., Talbot, J., Annable, L. and Pinard, G. (2007). Suitability for short-term cognitive-behavioural therapy. *Journal of Cognitive Psychotherapy*, **21**, 334–345.

Safran, J.D. and Segal, Z.V. (1990). *Interpersonal Process in Cognitive Therapy*. New York, NY: Basic Books.

Safran, J.D., Segal, Z.V., Vallis, T.M., Shaw, B.F. and Samstag, L.W. (1993). Assessing patient suitability for short-term cognitive therapy with an interpersonal focus. *Cognitive Therapy and Research*, **17**, 23–38.

Schmidt, N. and Woolaway-Bickel, K. (2000). The effects of treatment compliance on outcome in cognitive-behavioral therapy for panic disorder: quality versus quantity. *Journal of Consulting and Clinical Psychology*, **68**, 13–18.

Schulte, D. and Eifert, G.H. (2002). What to do when manuals fail? The dual model of psychotherapy. *Clinical Psychology: Science and Practice*, **9**, 312–328.

Waller, G. (2009). Evidence-based treatment and therapist drift. *Behaviour Research and Therapy*, **47**, 119–127.

Westbrook, D., Kennerley, H. and Kirk, J. (2007). *An Introduction to Cognitive Behaviour Therapy: Skills and Applications.* London: Sage.

Westra, H. and Stewart, S. (1998). Cognitive behavioural therapy and pharmacotherapy: complementary or contradictory approaches to the treatment of anxiety? *Clinical Psychology Review*, **18**, 307–340.

Williams, J.M.G., Watts, F.N., MacLeod, C.M. and Mathews, A. (1997). *Cognitive Psychology and Emotional Disorders.* Second edition. Chichester: Wiley.

Chapter 2

Using CBT with diverse patients: working with South Asian Muslims

Farooq Naeem, Peter Phiri, Shanaya Rathod, and David Kingdon

Cognitive behavioural therapy (CBT) has been developed primarily within Western cultures and the evidence for its effectiveness has mainly been focused on these cultures. Yet Britain is a multicultural society, with an estimated 4.6 million black and minority ethnic (BME) people, constituting nearly 9% of the total population—and there are arguments that CBT's philosophy and methods may not be straightforwardly transferable to patients from such diverse cultures and backgrounds. Some CBT therapists have described their experience of working with patients from ethnic minorities (e.g. Hays and Iwamasa, 2006, pp. 3–20), and in recent years CBT has become more popular in non-Western countries. However, this area remains underdeveloped: the evidence base for CBT with such patient groups remains sparse, and further research is needed with a wide range of BME and other minority groups to address issues of generalizability. This chapter therefore aims to introduce issues of ethnic and cultural diversity, using examples from South Asian Muslim patients.

Defining ethnicity can be complex and fraught with confusion, even for researchers in this field, but generally ethnicity is characterized by a sense of belonging, and determined by the identity of a group that shares common values and norms, including language, religion, culture, and racial background (Fernando, 1991; Tseng *et al.*, 2005). These authors agree that ethnicity is not stagnant, but amenable to change over time, and ethnicity does not apply only to ethnic minorities: the majority white group in the United Kingdom is an ethnic group just as much as any other minority group.

Adaptation of CBT

A large part of culture is the meaning given to experiences and behaviour, and such differences in meaning can interact with CBT in helpful or unhelpful ways.

For example, Western cultures usually interpret direct eye contact as indicating friendliness and, within psychiatric care, 'poor eye contact' is sometimes seen as a symptom of mental illness. However, South Asian Muslim patients might avoid direct eye contact out of respect, and some cultures will perceive direct eye contact as a sign of confrontation and hostility. Therapist awareness of such cultural differences is crucial in avoiding misunderstandings.

As another example, CBT's strong emphasis on the collaborative relationship tends to work well with Western patients. However, South Asian Muslims often expect a more paternalistic attitude when they see an expert, and they may well expect you to solve their problems for them, just like a spiritual or faith healer would. For example, when one of us asked a patient, *So what seems to be the problem*? the patient replied *But you are the expert—you tell me what is wrong with me!*. You therefore might need to make a gradual transition from one mode to the other, perhaps being more prescriptive and giving more expert advice than usual at the beginning of the therapy, but moving towards a more collaborative approach: for example, *OK, I'll make a suggestion, but then let's test it out to see how it works for you.* Patients may also expect that a professional working in a hospital will treat them with medication, and you may need to spend time educating them that a non-medical therapy can be effective. In other words, you need to be creative in finding ways to actively engage your patients in working towards their own recovery (however, once the patient is engaged you might not need to make major changes in common CBT strategies).

Developing Culturally Sensitive CBT Project

In Southampton, the Developing Culturally Sensitive CBT Project has been developing methods of modifying CBT for use in non-Western cultures, both in the United Kingdom and in Pakistan (Naeem *et al.*, in press). The UK project aimed to '...develop culturally sensitive CBT for psychosis for ethnic minority patients by exploration and incorporation of service users and health professionals' views and opinions' (Rathod *et al.*, 2009). The Pakistani project aimed to establish whether CBT can be an acceptable, accessible, and effective treatment for depression in a developing country. Both projects included interviews with psychologists, patients, and university students; therapy with patients; and field observations. We also developed a framework for adapting CBT to guide the treatment process. Our adaptation framework consists of three major areas:

- Culture and related issues
- Capacity and circumstances
- Cognitions and beliefs

The following sections describe this framework and provide practical examples of working with diverse patients. Each major area is subdivided into sections that you may need to consider when working with patients from similar background. We have used examples from our experiences in both Pakistan and the United Kingdom.

Culture and related issues

Culture, religion, and spirituality

Religion and spirituality are important aspects of people's lives in many Asian cultures. They influence people's beliefs, including those related to health and well-being, illness, and help-seeking in time of distress. Culture, religion, and spirituality can also give rise to myths and stigma attached to illness. For example, many people in Pakistan believe that depression can arise from not following religion (an idea based on a misinterpretation of some verses from the Holy Quran). You need to be aware of such beliefs and discuss the nature of depression and its treatment with your patients. It can also be useful to ask your patients to contact a religious scholar, or the Imam of the local mosque, to help clarify questions about the relationship between their faith and psychological difficulties. Talking to a respected member of the local community might also be helpful with non-religious issues. When a local community member is not available, it may be possible (with the patient's agreement) to arrange a conversation with a health professional who comes from the patient's background (see also 'Further reading' at the end of this chapter). The Internet can also be a valuable resource. For example, the first author found valuable information on Islam while developing an adapted manual for CBT for depression.

Culture and religion also influence beliefs about the causes and effects of day-to-day events:

> *A depressed woman believed that her adult son was under the magic spell of her daughter-in-law. Her son had married 6 months ago and the attention he paid to his wife had led his mother to conclude that he was ignoring her. She began to feel depressed, thinking that the change in her son's behaviour was due to a magic spell. Talking to other family members, it became clear that they did not share the woman's belief and the therapist encouraged them to talk to the mother about this between sessions. The therapist advised them on highlighting alternative explanations to her at least twice a day. This was very helpful and on her next visit she was less clear that her son was under a magic spell and more willing to accept therapy for depression.*

Religious faith is used to help people cope with distress in many cultures, so it can be helpful to ask if your patient is getting support from religious or spiritual healers, or is active in his/her religious practice. Such practices can be very helpful for many patients, and examples include reciting the Quran; using charm lockets, talismans, and *tavees* (armlets) to ward off evil spirits; and the repetition of religious mantras (called *wird* or *wazifa*) to sooth distress and instil hope.

Sometimes patients might reduce or even stop their previous religious activities and you might encourage them to gradually return to such activities. When planning behavioural activation, we advise patients with religious faith to get back to their religious activities as soon as possible. There is scope for more collaborative work with religious and spiritual leaders in order to embrace a holistic approach to meeting individual patient's needs in psychotherapy, and some psychiatrists are already involved in such collaborative work in the United Kingdom.

Saiqa was a school teacher who presented with symptoms of anxiety and mild depression. She had left her husband because he shouted and scolded the children, was controlling, and emotionally abusive to her. Our initial work focused on helping her with her feelings of anxiety, low mood, and difficulties in decision making. By the fourth session she had decided to give her husband a last chance provided he fulfilled certain conditions: she required that she be allowed to visit her parents regularly, to return to work and to continue her CBT for six sessions. The aim of joint sessions was to help the couple to address Saiqa's abusive experiences. The therapist carefully explored the husband's ideas about dealing with his family, and learned that Saiqa's husband thought it was his right and privilege to deal with his wife and family in this way, because this is allowed in Islam. The therapist asked Saiqa's husband to write the evidence for and against "controlling his wife and children" from the Quran and Hadis (sayings of Prophet Muhammad) as homework. The results were amazing when the couple returned next time. He brought with him a long list of verses and Ahadis (plural for Hadis) which contradicted his assumption. Saiqa returned to her husband's home after another 4 sessions. The couple came back for follow-up after 6 months, when they brought a huge basket of sweets!

Family

Family members of an Asian patient are often involved in a way that might seem *over*-involved to Western therapists. You can use the family's involvement to your patient's advantage, in several ways:

- To aid information gathering.
- To act as a co-therapist, especially if the patient is not literate but an educated family member is available (boundary issues and the limits of confidentiality need to be negotiated).
- By supporting the patient at home in a range of ways.
- By accompanying the patient for follow-up appointments.

Communication and language

Language barriers can lead to misinterpretation and even misdiagnosis of presenting problems. If patients cannot speak English, you need to work with interpreters to allow you to communicate effectively with your patient. Try not to use relatives or friends for this purpose, because it can inhibit self-disclosure and upset the balance of the existing relationship. Although working with interpreters can be enormously helpful to the therapeutic process, it is not always easy and requires careful consideration. For an excellent guide on using interpreters in CBT, see d'Ardenne and Farmer (2009).

Patients with depression and anxiety sometimes need help with interpersonal skills, and a good understanding of cultural differences in social behaviour is therefore helpful. For instance, respect for one's elders is an important part of Asian cultures and may mean that a son cannot disagree with his father, or that an employee cannot express his opinion when his/her boss is present.

Ahmed was referred for help with anxiety, low mood, sleep disturbance and headaches. The assessment revealed that, after completing his degree in another town, Ahmed had returned to live in the parental home because his father had told him that leaving the family home was against their religion as well as family and cultural values, and would bring shame to his parents. So, to comply with his father's wishes, Ahmed had taken a job in his home town that didn't utilize his training and offered little hope of progress in his chosen career, nor much opportunity to make new friends. Ahmed wanted to return to the city where he had attended university, to find better work and improve his social life. He was thus torn between respecting his father's wishes and pursuing his desire for change. To help address the resultant feelings of shame and guilt, his therapist asked Ahmed to consult a faith healer in the local community to help clarify his thinking. He was told that a man is allowed to express his opinion and disagree with his parents, so long as he is not rude to them. He was also told that he had rights as well as duties as a son. Finally he was able to discuss the issue with his father and in the end they both agreed that it would be better for Ahmed to move out.

Appropriate assertiveness needs to be culturally sensitive. Good communicators from Asian cultures often use an assertive strategy that we call the 'apology technique'. This strategy begins by apologizing and requesting permission to speak or disagree: for instance, 'I would like to seek your permission to disagree…'; 'If you allow me to express myself…'; or 'With due respect I would like to say that my opinion is…' People using this technique also present a humble appearance, especially lowering their eyes as a sign of respect. You can teach patients how to do this by using role-plays in session.

The therapeutic relationship

Developing a therapeutic relationship based on warmth and trust is of paramount importance in the therapeutic process, both for promoting engagement and for maintaining therapist-patient rapport. This becomes even more important in the context of Asian cultures, where people often go to see healers because of faith, and where word of mouth is an important way in which good or bad news is spread in the community. If your patient and his/her family are convinced that you have 'healing powers', he/she is much more likely to attend future sessions. This faith is built by providing some relief in the first few sessions, for example, by using simple strategies for managing an important symptom your patient is concerned about. Involving patient's family (with the patient's consent) might also be helpful in this regard.

Just like their Caucasian counterparts, Asian patients expect courtesy, careful listening, warmth, and genuineness. Adaptations of CBT might need to take account of some patients' preference for direct advice, and a greater reluctance to disagree with the therapist due to the respect they may hold for figures of authority. Disagreement may instead be shown by not attending appointments, or prematurely ending treatment. You should therefore pay particular attention to your patients' body language, or other subtle changes in language and expression, and make sure you get regular feedback, especially at the beginning of therapy. Questions that frame feedback positively are also helpful, for example:

- What part of our conversation has been most useful to you?
- How might I respond in a way that would be useful to you?
- As we talk about this, would you prefer to focus on X or Y?
- Would you like me to go along with your thoughts on this issue or would you like me to suggest other ways of thinking about this?

Expression of distress and symptoms

Many Asian patients with anxiety or depression present with physical complaints. You should thoroughly understand the nature of the physical symptoms, especially during the first sessions, before moving on to other aspects of the CBT assessment. Begin by using your patients' formulation of their difficulties and gradually, as the therapeutic relationship permits, reframe problems using a wider, more CBT-based, understanding of the problems and their maintenance. A CBT formulation can easily include linking somatic complaints with thoughts, emotions, and behaviours, and we often use an extra column in our patients' first thought diary for them to write about physical symptoms. However, you need to be careful that your patient does not see your linking his/her physical symptoms with thoughts as meaning you are not taking them seriously, or as implying that the physical symptoms are only in his/her mind.

Focus of therapy

A therapist who is trained in Western therapy techniques alone might find himself out of his depth when dealing with patients who present with somatic complaints, especially since techniques to address somatic or dissociative symptoms are not well developed. You should spend plenty of time in preparing patients for therapy. Start by simply talking to them about their somatic symptoms, and show genuine concern and respect. Previous health professionals may have not shown much interest in the patients' physical complaints, so merely by listening to them you might gain their trust.

The two-stage rule we use can be described as 'focus and connect':

- In the first stage, you *focus* on the patient's main concern, whatever it is (e.g. somatic complaints).
- In the second stage, you *connect* your patient's concern with what you think is clinically important and will need addressing (e.g. depressed mood, anxiety, or reduced activities).

This approach applies not only to somatic symptoms but also to other issues that are on the patient's mind, like communication, social problems, or relationship difficulties.

Mrs Khadeeja presented with recurrent headaches as well as symptoms of anxiety and depression. She felt angry and frustrated because she believed that her family doctor had not been interested in her headache and had not examined her. The first two sessions therefore focused on assessing her headache; we even arranged for her to be examined by a physician, which she found reassuring. She was then advised to use breathing exercises and muscle relaxation to help the headaches. She asked whether Indian head massage might be useful, and the therapist encouraged her to pursue this idea. When she returned the next week, Mrs Khadeeja reported some recovery. Her therapist began educating her about anxiety and depression, describing her symptoms and using her response to relaxation as evidence that her headache might be due to anxiety and not an underlying physical illness. She was happy to consider this alternative hypothesis further.

Traditional healing practices

In the UK project's qualitative study, South Asian Muslim groups reported consulting faith healers, Imams, and community leaders as part of their health-seeking behaviours and pathways (Rathod *et al.*, 2008). It was also apparent in these patients' reports that they tended to use a multi-dimensional approach, that is, they often used multiple sources of help simultaneously. For instance, a patient might consult a *general practitioner* (GP) and also see the Imam for prayers. Sometimes a patient would use traditional remedies; and in some instances, following consultation with the extended family members, the family would send the patient back to Pakistan or Bangladesh for healing. Most of these sources of help are likely to be at worst harmless from a CBT point of view. It is also worth bearing in mind that the patient might be seeing you because of a suggestion from a faith or religious healer. You need to acknowledge and accept such pathways as apart of the healing process. In fact, the multidimensional nature of this approach has some similarities to the biopsychosocial model often used in Western mental health practice.

Capacity and circumstances

In the later sections we describe issues of capacity and circumstances, first on an individual level and then on a system level (i.e. the medical or traditional health system, as well as the system of support available to the patient). Although some of the areas in this domain may not be new to you, they are probably different in their significance.

Individual level

Gender

Women from a South Asian Muslim background often have less autonomy than many other patients. They may have to seek permission from their husband or father to see a therapist or to change the way they do things, and are commonly brought to appointments. It is important that you acknowledge this cultural difference and take care to involve the accompanying person in the assessment process, and thereafter talk to him on how the mental health of the woman can have an effect on the health of the family and especially children. Some female Muslims might feel uncomfortable with a male therapist, so try to offer a choice of therapist gender where possible.

Mental illness carries significant stigma in these cultures. It is a common belief that mental illnesses are genetic and can pass on to the next generation (Rathod *et al.*, 2009). This belief causes enormous distress in the families of female patients because of likely consequent problems in arranging marriage. You should therefore explore patients' and families' understanding of the illness and its transmission, and educate them to reduce their anxiety.

Differences in cultural expectations of men and women tend to vary by generation and by degree of acculturation. First generation South Asian Muslim patients will often prefer to be seen by a therapist of the same gender. However, the second generation are often more flexible and may not mind being seen by either a female or male therapist, so long as the therapist is aware of and respects their cultural background. Of course, not everyone is the same, and therefore it is important to be flexible where possible.

Age

Age of the patient can be important as it often correlates with level of acculturation. In our experience, younger patients are more likely to benefit from therapy (Naeem *et al.*, in press). Higher levels of education and access to electronic and print media may contribute to changed attitudes, and of course younger patients also tend to be more aware of Western concepts of mental illness and its treatment.

Educational level

A significant part of CBT practice is homework, and some homework tasks usually demand reading and writing skills—for example, keeping a thought record or reading a self-help book. Patients who cannot read or write English might be able to read and write their native languages, and Urdu versions of reading and practice materials (such as thought diaries) can be obtained from the authors of this chapter. It is still common to come across patients, especially women, who are not literate at all. This needs to be sensitively addressed, and there are many alternatives to reading/writing that can be used: audio tapes, CDs, MP3 players, mobile phones, or digital recorders can be used to record thoughts and to record sessions for patients to review. Audio diaries and beads, counters or symbols can be used for counting thoughts or other data gathering (beads and counters are commonly used in Pakistan for repeating religious verses or words). Involving a family member as a co-therapist can also sometimes be useful. In the last resort, detailed recall may substitute for diaries, as many people with limited literacy seem to be able to train and improve their memory capacity to compensate.

Coping strategies

Although an important component of CBT is to reactivate old skills, new skills can help build useful coping resources for dealing with the difficulties that patients face. Such coping skills need to be compatible with your patient's cultural, religious, or spiritual background. As noted earlier, Asian patients are more likely to use religious and spiritual coping skills. Careful discussion with your patient will help you utilize new coping skills that are helpful to your patient as well as culturally acceptable.

System level

Capacity of the health system

Necessary adjustments might involve negotiating with your patients about how frequently they can attend therapy sessions. It may not be practical for your patient to attend weekly 1-hour session, when she has a social role that extends to supporting the entire extended family. You will need to assess for this and collaboratively agree on a frequency that is acceptable to your patient.

Pathways to care and help-seeking behaviours

Pathways to care and help-seeking behaviours are related to multiple factors, for example, socio-demographic factors, social structures, level of education, cultural beliefs and practices, gender discrimination, the status of women, economic and political systems, environmental conditions and disease patterns, as well as the health system itself (Shaikh *et al.*, 2004). In the UK project, the moderators influencing help-seeking behaviours were those shown in Box 2.1.

Cognitions and beliefs

Under this heading we refer not only to the usual cognitions and beliefs that are directly addressed in CBT, but also to what patients think about health, healers, and the healthcare system.

Box 2.1 Moderators influencing help-seeking behaviours

- Type of psychological problem
- How it is dealt in the family/extended family
- Advice given by GP
- Symptom severity/extent of illness
- Stigma/shame
- Community pressure (e.g. stigma attached to illness) and the knowledge and attitude of community members towards the illness
- Faith healer's/Imam's knowledge of the problem
- Being sent back to country of origin for healing or arranged marriage (it is a common belief that marriage will bring a sense of responsibility as well as emotional support, which might help with the illness)
- Religiosity
- Level of education and awareness of mental illness
- Whether first or second generation migrant

Source: Rathod, S., Kingdon, D., Phiri, P. and Gobbi, M. (2009). *Developing culturally sensitive cognitive behaviour therapy for psychosis for ethnic minority patients by exploration and incorporation of service users and health professional's views and opinions.* Report to Delivering Race Equality, DOH Clinical Trail Blazers programme.

Beliefs about health and illness

It is important to explore a patient's beliefs about health and illness. Your patient's ideas of good and bad health might be different from your ideas. For example, the patient who believes that feeling tense and depressed is a normal reaction in certain circumstances is not likely to seek help (even if you might think he/she has clinical depression). Similarly, some people think of normal health as consisting only of physical health. Only a small number of depressed or anxious patients present to the medical system, perhaps because of a belief that only people with somatic symptoms go to medical healers, while those with psychological symptoms should seek help from faith healers or spiritual healers.

Beliefs about causes of illness

In the UK project, the emergent themes relating to the participants' explanatory models of what causes mental illness (in particular psychosis) were very varied, and included: previous wrongdoing; supernatural factors such as magic, the 'evil eye', *saya* (being under the influence of an evil spirit), and *taweez* (a spell done by writing on paper); social factors; biological factors; being arrested by the police; and drugs (Rathod *et al.*, 2008). In contrast, depressed patients in the project were found to hold a more ordinary psychosocial model of illness, with depression being caused by relationship difficulties, ongoing problems, and losses. This model is of course consistent with CBT, and you can start by helping your patients deal with these problems early on in treatment. We often use problem-solving and coping skills training at the start of the therapy to foster engagement in CBT.

Beliefs about treatment

Beliefs about the causes of an illness can strongly influence treatment choice, and therefore asking patients about their expectation of treatment is important. Talking to patients about their concept of illness and its treatment can be helpful, and can guide you in delivering therapy. Educating patients about medication side effects, and the indications for and limitations of medication, can result in increased confidence in the therapist's abilities and thus improve engagement. This also helps in monitoring the effects, side effects, and dosage of medication, as well as the patient's adherence to treatment. You can then slowly introduce the concepts of CBT and proceed with more psychological therapy.

Beliefs about the health system

Patients' knowledge of the health system, available treatments, and their likely outcomes are important factors determining service utilization and engagement.

As noted, patients from a Muslim background may be more likely to expect medication and may have less knowledge about psychological interventions. Patients may also be more likely to seek help from a doctor who belongs to their own sectarian, religious, or linguistic group.

Simply being aware of these beliefs at an early stage will be helpful, and you may realize that you don't need to challenge most of them. You can then keep your focus on relevant issues, avoiding conflict with patients over trivial issues.

Beliefs about healing and the healer

At the start of this chapter we mentioned the patient who seemed to believe that the therapist should understand his/her problem just by looking at him/her. Patients and their families talk about *Hakims* (practitioners of Greek-Indian medicine) who can diagnose you just by looking at you, and about faith healers or spiritual healers who can change the way you feel in the same way. It is therefore important to identify patients' beliefs about healing, their faith in other healing systems, and their expectations about treatment and what it can do for them, so that you can identify and work with these beliefs.

Abdul had a long history of schizophrenia that had only partially responded to medicines. His family were very excited when they met his therapist. They had been told by his psychiatrist that he was being referred for treatment that did not involve medicines. When the therapist explored their expectations from therapy, the father said "Abdul's cousin in Bangladesh had a similar illness two years ago and was cured by joint treatment by a psychiatrist and a religious healer. He was married a few weeks ago. We think you can also cure Abdul". On detailed inquiry it appeared that the cousin's illness was more likely to be an episode of bipolar illness. However the therapist was careful and did not immediately spell out his conclusions. He asked them to get more details of the cousin's illness and its diagnosis, and started working with Abdul.

Abdul's family brought back more information in the 5th session. As expected, the diagnosis was bipolar disorder and the cousin was on a mood stabilizer. The therapist carefully pointed out the differences between this and schizophrenia. Although the family were a little disappointed, they were reassured by the fact that Abdul liked to talk to his therapist and had shown some signs of improvement already. They therefore continued with the therapy.

Cognitive errors and dysfunctional beliefs

Cognitive errors and dysfunctional beliefs may vary from culture to culture (Padesky and Greenberger, 1995). There is some evidence from Hong Kong (Tam and Wong, 2007) and Turkey (Sahin and Sahin, 1992) of such variation. You may therefore have to consider some modifications for working on these areas in therapy.

We have already described changes in thought diaries that you might find useful. Some kinds of thinking errors may also not be readily understood. For example, the idea of 'black and white thinking' might not need much explanation to a Western patient, but it might be a totally new concept for a South Asian Muslim patient. Culturally adapted description of cognitive errors, as well as their translation in colloquial terms for patients of Pakistani origin, can be obtained from the authors. Remember also that in Asian cultures, mind and body are not considered separate, and patients might mix cognitions with emotions. Therefore, before you start cognitive work you will have to spend some time trying to educate your patients about cognitions, emotions, and the cognitive model. Putting together a list of commonly experienced emotions and including some of these in a thought diary might be helpful.

When working with patients' beliefs you need to be mindful of the fact that some of their apparently dysfunctional beliefs might be normal beliefs in their culture, or might even be seen as positive traits. Role performance within the family, familial harmony, fate, 'face', and fairness were described as culture-specific themes in the study from Hong Kong (Tam and Wong, 2007). In our work, we found that some of what may be seen as dysfunctional beliefs in the West (e.g. dependence on family, giving up personal needs for the good of the family, or the need for acceptance by others) are widely shared by healthy individuals in other societies. You will have to weigh the advantages and disadvantages of changing such beliefs. The problem is compounded by the wide variations that exist *within* these cultures, in the degree and the expression of such beliefs among different people. The best way forward is to consult a family member and enquire how acceptable that belief is within that particular family. This might be easy if you have already involved a family member in therapy. You also need to be mindful of your own beliefs, especially about the way your patients from these cultures might live; for example, arranged marriages, the use of a head scarf by a female, or an adult living with his parents (although social services might look after elderly parents, for many Asian Muslims it is a sin to leave their parents alone).

You need to be very careful when using some of the commonly used CBT techniques for dealing with beliefs, for example, downward arrow technique or Socratic dialogue. Patients often expect you to be a master, a teacher, or a guru, who will advise them rather than use a long Socratic dialogue to help them to achieve insights. Be comfortable with dealing with them like a teacher who points out certain insights to the patient. Socratic dialogue in particular can make patients uncomfortable as they may be more likely to interpret it as criticism of their thinking. You can deal with this by preparing your patients for the Socratic approach and reassuring them that you want to help them, *not* to start an inquisition!

Key points

The framework in this chapter provides some initial guidelines, but therapists should be cautious in generalizing these. As with all forms of CBT, patients are likely to benefit most when their treatment is tailored to their specific needs and style.

- Be sensitive and listen carefully to understand your patient's culture.
- Be mindful that your own speech can reflect attitudes and beliefs you hold about others' culture.
- Consult therapists with cultural expertise.
- Consider addressing language issues by using a trained interpreter.
- Avoid misinterpretation of patient's behaviour by not making cultural assumptions.
- Be aware that patients are sensitive to stereotyping.
- Be sure to remain validating and non-judgemental.
- Do not react defensively to apparently resistant patients: instead find a common ground to work from, and always link with your patient's goals.
- Try to understand how your own cultural background may interfere with that of your patient. Use supervision to address this.
- Remember that core beliefs or schemas are strongly influenced by culture and will impact how your patient responds to therapy. Always check with a family member whether the dysfunctional belief is shared by other members of the family or not.

Further reading

Hays, P.A. and Iwamasa, G.Y. (eds.) (2006). *Culturally Responsive Cognitive Behaviour Therapy. Assessment, Practice and Supervision.* Washington, DC: American Psychological Association.

Mason, B. and Sawyer, A. (2002). *Exploring the Unsaid: Creativity, Risks and Dilemmas in Working Cross-Culturally.* London: Karnac.

The Developing Culturally Sensitive CBT for Psychosis project website. Available at: www.its-services.org.uk/equalities/en/our-work/delivering-race-equality/clinical-trailblazers/mid-hampshire-and-eastleigh/ (accessed on 26 February 2010).

Williams, M.W., Foo, K.H. and Haarhoff, B. (2006). Cultural considerations in using cognitive behaviour therapy with Chinese people: a case study of an elderly Chinese woman with generalised anxiety disorder. *New Zealand Journal of Psychology*, **35**, 153–162.

References

d'Ardenne, P. and Farmer, E. (2009). Using interpreters in trauma therapy, in Grey, N. (ed.), *A Casebook of Cognitive Therapy for Traumatic Stress Reactions.* Hove: Routledge.

Fernando, S. (1991). *Mental Health, Race and Culture.* Basingstoke: Palgrave.

Hays, P.A. and Iwamasa, G.Y. (eds.) (2006). *Culturally Responsive Cognitive Behaviour Therapy. Assessment, Practice and Supervision.* Washington, DC: American Psychological Association.

Naeem, F., Ayub, M., Gobbi, M. and Kingdon, D. (in press). Development of Southampton Adaptation Framework for CBT (SAF-CBT). A framework for adaptation of CBT in non-Western cultures. *Journal of the Pakistan Psychiatric Society.*

Padesky, C. and Greenberger, D. (1995). *Clinician's Guide to Mind Over Mood.* New York, NY: Guilford Press.

Rathod, S., Naeem, F., Phiri, P. and Kingdon, K. (2008). Expansion of psychological therapies. *British Journal of Psychiatry*, **193**, 256–257.

Rathod, S., Kingdon, D., Phiri, P. and Gobbi, M. (2009). *Developing culturally sensitive cognitive behaviour therapy for psychosis for ethnic minority patients by exploration and incorporation of service users and health professional's views and opinions.* Report to Delivering Race Equality, DOH Clinical Trail Blazers programme.

Sahin, N.H. and Sahin, N. (1992). How dysfunctional are the dysfunctional attitudes in another culture? *British Journal of Medical Psychology*, **65**, 17–26.

Shaikh, B. and Hatcher, J (2004). Health seeking behaviour and health service utilization in Pakistan: challenging the policy makers. *Journal of Public Health*, **27**(1), 49–54.

Tam, P.W.C. and Wong, D.F.K. (2007). Qualitative analysis of dysfunctional attitudes in Chinese persons suffering from depression. *Hong Kong Journal of Psychiatry*, **17**, 109–114.

Tseng, W. (2004). Culture and psychotherapy: Asian perspectives. *Journal of Mental Health*, **13**, 151–161.

Tseng, Wen-Shing., Chang, S.C., and Nishjzono, M. (2005). *Asian Culture and Psychotherapy: Implications for East and West.* USA: University of Hawaii Press.

Chapter 3

Looking after yourself

Helen Kennerley, Martina Mueller, and Melanie Fennell

Eighteen months after taking the job, Mathew found that he had lost enthusiasm and optimism. He felt overburdened and out of his depth and unsupported by colleagues.

Introduction

As CBT (cognitive behavioural therapy) therapists we are well trained to enable our patients to care for themselves; to appreciate when they need to rest, to find simulation, or to tackle problems that wear them down. We teach them to notice difficulties and to find ways to resolve them. Yet all too often we ignore our own needs, ploughing on regardless of signs that we are exhausted, stressed, or cranky. We then get less pleasure and fulfilment from what we do, we are less likely to accomplish what we set out to achieve, and we become less effective therapists. Our ability to care for others is compromised if we do not take care of ourselves.

In this chapter, we hope to dispel common myths that lead us to adopt this 'looking after yourself is for patients' assumption. Instead we encourage you to think about your physical and psychological well-being by considering the practical and emotional issues that might affect you, and to explore how you might use your understanding of CBT to look after yourself. We highlight:

- Beliefs which can fuel therapist self-neglect
- Sources of stress
- Tools for dealing with stress
- Special challenges: namely, coping with emotionally demanding patients and dealing with work pressure, harassment, and complaints

Common myths about looking after yourself

- **Self-care is optional.** This conflicts with the message we give to our patients when we stress the importance of ongoing self-care in our blueprints and relapse management plans—yet we consider it optional for ourselves. For example, in a study on vicarious trauma, Bober and Regehr (2006) found that 259 therapists surveyed generally endorsed the value of self-care and supervision but many therapists did not actually practice them.
- **Knowing how to look after yourself is as good as actually doing it.** This is the self-care version of the belief that photocopying academic papers is as good as reading them! We know that we need to balance activities that drain our resources with those that replenish us, we know how to problem-solve and the importance of sharing worries and concerns: so why don't we apply this knowledge to ourselves more often? Perhaps we believe that we don't (or shouldn't) need to. Perhaps we think that we really will get around to looking after ourselves—as soon as we finish this pressing task or survive this cluster of demands.
- **I'm a therapist—I can cope.** At one time or another we all have to deal with problems in our personal or professional lives which make it hard to function effectively or well. We might become ill, have to cope with losses or problems in our relationships, or our children might get sick. Life events and chronic life stresses can take a psychological toll on anyone, and CBT therapists are not immune to their impact. Yet, how often do we assume that we can get by simply because we are therapists?

The American Psychological Association code of ethics (APA, 2002) sets out the ethical imperative of self-care for their members, namely to be aware 'of the possible effect of their own physical and mental health on their ability to help those with whom they work' (p. 1062). We all need to recognize the hazards we face and replace denial with acceptance and self-criticism with self-compassion.

The hazards we face: sources of stress

Over 50 years ago, Abraham Maslow developed his 'Hierarchy of Needs' in the workplace (1954). This illustrated five areas which need to be attended to if employees are to feel encouraged and able to fulfil their unique potential (self-actualization). He described them as a hierarchy because they build on each other—initially we look to meet our needs at one level and once that is achieved we look to the next and so on. Failure to meet our needs at any level is a source of stress. Box 3.1 summarizes the five areas and what this means with regard to

Box 3.1 Maslow's hierarchy of needs

1. **Basic environment**: your workplace should meet your fundamental needs for comfort. It should afford you warmth, privacy, access to refreshments, satisfactory equipment, and so on.
2. **Safety:** you need to be protected from danger (structural and interpersonal) and to have a sense of security regarding your job and income. This should be explicit from your induction package, your work contract, and from regular meetings with your line manager.
3. **Sense of belonging**: you should feel part of an organization and be able to form relationships within it. You should feel supported and able to express yourself and state your needs.
4. **Self-esteem**: you need a sense of achievement, mastery, independence in order to meet esteem needs. This will be reflected in your gaining status within the workplace and possibly taking on managerial responsibility, etc. Therefore, you need access to further training.
5. **Personal growth**: this is the stage of 'self-actualization' and reflects your need to realize personal potential and self-fulfilment. This means gaining further training and career progress, helping you maximize opportunities for personal development.

your workplace: review them and consider if your workplace enables you to meet your needs at each level. If you work independently, then ask yourself if the working conditions which you have developed are adequate.

As you read through, did you feel that some of your needs were not met? If so, you will have identified sources of stress.

Mathew considered his working environment: his office was warm and at least he and the therapist with whom he shared had privacy, which some of his colleagues lacked. However, the furniture was old and his back ached after he had spent an afternoon at his desk, and his eyes hurt because his ancient computer flickered too much. He was also often frustrated because it was so slow. He thought about his sense of safety and realized that he had not been given an induction which clarified safety procedures within the building—he did not know how to deal with a potentially dangerous patient or where the fire exits were, which unnerved him. However, he did feel able to ask other staff members about this as the department had an atmosphere of friendliness and he felt supported within in. He also felt able to approach his immediate line manager and Mathew now realized that he needed to do this in order to protect himself from physical discomfort, over-working and to establish the opportunities for personal development which might be available within his department. Over the past eighteen months he had been carrying a significant work-load which had now become top-heavy with "difficult" patients and this was creating stress without much reward. As one of the few men in the department, the majority of referrals for anger management and the majority of abused male patients seemed to come Mathew's way and it was taking a toll on his well-being. This was made worse by the fact that Mathew did not feel particularly skilled to rise to the challenge. He also felt that he had not been developing a career path since he took the job and this was frustrating.

Once you have identified *your* sources of stress, they need to be addressed, and this is what we consider next.

Physician heal thyself: putting our knowledge into practice

As a cognitive therapist you are in a good position to deal with stress: you are skilled in developing awareness of psychological barriers to progress, putting this into context and using problem-solving to resolve difficulties. How often do you systematically address work-related or personal problems that are impacting on your work? Through training you will have developed self-reflection skills: are you still setting aside time for this? Your training will also have enhanced your ability to formulate difficulties and to devise appropriate interventions based on that understanding: do you make and justify the time to formulate your own occupational problems?

Consider your abilities:

- Self-reflection
- Formulating difficulties
- Using CBT to identify and address cognitive distortion
- Problem-solving and flexibility in dealing with change
- Resourcing yourself through supervision and training and modifying your environment
- Knowledge and skills of particular clinical problems

The rest of this chapter will help you consider how you can use your skills and knowledge to look after yourself at work.

Self-reflection

Although it can be tempting to assume that if we ignore a problem it will go away, step one in dealing with our own difficulties is to look at them: to reflect on what doesn't work or causes distress and to consider what factors, both environmental and psychological, contribute to this. Self-reflection has long been considered part of good practice in psychotherapy (see Chapter 20) and in order to ensure that you look after yourself as well as your patients, try to find time to reflect on your needs and evolve ways of working which accommodate them. This is perhaps stating the obvious, but if you are neglecting self-reflection then you need to devise ways to makes it easier.

Make time for self-reflection

Many of us find it difficult to make enough space for everything we need to do: clinical demands from patients, targets we have to reach, meetings we need to attend, the demands of excessive paperwork, and seemingly endless emails. For some of us, making time for lunch can be a real challenge never mind time for self-reflection, but neglecting this can worsen our stress. You might have heard the story of the woodcutter who managed to fell a great many trees on the first day of his job, but felled fewer and fewer as time went on because he was too busy to sharpen his axe. It is particularly important to reflect on therapy sessions or therapeutic tasks which are especially demanding.

It can be hard to spot these self-defeating patterns in ourselves unless we deliberately make time to do so. So make a date with yourself, book reflection time in your diary as a regular slot and guard the time as fiercely as a patient session or a meeting. You could do that right now.

Mathew put a regular "appointment with himself" in his diary: he allocated one of his weekly clinic slots to himself so that he could dedicate sufficient time to review and plan his work. He also resolved to make sure that he left some time for reflection between patients—a practice which slipped when he felt under clinical pressure.

Once you have time, reflect on your reactions both during and after a session, critically listen to a recording of the session and discuss your reactions and concerns in supervision.

Formulating the problem(s); assessing your need(s)

When you reflect on your work try not to suppress or dismiss your reactions, instead take time (however brief) to consider:

- What am I feeling and thinking?
- What caused me to react in this way? Why am I upset?
- How is this impacting on my behaviour? (Towards myself or my patient, in or outside of the session).
- What conclusions am I drawing from this?
- What do I know about my attitudes towards my work and myself as a therapist that might be relevant here?
- What is/is not working well?
- What do I want/need to change?

This puts you in a position to formulate what might be maintaining your problems and to decide what you can do to try to change things. If you get stuck in this process use supervision or an informal chat with a colleague to help you gain a clearer understanding of your feelings and reactions. You might also find that using thought records will help you better understand and formulate your work challenges.

Mathew realized that there were several factors maintaining his problems. Some lay outside his control, such as, the ever diminishing staff levels in his unit, but others were within his control. For example, he realized that he was not asking his line manager for enough support or making his CPD needs clear, and self monitoring had revealed some exaggerated and catastrophic thinking which he could begin to address. Once he had clarified the sources of his difficulties he could begin problem solving.

It is helpful not only to consider the difficulties you face, but also to identify and appreciate your strengths and preferences. Even if you have never completed personality questionnaires or learning style assessments and you may already have a sense of your preferences for:

- Social interaction (introvert/extrovert)
- Task management (organized/disorganized; creative/concrete, etc.)
- Learning style (active learning/reflecting and theorizing—there is a more detailed description of learning styles in Chapter 15) and so on

This awareness creates a foundation for building on your strengths and compensating for your needs. For example:

- If you are creative but disorganized—embrace your creativity and at the same time compensate for your disorganization by learning to keep lists, memos, and a detailed diary.
- If you are extraverted and work best with others to bounce ideas off—aim to work in forums that allow discussion.
- If you are poor at task-completion—compensate by delegating or ensuring you always plan time to finish before moving on to the next thing.

Mathew knew that he tended towards introversion and avoidance of conflict and that he was a resourceful and creative problem-solver who worked well alone, but he had not considered how this impacted on his work difficulties, nor how he might best use his strengths in the workplace. Mindful of his strengths, he set aside solitary time to consider solutions to his difficulties and discovered that he rapidly came up with ideas. One of his ideas was to revise his assertiveness skills as he knew that being unassertive was contributing to his occupational difficulties as it prevented him from saying "no" when asked to take on extra patients.

When you are clear about how you can best use your strengths and preferences, to maximize the benefits of your personal style, incorporate this into concrete action plans and put a review date in your diary. Even good plans can flounder—following through is a real challenge so consider asking a colleague or supervisor to encourage you.

Using CBT approaches to resolve problem(s)

You are experienced in helping patients deal with problem emotions and behaviours: you have used thought records and activity scheduling, challenged unhelpful thoughts, and learnt problem-solving with them. Thus, you already have a powerful and flexible set of tools to help you make changes and resolve your difficulties. Of course, an additional advantage of applying CBT interventions to yourself is that it will make it easier for you to empathize with your patients who use them.

A good starting point for coping is to ask: 'What would I suggest to a patient in this situation?' This will tap into your skills base and help you generate coping strategies such as the ones below.

- Give yourself space to process your emotions.
- Maintain nurturing relationships in and outside of work and regularly engage in restorative activities.
- Consider your caseload and workload. Try to see a mix of patients with different presenting problems and experiences if you can. If you work with only one type of presentation you may struggle to maintain a balanced perspective. Try to see patients with 'straightforward' problems as well as complex difficulties and balance out the phases of treatment so that some of your patients will be beginning treatment while others are getting nearer the end. This will ensure a more balanced spread of demands on you as a therapist and reduce the likelihood of feeling overwhelmed.
- Consider the overlap between your own life and the clinical work you do. For example, if you have recently been bereaved it might be hard to hear about loss and grief from your patient, or if you have experienced violence in your own life you may reasonably choose not to see someone who is recovering from a physically abusive relationship. On the other hand, your experience of coping with personal difficulties might help you be particularly empathic and constructive. You need to be aware of your own strengths and needs.
- Keep an eye on your expectations of yourself. Although your job description or contract, or your need to generate a certain income, mean that you do not have complete control over what and how much you do, be aware of your own beliefs and expectations which could contribute to your working at unsustainable levels. You may feel you are doing the right thing by squeezing in another patient into your already stretched schedule, but seeing too many patients will reduce the effectiveness of your CBT because you

will not have enough time to reflect and prepare or process your emotional responses. This will have an impact on you.

Not every strategy listed here will be useful at any given time, consider the best one for you for a particular situation.

Sound strategies will go some way towards stress-proofing you but your own unhelpful beliefs may still generate stress or get in the way of persisting with changes. Supposing your patient was struggling to find time to carry out an important task—what would you do? You would probably hypothesize that some beliefs were getting in the way. You would check out your hunches through Socratic questioning and perhaps by encouraging your patient to catch and record unhelpful thoughts. How about attempting the same thing for yourself?

Mathew found that although he had planned to use a thought record to identify and challenge the beliefs behind his unassertiveness at work, days slipped by without his making any entries. When his supervisor asked him to cast his mind back to a time when he had thought about making an entry but didn't, Mathew was able to better understand the obstacles to keeping the record. He identified thoughts such as: "I should be able to resolve this without regressing to diary keeping"; "I'll think about it more when I've time", "there's a difference between patients' needs and mine". Catching these thoughts enabled him to stand back and search for more helpful alternatives. This, in turn, freed him up to use helpful CBT strategies to address his own difficulties.

Next time you fail to prepare for a meeting, despite appreciating that you are the sort of person who is not readily creative and spontaneous, or the next time you fail to delegate, despite knowing that you tend to overburden yourself, try to set aside time to identify the thoughts that drive that behaviour. For example: 'If I think about it in advance I'll get nervous so I just deal with it at the time'. Or 'I couldn't possibly ask her to take this on—she'll think I'm lazy or bullying her'. Consider how you help your patients make identifying NATs (negative automatic thoughts) part of their daily routine. Can you apply the same advice to yourself? Assumptions, in particular, often lend themselves to behavioural testing and each of these therapist predictions could be subjected to behavioural scrutiny. See if you can devise a behavioural experiment to check out whether or not your predictions are valid.

In this section, you have considered how to use your professional skills to address work stress, but making changes in work patterns can still be hard to do on your own, so it is important to ensure that you have the resources you need to follow through.

Resource yourself: create a comfortable and safe working environment

Maslow's hierarchy puts comfort and safety firmly at its base, so do not overlook this.

Comfort: Look around—is your working environment satisfactory? For example, is your equipment reliable and ergonomic? Are you afforded privacy for your clinical sessions? Can you access the administrative support that you need? If your basic working conditions are lacking then use your problem-solving skills (see previous section) to rectify this. Like Mathew, you might need to overcome interpersonal obstacles such as being assertive, but this is not insurmountable.

You also need to consider your physical safety and, although *it is rare*, patients have been known to threaten, intimidate, harass, stalk, or even attack therapists. Therefore, you need to be able to assess risk to yourself and to implement management strategies.

Assessing risk: It involves knowing the patient and the environment within which you work and it is wise to keep these under review.

Ask yourself:

- Are there aspects of this patient's history which suggest risk—a history of violence or drinking and disinhibition; or a history of overattachment, violation of therapist privacy, making complaints?
- In this particular setting, are there patients who could pose a risk to me?
- Does the setting itself pose risks—is it safe to being alone with this patient during a home visit? Are these areas well lit? Are other staff members around at this time? Is it safe to carry out behavioural experiments *in vivo* with this person?
- Is my office seating arrangement safe—can I exit the room and/or reach an alarm swiftly?
- Am I sufficiently skilled to deal with an aggressive outburst or an overdependent patient?

If you have doubts do not take risks. Although dangerous incidents are rare they can happen. It is also wise to ensure that your personal details (where you live, a description of your car, and so on) are not disclosed to your patients either by you or others, such as administrative staff.

Managing risk: If you carry out a realistic assessment of risk you can then consider ways of avoiding it and you can develop contingency plans.

Mathew feared that a particular patient would become aggressive towards him. He had reviewed the patient's history and knew that he had been verbally aggressive in the past. Now that the patient was drinking more his angry outbursts were increasing. Thus, Mathew's fears were valid and he knew that he must act on them. Although he did not see this person out of hours, he tended to give him an appointment on Friday afternoons when there were very few staff members around. This added to his discomfort, so he shifted the appointment to a time when the department was busier. He also checked that the alarm in the treatment room was working. He sought advice from his line manager who offered support and focused his thinking on risk assessment and prevention of an unwanted incident. This improved his confidence so that he could better appreciate when a situation was dangerous and was better able to manage it. This increased confidence helped him consider how he might address the difficulty with his patient. His clinical supervisor helped him develop a formulation of the interaction between him and his patient and discussed with Mathew how this could be developed with the patient in a respectful, sensitive and collaborative way. He then successfully broached the issue with his patient. With hindsight, Mathew realized that it would have been useful for his supervisor to have carried out a joint assessment with him, so that she was better able to assess risk.

- **Formulate difficulties with the patient:** If you think that there is an issue with your patient, bring it up sooner rather than later and as sensitively and empathically as you can. If you avoid addressing it or address it insensitively you might be putting yourself at greater risk. An awareness of your patients' inner world, their vulnerabilities to episodes of anger or obsession, for example, might put you in a position of being able to pre-empt the problem behaviour. Thus, a detailed formulation could help you both appreciate possible triggers and early warning signs, and facilitate developing a shared management plan.
- **Use colleagues for support:** In addition to using supervision sessions and seeking support from your line manager, turn to colleagues to air your personal safety concerns, make sure colleagues know when you are seeing a patient who might pose a risk, ask for a professional chaperone if necessary and benefit from the experiences of others.
- **Challenge thoughts that get in the way of your safety:** Identify and tackle thoughts that might put you at risk such as: 'I should know what to do, it's embarrassing to admit that I don't' or 'I don't want to look like a wimp' or 'the patient's needs are more important than mine' or 'I have to do this home visit because my team has suggested it/my patient has asked me to'.
- **Put your concerns in writing:** Ensure that key others know of your concerns so that they are aware of the potential danger to you or others.
- **Make practical changes:** As Mathew did, consider the timing and venue of patient contacts. Review your office layout and your access to an alarm.
- **Misinterpretation:** You also need to feel confident that you are safe from misinterpretation of your clinical work. If a patient or a colleague accuses you of misconduct, or even goes as far as filing a complaint, you need to be able to defend yourself. So make sure that your note-keeping is of a standard that is easily interpreted by others, and you might find it useful to routinely record your sessions (remember to get consent from your patient to do this) or, if you think that there is a particular risk of misinterpretation ask a co-worker to sit in.

Resourcing yourself: ongoing training

Keeping up-to-date with the necessary skills and knowledge required for your particular area of work and having access to sufficient supervision and support for you to carry out your work safely is a matter of ethical practice and should be prioritized as such. However, creating and taking opportunities for further training and development is the means of meeting our needs for self-esteem and personal growth, which sit firmly at the top of Maslow's hierarchy.

The BABCP accreditation criteria include guidelines on the minimum CPD (continued professional development) and supervision that is acceptable for a CBT practitioner which you can use as a framework for identifying and prioritizing your own particular needs—which will depend on your working environment, your specialist area, and your level of experience.

This will require you to set aside time for:

- Self-reflection
- Identifying your needs
- Prioritizing them

Confidence in your knowledge and skills This will reduce your work stress and you should consider both revising existing CBT skills and developing new ones. This can only be done by dedicating time to your CPD, so, you need to create time for reading and for attending workshops and conferences. Visit websites which advertise training opportunities (e.g. BABCP, OCTC; see websites listed at the end of this chapter) to find out what is available to you.

General mental health and psychological knowledge can be invaluable, too. For example, familiarity with the Mental Health Act (2007) and the Children Act (2004) will allow you more confidently and reliably to manage risk; familiarity with the effects of certain drugs can help you formulate your patient's difficulties more accurately; understanding psychological processes—for example, knowing how memory works—will help in working with intrusive memories.

Confidence that your practice is of good standard will further reduce your work stress. Therefore, be familiar with the BABCP 'Guidelines for Good Practice of Behavioural and Cognitive Psychotherapy' (which are also accessible from their website). Many of you will also have guidelines for ethical practice issued by your professional body (e.g. the Royal College of Nursing or of Psychiatry, the British Psychological Society, or the American Psychological Society) and knowing that you abide by them can enhance your confidence.

Finally, being vigilant about professional insurance and union membership may help reduce your work stress because knowing that you will be supported in a crisis is reassuring. Some of you will find that your union or employer will cover legal costs incurred in the event of a complaint involving legal action; others will find that you are responsible for insuring against this yourself.

Resourcing yourself does not just mean increasing your knowledge—you also need to create a restorative environment both inside and outside the workplace. Ensure that you have access to support amongst colleagues and friends, balance your work activities so that stimulating and relaxing tasks balance the stressful and less rewarding ones and balance your lifestyle so that the stresses of work are offset by pleasurable activities at home.

Mathew attended a training session on dealing with potentially violent patients which was organized by his trust. He was very relieved to learn that his employers were extremely conscientious about safety and he was reassured by knowing how to make the most of the procedures which were in place. However, he was not confident that this training had entirely met his needs so he found an additional workshop on Anger Management via his local branch of the BABCP.

Using supervision Supervision can make an enormous difference to your success in using CBT on yourself and with your patients. A good supervisor will have an eye to your needs as well as your patient's and can direct you towards, and support you in, self-reflection and problem-solving. In this book, we consider 'How to be a supervisor' (Chapter 16) but it is also worth giving some thought to how you make most of the supervision that you receive. Westbrook *et al.* (2007) provide some guidelines:

- *Choosing a supervisor*: consider compatibility, level of expertise, commitment;
- *Negotiating supervision arrangements*: ensure your supervision contract meets your needs and be clear about what you want from supervision. Build in regular reviews of your work issues;
- *Preparing for supervision*: have a clear supervision question, prepare recordings and background information for your supervisor;
- *Using a supervision session*: attend to structure, focus, and be honest in expressing difficulties and open to feedback.

Sometimes, in addition to formal supervision, you may need support from peers and colleagues. For example, when you are learning something new it is helpful to share experiences with colleagues who are in a position to understand your needs and concerns. Or perhaps you are working with a stressful case and need the opportunity to debrief more frequently or spontaneously than supervision allows.

Even when you have attended to your psychological and physical well-being (and progressed through Maslow's hierarchy), you need to remain aware of particular stresses that can impair your enjoyment of your work or even your performance. Therefore, we will now consider some of the most common clinical and organizational sources of additional stress.

Coping with the emotionally demanding nature of your clinical work

Working with patients can be very rewarding, and well-executed CBT is intellectually and emotionally stimulating, affording opportunities to be creative. Thus, it not only helps others but also provides you with a rich opportunity for personal and professional growth. That said, practicing CBT can still be emotionally demanding. As therapists, we need to remain empathically attuned to a wide range of difficult emotions ranging from fear, grief, and shame to profound hopelessness. We sometimes must tolerate hearing of injustices and depravations that we cannot fix or change. This is particularly so if we work with survivors of chronic trauma, patients who suffer extreme social deprivation or severe disability, patients who are profoundly hopeless or suicidal. Although the focus of your attention must be on helping your patient, it is not unusual to feel upset by what you hear and to need a way of dealing effectively with the emotional demands. If you do not they can interfere with the quality of therapy and may cause disruption in other areas of your life.

Strategies for addressing your emotional reactions: use CBT

The key in addressing unhelpful emotional reactions is to achieve and maintain a balanced perspective which helps us function well as therapists and in other areas of our working and private lives. Remember that strong reactions to patients' accounts are normal: it is how we deal with these reactions that determine our functioning as therapists and our well-being. To summarize what we have already stated, you will do well to:

- Clarify your problem
- Understand your reactions
- Plan and try out a solution or strategy
- Seek supervision, support, and training

The first time a patient disclosed a history of childhood abuse, Mathew was shocked. He was not anticipating the revelation and at first, he felt disbelief—surely no adult could do this to a young boy; surely no parent would ignore a little boy's injuries and pleas for help. He was unable to put this patient's story out of his head. As Mathew came to accept that the abuse had very probably happened he felt numb and sickened at the same time and he found his own anger was interfering with his ability to deliver therapy and he began to feel hopeless to help.

Mathew asked his supervisor to see him before his next appointment with his patient. Together they formulated his reactions to learning of the abuse, she directed him towards literature which might help him better understand how to help survivors of trauma and they discussed ways in which he could maintain a more decentred position during therapy sessions and ways in which he could avoid reflecting too much on his work once he went home. All of this helped him regain a professional perspective which improved his therapy and his sense of well-being. In addition to feeling safer in his workplace and having his confidence restored he began to see an opportunity to develop his skills in a specialist area.

Also, remember to help your patient use the skills and resources available to them. This is especially important if you have an inclination towards taking excessive responsibility for your patients. By paying careful attention to what your patient can do to cope and encouraging them to use their own resources and support you will nurture their resilience and protect yourself from having to fix everything.

Working with particularly challenging patient behaviour

Some patients are more challenging than others to work with and this might be for a variety of reasons. Some challenge our sense of safety, for example, those who threaten violence or complaint. Others challenge our sense of efficacy, for example, those whose interpersonal styles make it hard to achieve and maintain a collaborative relationship; or whose hopelessness is so profound that we question our ability to help; or those whose expression is incomplete, subtle, or veiled and hard to pin down so that we cannot develop a good dialogue or formulation; or those who simply 'press our buttons' so that we become less effective therapists.

This can be taxing and wearing and, again, you need to reflect on the impact this work has on you and the ways in which you can deal with it. If appropriate, consider how you can share, with your patient, the therapeutic problems that it poses. Safran and Segal (1990) offer guidelines for achieving this in a respectful and Socratic manner which is very consistent with the ethos of CBT.

We really do need to look after ourselves because longer-term exposure to difficult therapeutic work can lead to 'burn out' or what Figley (1995) termed 'compassion fatigue'. This makes it hard to empathize, we feel emotionally stretched and depleted, take less satisfaction from what we achieve, and often struggle to work efficiently. It takes its toll on us, on our therapeutic relationships, and other aspects of our work.

There is a good chance that the most clinically challenging presentations that you will encounter are chronic or severe depression and trauma. Either of these can leave you feeling exhausted, hopeless, fearful, or even traumatized. Therefore, the next section addresses ways in which you can 'stress-proof' yourself against their potentially debilitating impact.

Working with depression

There's no point—nothing's going to help.
I feel so terrible. I wish I was dead.

CBT for depression asks patients to engage actively in treatment, to take action on their own behalf, and to carry out assignments between sessions. Yet the symptoms of depression include loss of motivation, difficulty initiating action, low energy, and hopelessness about change. Its relentless negativity drains patients' resources and undermines their desire to help themselves. You can find yourself feeling extremely frustrated. The global nature of depressed thinking colors their responses to treatment/and to you (see Fig. 3.1). The more severe the depression, the more so. Furthermore, depression is infectious. Its voice is powerful and, unless you can remain decentred from it, you may become 'contaminated', losing CBT's optimistic, problem-solving stance. How can you best take care of yourself in this difficult situation?

The key is metacognitive awareness: This capacity to experience thoughts as thoughts, passing events in the mind, rather than necessarily a reflection of objective truth is not just theoretical understanding, but feeling and acting from a decentred perspective. If you can experience thoughts in this way, no matter how compelling and emotionally charged, instead of being overwhelmed (sucked into the whirlpool), you can perhaps stand back, choosing how to respond (standing on the bank and watching it go round). This is what you teach depressed patients when you do CBT: all cognitive-behavioural treatment methods tend towards this point. Equally, metacognitive awareness will help you, the therapist, to remain uncontaminated.

How do I achieve metacognitive awareness? Hold on to the cognitive model of depression. This means that when your patient is lost in negativity, you recognize the voice of depression speaking, knowing it is often economical with the truth. This will help you to move from 'Oh goodness, what now?' to 'Aha, there's another one of those!', from shared hopelessness to curiosity. Your patient *will* expect the worst and feel hopeless about change; that's the nature of the beast. And that's precisely what you are there to work on.

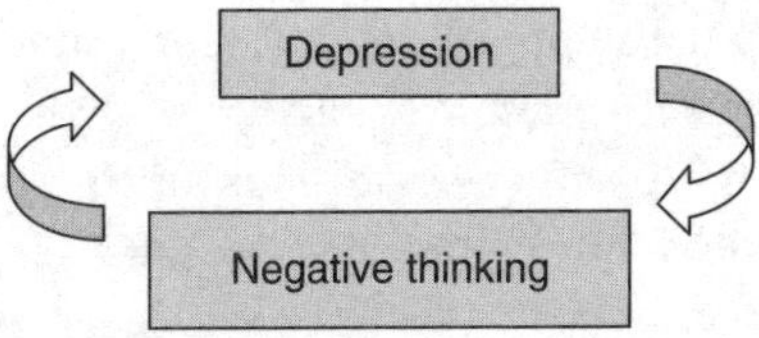

Fig. 3.1 The cycle of depression.

Share the cognitive model: Right from the first session, educate the patient about depression. You can use a simple vicious circle, to which you can return again and again as a means of identifying unhelpful patterns and exploring their impact.

Most people have no idea how to deal with depression. Their thinking seems absolutely convincing to them. Many patients, simply given the CBT rationale, will experience a lightening of mood: so this is something that can be understood and worked with—there *is* something they can do.

Be persistent: Depressed patients often find it difficult to formulate suggestions during sessions, or to carry out self-help assignments. This is not a signal to give up. Stick with it—each difficulty further illuminates what is maintaining the problem.

Leaven the lump: If possible, intersperse depressed patients with patients who have other difficulties and whose thinking is less globally negative. This will refresh you and help you to keep your balance. It can also be helpful to take short breaks after working with a difficult depressed patient. Go and do something which allows you to access a different mood—a walk, a chat with a friend, a computer game. Finally, find a supervisor who is used to working with depression and suicidality and who is not intimidated by it, someone who will be able to keep you optimistic and problem-focused when you begin to lose that capacity yourself.

Working with suicidal patients

Suicidal thoughts, plans, and actions are expressed by about 50% of depressed patients but not all suicidal thinking and behaviour are associated with depression; even if you do not regularly work with the depressed, you may still encounter suicidal patients.

No matter how knowledgeable and competent a therapist you are, you may at some point be faced with the distressing news that a patient of yours has committed suicide. Even knowing that a patient is contemplating, it induces a clutch in the gut and heart of the therapist—especially if this is someone you know well, like, and are fond of (yes, we do develop person-to-person relationships with our patients), or if it is a young person with the whole of life ahead of him/her. When someone kills themselves, it is inevitable and proper that we will ask ourselves: 'Was there something more I could have done? Something different? How could I have stopped this from happening?'

Of course it is possible that, yes, we could or should have done more, could have stopped this from happening—at least for the time being. But oftentimes therapists have genuinely done all they can, perhaps going to great lengths to protect patients' safety and well-being, and still it happens. The sad truth is that, unless we are with a patient 24 hours a day, we cannot prevent it. Even patients under close observation in inpatient units sometimes succeed in harming themselves. It is absolutely ethical to investigate what our role may have been in the time leading up to the suicide, and to learn from it in the interest of future patients, but we also need to recognize the limits of our power and influence.

So:

- Ensure that you are up-to-date on theory and research related to suicide. This will help you to identify subtle signs, to explore the subject with sensitivity, to know what sort of thinking patterns to investigate (e.g. loss of effective problem-solving skills, loss of a perceived viable future, hopelessness), and what interventions may be of help (e.g. questioning hopeless thoughts, developing a 'hope chest' with reminders of what makes life worth living, problem-solving training).
- Remember that, as you work with suicidal patients, carefully exploring their distress, you are communicating invaluable non-verbal messages which can potentially counter their hopelessness and sense of worthlessness and disconnection (e.g. 'This person cares about me', 'She thinks there may be a better solution', 'Perhaps it's worth hanging on'). Use all your generic therapeutic skills (empathy, warmth, careful listening) to maximize these 'meta-messages'.
- Hendin *et al.* (2004) found that one-third of therapists suffered from 'severe mental distress' following a patient's suicide. If the worst comes to the worst, and you are unable to prevent a patient's suicide, then accept that you may well feel at least some degree of pain—sorrow, regret, grief, a sense of waste. You may even feel other, apparently less acceptable emotions—anger for instance ('How could they do this, after all you've done for them?'). Just as you would in the face of any other loss, seek out whatever support you need, at work and from friends and family. Give yourself time and space to recover.

Working with trauma

Trauma-focused CBT makes considerable emotional demands on you as a therapist, because you will hear potentially distressing information and will often need to guide your patient through a detailed account of traumatic events in order to work with the associated meaning. You might also be faced with significant dilemmas, such as what you do if you learn that a child abuser is still active, or if ongoing adult abuse is revealed to you?

Impact on the therapist

Despite several studies, the impact of trauma work on therapist remains unclear and potential negative effects on therapist functioning may have been overestimated (for a review see Sabin-Farrell and Turpin, 2003). For example, van Minnen and Keijsers (2000) found that although exposure treatments can distress therapists, they coped well with these treatments. That said, some aspects of trauma-focused CBT can still be more demanding and potentially distressing than many other areas of clinical work. For example:

- You might see the traumatic event from your own perspective rather than how the patient views the experience. This can add to your distress of listening to difficult and sometimes harrowing accounts, because you may become personally entwined with the unfolding events. It may also result in your not talking about the trauma as a whole, or not detailing specific aspects of it, thus diluting the therapeutic effect of your intervention.

  Listening to the young woman describe the out of control car fatally injuring her mother, Jo's therapist began to see the events through her own daughter's eyes. This left her feeling sad and upset, both during the session and afterwards, and made it hard to focus on the feelings and thoughts of her patient. Indeed, she felt reluctant to explore the details of Jo's traumatic experience.

- Alternatively, empathy can be compromised if your perspective is different and this can make it difficult to support your patients in developing a clear and coherent narrative of their experiences, and to work with unhelpful thoughts and beliefs about them.
- Exposure to traumatic material can sometimes make you vulnerable to experiencing unwanted intrusions and you might find yourself recounting your patient's traumatic experiences—which can cause you distress. Fortunately, this is often self-limiting and as your patient becomes less distressed by the memory and associated reminders so will you. Very rarely will intrusions persist.

  Ruth had completed her work with a survivor of rape six months earlier but continued to avoid movies which depicted sexual violence because this tended to trigger vivid memories of her patient's experiences and distress at the time of the rape. An otherwise previously neutral phrase which had been used by therapists triggered a vivid image and feelings of fear.

- If you regularly work with traumatized patients you may be vulnerable to gradual changes in your own beliefs about the world, especially in your assessment of risk and your faith in human nature. This can have an insidious effect on your life, leading to a narrowing of your activities, and a persistent tendency to overprotect people you care about.

Whilst on holiday in Italy Beth went to see a popular horse race which takes place annually in the streets of Sienna. The town centre was crowded and the balconies of the picturesque old houses were packed to overflowing with spectators in raucous humour. Instead of watching the spectacle Beth had come to see, she found her attention drawn to the balconies, searching carefully for signs of structural weakness and seeing collapsing balconies in her mind's eye, thinking: 'why doesn't someone limit the number of people on these rickety balconies, this just isn't safe!'

- The particular dilemmas and challenges of working with survivors of trauma can render you feeling insecure and worried about the safety of others and your competence to practice.

  Jon felt out of his depth. His patient's account of her abusive experiences was inconsistent—was she lying or was this a normal distortion of distant memories? She hinted that her father, who abused her, was abusing her nieces—was this true, how could he be sure? What should he do—should he break patient confidentiality? He was confronted by dilemmas: should he confront her about the discrepancies in her accounts and perhaps risk the therapeutic relationship and should he break confidentiality in case her nieces were at risk? She had also disclosed that she managed her flashbacks by cutting herself and he had not anticipated this, so it added to his distress.

Managing the impact of hearing about trauma

During a session: There are several things you can do to help regulate how distressing and difficult trauma-focused CBT will be for you.

- Develop a metacognitive perspective (see section 'Working with Depression').
- Be aware of the images you see in your mind's eye when you are listening to the details of a traumatic experience and of the differences between your own elaborations of what you have heard and what you actually know. Remain aware of the 'here and now'. As Alfred Hitchcock knew very well, it is normal to add detail in imagination when information is lacking. For example, if you hear about an assault you may well 'see' it in your mind; where it took place, what the assailant might have looked like, how something might have felt or smelled. Try to recognize these as elaborations and not accurate representations of the event and identify those that trouble you and restructure them.
- Focus empathy thoughtfully as the focus of your empathy will influence how burdened and distressed you feel. Pearlman and Saakvitne (1995) suggest we consider four types of empathy:
  - Empathy with past experience
  - Empathy with the here and now experience of the patient
  - Cognitive empathy
  - Affective empathy

How and when we adopt these different types of empathy can not only make a difference to how supported our patient feels and help with identifying traumatic hotspots and their associated emotions and meaning, but can also contribute to our looking after ourselves in sessions. Empathy with how your patient *felt* during the trauma is likely to cause you most distress, so try to keep your focus on understanding your patient in the 'here and now', with occasional 'empathic dips into the past' to make sure that you're not misunderstanding things or missing bits. This also means you more clearly remain in the moment with your patient which will help you remain collaborative and focused on difficulties your patient might be having in the session.

After a session: Remember that it is normal to experience some symptoms akin to post-traumatic stress disorder (PTSD) when you are working with traumatized people. It does not mean that you are 'losing it' or that you are bad at this kind of work.

- Get a balance: try not to dwell on intrusions or upsetting memories, but do not try to suppress them either. Accept that they happen, without pushing the pictures, thoughts, and feelings away, but resist urges to dwell on the work you are doing or what you have heard.
- Ensure you have adequate supervision and training. Becker *et al.* (2004) found that perceived lack of training was an important factor in deterring experienced clinicians from using exposure-based treatments when working with patients with PTSD, thus leading to suboptimal treatment for some patients. Although this is obviously undesirable for your patients, it also means that you are more likely to feel burdened by the work that you do and miss out on the sense of achievement of helping a patient towards recovery from trauma.
- Seek out *informal* support after a difficult session. It is often helpful to have a diverting conversation or to talk about the meaning something has for you, rather than the details of a trauma itself. If you do feel the need to talk about details of a trauma with a colleague ask permission first—springing traumatic material on colleagues just spreads the upset around.
- Reflect on your needs and act on this. Your concerns in a session are likely to highlight a need for more support, supervision, and/or training. In the example above, Jon's experience eroded his confidence (and competence) but he could have protected himself if he had taken the time to learn more about trauma and memory, the range of cognitive and behavioural sequelae that patients present with, and been familiar with the Children Act and child protection procedures.

In the longer term: There are longer-term challenges when you regularly or primarily work with traumatized patients. You will need to protect yourself from a gradual erosion of positive beliefs about yourself and the world and the confirmation of pre-existing unhelpful beliefs you might already have. This presents you with an opportunity to try out and reflect on specific cognitive therapy techniques: especially strategies that we commonly use when working with assumptions and core beliefs such as continua and positive data logs (Padesky, 1994). For example, you may increasingly come to think that: 'Terrible things could happen at any moment so I must be extraordinarily careful to protect myself and family', or 'I'm responsible for undoing the damage that has been done to my patients'. Just as you might do with your patients, you will need to identify how these appraisals are maintained and to try to widen your narrowing perspective. To help you do this:

- Identify your own information processing biases, for example, scanning for danger.
- Recognize positive information that doesn't fit with your unhelpful belief: keep a positive data log. This can be very specific, for example, noting the times you see altruism or courteous and safe driving, or much broader to include the good things in life that counterbalance the terrible things you hear about: a great sunset, the smell of freshly mowed lawn, the love and affection of your family.
- Use what you know: for example, guided discovery to help you look for evidence that doesn't support your current view or a continuum to help you evaluate unhelpful beliefs and rules.

  George was always drained and distressed after his sessions with a particular patient who had suffered trauma. He decided to keep a thought record and soon realized that his belief: "I'm responsible for undoing the damage that has been done to my patients" could account for his feelings. He also realized that his thinking had became very dichotomous and he held the belief 100%. To help him regain a more balanced perspective of his role in therapy, he drafted a continuum of responsibility for change in CBT and (see Fig. 3.2). He then devised a behavioural experiment to test out the prediction that it would be therapeutic to: "help the patient learn and use helpful skills". This went well and helped establish his confidence that shared responsibility was optimal, not only for him but also for his patient. When he reviewed what he had achieved by using CBT approaches to resolve his own difficulty he realized that his success had rested on diligently carrying out an intervention and that an intellectual familiarity with CBT strategies had not been enough to help him.

- Reflect on and formulate what is happening to you and, where relevant, devise behavioural experiments to challenge fears and insecurities which have arisen from your work. Act as if you did not have a heightened concern or belief.

Belief: I'm responsible for my patients' recovery

0%		50%		100%
Nothing that happens in treatment is my responsibility: it is all my patient's responsibility	The onus is on my patient to do the work	I help patients learn and use helpful skills: it's a collaborative endeavour	The onus is on me to do the work	Nothing my patient contributes makes any difference to outcome: it is all my responsibility

Fig. 3.2 George's continuum.

For example, be driven as a passenger from time to time even if you generally prefer to stay in control of driving yourself, or allow your 8 year old to go to a sleepover with a friend. By doing so you engage in helpful behaviours that can help you to disconfirm your fears and other negative beliefs.

Thus far, we have focused on clinical issues, but work-related difficulties do not just apply to clinical experiences. A common source of stress is organizational so this is addressed in our final section.

Coping with organizational difficulties

It is always good to be aware of these stresses before they present problems for you, so we have highlighted three common causes of organizational stress for you to consider:

- Pressure of work
- Harassment
- Complaints

Pressure of work

Reiterating an earlier theme—when you sense there are problems stand back and review your situation, then formulate your difficulty, set goals, and challenge unhelpful beliefs. Ideally, you and your supervisor or line manager should review your level of work pressure regularly in order to avoid your becoming overstretched at work and to identify the situations, cognitions, and behaviours that might render you vulnerable to becoming overpressured. For example, do you overestimate what you can manage? Do you have beliefs that you have to please everyone? Do you find it impossible to say no? You would probably have good advice to give to a patient who harboured unhelpful beliefs or who was unable to be assertive or who needed prompting to problem-solve—you need to use this advice on yourself. In some instances, it is impossible to avoid working more than is ideal from time to time but you need to monitor your activities closely to ensure that you are not chronically overworking—if you are, try to understand why and take help in rectifying the situation. If necessary keep 'work-load review' as a standing item with your supervisor and/or manager.

Harassment

Harassment can take many forms, overt and covert, for example: intimidating behaviour, insult, misuse of power or position, the display of offensive materials, discrimination on the basis of sex, race, disability, sexual orientation, religion, belief, or age. However, since 1997, the Protection from Harassment Act has provided legislation specifically prohibiting occupational harassment, and thus protecting you from this source of occupational stress. You can also take additional steps to ensure your protection.

- **Familiarize yourself with the policies of your workplace**: The NHS (2006) has clear policy on the management of harassment and bullying in the workplace, and if you work in the NHS you will have ready access to this via your trust intranet. However, where can you go for help if you are a non-NHS practitioner? It is likely that your organization has its own policies with which you should make yourself familiar and you can also obtain advice from your trade union, legal advisers, Citizens Advice Bureau (CAB) and in relevant cases, the Commission for Racial Equality, the Equal Opportunities Commission, and the Disability Rights Commission. In addition, bullying and harassment help sites can be found on the Internet. If you are an employer, **you** are responsible for preventing bullying and harassing behaviour in your workplace. Thus, you should have a harassment policy which is made clear to employees during induction programmes and your staff should receive bullying and harassment awareness training.
- **Familiarize yourself with relevant procedures:** If you are accused of harassment, you should know what procedures are usually followed so that you can prepare yourself. If you feel that you are being harassed, be aware of the actions that you can take. Essential action in either case is to document key events: keep a diary of all incidents—records of dates, times, any witnesses, your feelings, etc. Keep copies of correspondence that may be relevant, for example: reports, letters, emails, memos, notes of meetings that relate to you. The procedure for tackling harassment is usually at an *informal* level when issues are resolved by communication between the two key parties. If this is not possible then the procedure becomes *formal* and the investigation is carried out by a committee.
- **Keep yourself safe:** As far as you can, avoid being alone with the person who is harassing you or accusing you of harassment. Discover what support

your organization offers and use what supervision, managerial, and informal support that you have available. Also, talk to colleagues to find out if anyone else is suffering, or if anyone has witnessed what has happened to you. You can also seek legal advice at an early stage.

Feeling harassed, being accused of harassment, or having a complaint lodged against you (see section 'Complaints') are situations which are likely to trigger strong emotions and cognitions. Once again, give yourself time to reflect on them and consider what support you need to help you manage them.

Complaints

A situation we all hope to avoid, and one which can come as a shock, is the discovery that a complaint has been lodged against us. We hope that the contracts that we form with our patients and the quality of our therapeutic relationship will enable a dissatisfied patient to articulate and resolve therapy issues within the confines of the sessions. However, in some cases patients might lodge a complaint via a relevant organization, such as BABCP or the NHS or the General Medical Council, or may take direct legal action against us or the service in which we work.

Complaints must be fully investigated regardless of anyone's belief about their validity and within statutory and non-statutory organizations there are usually clear complaints procedures which complainants are instructed to follow. Are you familiar with them and the support that is available to you as practitioner?

If a complaint is lodged against you:

- Involve your line manager as soon as possible.
- Establish the support you can expect from your supervisor, your employer, your union, and your professional body.
- Gather evidence that you have acted professionally: session recordings, therapy notes, supervision notes, and witness statements.
- Consider your psychological and emotional needs during this time. Again, you may benefit from the stress management strategies that you teach patients.

In general, attempts are made to resolve complaints swiftly and locally and the chances are that this will be the case. In many instances, the complaint will be handled by a dedicated complaints officer who should be able to inform you of procedure and advise you on your best action.

If a complaint cannot be resolved locally, it may become subject to more formal procedures such as independent review, referral to an ombudsman, or legal action might be taken. When this happens it can be frustrating because procedures are remote and you often simply have to await decisions.

Nonetheless, you can elicit help in preparing your statements or appeals and make sure that you maximize your support during a difficult time.

Having to endure harassment, bullying, or having complaints filed against you can be harrowing and demoralising—even if cases are resolved in your favour. The most resilient clinicians can find themselves losing confidence as a result of such experiences. You may well need time to recover a positive mind set, to review unhelpful assumptions which have been revived, exaggerated, or developed as a result of these organizational stresses. Be realistic about your needs and take the time and support that is necessary to recover.

Conclusion

The aim of this chapter has been to help you better look after yourself as a CBT therapist by drawing on your existing skills and knowledge and by resourcing yourself emotionally, intellectually, physically, and procedurally. We realize that you will be busy and it might well be impossible to follow all of our recommendations all of the time, however, if you do nothing else do make sure to take the time to reflect and get good supervision and support and remember that the more you put into looking after yourself the more you (and your patients) with get from your work.

Key points

- Resource yourself psychologically and physically by:
  - Engaging in replenishing activities inside and outside of work
  - Using CBT strategies to work with your own unhelpful thinking
  - Seeking supervision and support
  - Meeting your environmental and training needs
- Make sure that your working conditions are safe.
- When working with depressed patients metacognitive awareness and a real appreciation of the cognitive model will help you avoid becoming 'infected' by depressive thinking.
- Working with survivors of traumatic experiences can be distressing at times. If you have appropriate training and you receive regular supervision, the distress is likely to be relatively mild and transitory.
- Manage your time and your caseload.
- Be familiar with the procedures for dealing with harassment and complaints in your workplace.

Further reading

British Association of Behavioural and Cognitive Psychotherapy (BABCP) advertises training events and publishes good practice guidelines which are available at: www.babcp.com (accessed 1 March 2010).

NHS Direct's *Dignity at work policy* is available at: http://www.nhsdirect.nhs (accessed 29 June 2009).

Norcross, J.C. and James, D.G. (2007). *Leaving it at the Office: A Guide to Psychotherapist Self-care.* New York, NY: Guilford Press.

The Office of Public Sector Information provides details of relevant Acts of Parliament: The Protection from Harassment Act (1997), The Children Act (2004), and The Mental Health Act (2007) are available at: www.opsi.gov.uk (accessed 23 August 2009).

Oxford Cognitive Therapy Centre (OCTC) has many training events which are available at: www.octc.co.uk (accessed 1 March 2010).

References

Becker, C., Zayfert, C. and Anderson, E. (2004). A survey of psychologists' attitudes towards and utilization of exposure based therapy for PTSD. *Behaviour Research and Therapy*, **42**, 277–292.

Bober, T. and Regehr, C. (2006). Strategies for reducing secondary traumatic stress or vicarious trauma: Do they work? *Brief Treatment and Crisis Intervention*, **6**, 1–9.

Figley, C.R. (1995) *Compassion Fatigue: Coping with Secondary Traumatic Stress Disorder in Those who Treat the Traumatized.* London: Brunner-Routledge.

Hendin, H., Pollinger Haas, A., Maltsberger, J., Szanto, K. and Rabinowicz, H. (2004). Therapist's distress after the suicide of a patient. *American Journal of Psychiatry*, **161**, 1442–1446.

Maslow, A. (1954). *Motivation and Personality.* New York, NY: Harper.

Padesky, C.A. (1994). Schema change processes in cognitive therapy. *Clinical Psychology and Psychotherapy*, **1**, 267–278.

Pearlman, L.A. and Saakvitne, K.W. (1995). *Trauma and the Therapist: Countertransference and Vicarious Traumatization in Psychotherapy with Incest Survivors.* London: W.W. Norton.

Sabin-Farrell, R. and Turpin, G. (2003). Vicarious traumatization: implications for the mental health of mental health workers? *Clinical Psychology Review*, **23**, 449–481.

Safran, J.D. and Segal, Z.V. (1990). *Interpersonal Processes in Cognitive Therapy.* New York, NY: Basic Books.

van Minnen, A. and Keijsers, G. (2000). A controlled study into the (cognitive) effects of exposure treatment on trauma therapists. *Journal of Behavioral Therapy and Experimental Psychiatry*, **31**, 189–200.

Westbrook, D., Kennerley, H. and Kirk, J. (2007). *An Introduction to Cognitive Behaviour Therapy.* London: Sage.

Chapter 4

Ethics

Tony Hope

The unexamined life is not worth living.
Socrates, see Plato (1977)

A patient of yours, a teenager, who is at some risk of suicide, does not want his parents to know that he is having therapy. Another patient seems trapped in a damaging marriage. You believe it would be best for her to break from the relationship. You could encourage her to explore this possibility. A third patient, who trusts you, spends a great deal of time with people engaged in criminal activity. A fourth, timid, and with an obsessional fear of dirt might be persuaded to undertake the behavioural experiment that could help him but you would need to be pretty forceful. One patient who has almost completed the ten sessions that the NHS generally allowed in your service would make very good use of some further sessions. Another patient has said that she would like a little more affection from you.

These situations, and many others, may raise difficult questions for the therapist about what is the right thing to do, questions that cannot be answered by looking more deeply into the nature of cognitive behavioural therapy (CBT), nor avoided simply by developing your therapeutic skills. To be a health professional is to have ethical as well as clinical standards. That is why there are professional guidelines.

Can the ethical issues therefore be solved simply by turning to your professional guidelines or to the law? Fortunately not. Guidelines, useful though they can be, need to be interpreted and applied to the specific situation. No matter how carefully or cleverly they are formulated they cannot be applied unambiguously to the variety of situations that reality throws up, and if they could they would be too inflexible. Besides, guidelines may be wrong. Although, as a professional you must normally follow the relevant guidelines, you may, as you become more senior, be able to influence what guidelines say. A profession, as well as a person, creates and defines itself in part through its moral choices.

Society expects health professionals to be able to give reasons for their decisions and actions as part of transparent decision-making. Your reasoning about the ethical aspects of care will need to stand up to scrutiny—in a court if necessary—just as much as the scientific and therapeutic aspects.

In this chapter, I will outline two ethical principles and then discuss some problematic situations that can arise in the course of CBT in relation to three main areas: confidentiality, autonomy, and the allocation of resources.

Ethical theories

Ethics is concerned with the issue of how we should live. It is the systematic study of moral questions: questions about how we should act and think.

There are various ways of approaching the question: how should you live? One might say that one should be kind, or compassionate, or hard working, or fun. These are answers in terms of the virtues of character. Alternatively, one might answer in terms of duties, for example one should not lie, or should try and preserve life, or respect others. Duties are focused on actions. Or one might give an answer based on outcomes or consequences, for example, one should maximize happiness in the world to the best of one's ability.

Each type of answer relates to a different approach to ethical theory: virtue ethics; duty-based (deontological) ethics; and consequentialism, respectively (Hope *et al.*, 2007; Singer, 1991).

Two key ethical principles

Although there are times when it is helpful to use the ideas highlighted by different ethical theories, for many practical purposes these theories are too abstract. There are several ethical principles that are useful for health professionals. Two of the most important are: promoting your patients' *best interests* (*principle of beneficence*) and promoting their *autonomy* (*principle of autonomy*).

Promoting patients' best interests

One way of thinking about well-being is to imagine that at any one time we each have a certain level of happiness or misery, let us call this level the 'moment utility' (Kahneman and Riis, 2005). Total well-being over time is the integral of these moment utilities. A person's best interests, using this approach, lies in his/her enjoying the highest possible level of overall (integrated) moment utilities.

A limitation of this approach is that certain achievements may be important for well-being over and above their effect on happiness. It is perfectly coherent, although not perhaps very plausible, to say that my overall well-being is greater if I write this chapter, because of the value I put on the achievement, than were I to spend the time eating strawberries and watching DVDs. *Desire fulfilment theories* (Hope et al., 2007) highlight this aspect of well-being.

A further perspective sees some activities as intrinsically good, such as engaging in deep personal relationships and developing one's abilities, and some as intrinsically bad such as being deceived, or gaining pleasure from cruelty, even if they do not have an effect on happiness or desires.

Reducing a patient's problems of anxiety or depression, for example, may increase well-being on all the above accounts, but issues may arise in therapy where judging best interests is problematic: in the context of relationships, for example. And sometimes curing symptoms can negatively affect best interests. Best interests provide a broader perspective for you and your patient than problems and symptoms.

Respect for patient autonomy

The principle of respect for patient autonomy has had enormous effect in changing attitudes to the doctor-patient relationship over the last 30 years. It could be seen as central to CBT (see section 'CBT theory and ethics'). One definition of autonomy is: 'To regard himself as autonomous…a person must see himself as sovereign in deciding what to believe and in weighing competing reasons for action' (Dworkin, 1988, p. 5).

The concept of autonomy in modern medicine emphasizes the right of competent adults to refuse any specific treatment. The classic account of this view of autonomy was given by Mill, written in 1859:

> …the only purpose for which power can be rightfully exercised over any member of a civilised community, against his will, is to prevent harm to others. His own good, either physical or moral, is not a sufficient warrant.
>
> (Mill, 1859, Chapter 1)

This account is insufficient in the context of CBT. Therapy changes people and the question arises: what change, and what ways of affecting such change, most respects autonomy? To answer these questions it may be helpful to picture the ideal autonomous person. Young (1986) describes such a person: *she forms desires for how her life is to go (life plans) and can act on those desires.* In order to create such a life plan for ourselves we need to make evaluations, in particular about what kind of life we think we should live. In the ideal of autonomy day-to-day decisions should be rational, that is, consistent with the person's life plans.

CBT theory and ethics

CBT has embedded within its methods, theory, and development two central values: rational self-examination and effectiveness. The first is related to respecting autonomy, the second to best interests.

CBT and patient autonomy

CBT aims to alleviate psychological distress through helping patients undertake rational self-examination. Through such techniques as Socratic questioning the therapist enables the patient to see inconsistencies in his/her thinking. A prominent view of CBT is as 'guided discovery': a good therapist enables the patient to discover what is already latent within him/her. But this is too simplistic. Therapy can lead a patient to create, and not simply discover, new ways of thinking and behaving. Padesky (1993) asks a patient: 'What things would you do if you were ... a better father in your eyes?' This question is most significant for patients who are stimulated to new thinking and who create their views about what it is to be a good father.

How patients will change during therapy and the control they have cannot be known at the start. Although the emphasis in CBT on rational self-examination, openness, honesty, and allowing the patient control over therapy are all values based on respect for autonomy, it is naïve to conclude that the patient is in full control of the changes that occur. One way of deciding what intervention to make is to think how best to enhance patient autonomy.

CBT and patient best interests

CBT prides itself on concern for effectiveness. If it is in the patient's best interests to cure his/her mental disorder then an intervention that is effective in doing so is in his/her best interests.

If a practice, however, is guided by two or more principles there will be situations when the principles conflict. What should be done when what is most effective conflicts with what most respects autonomy? For example, an obsessional patient may wish to reduce the frequency of rituals, but not eliminate them altogether. Evidence may suggest that relapse is less likely if the rituals are completely eliminated. How far should the therapist go in trying to persuade the patient to persist rather than simply informing him/her of the risks of relapse? What, at first sight, might look like a purely technical issue in CBT involves ethical values because such values are embedded in the practice and theory of CBT itself.

Confidentiality

Why is confidentiality important?

Three different reasons can ground the importance of confidentiality in a clinical setting.

Respect for patient autonomy

The principle of autonomy emphasizes patients' right to control their own life and to decide who should have access to their personal information.

Implied promise

Professional guidelines, and patient expectations, can be seen as amounting to an implied promise that therapists keep information about their patients confidential. This view of confidentiality, unlike that of respect for autonomy, does not depend on what the patient would want but on a concept of the patient-therapist relationship.

Consequences of the breach

Unless therapists maintain high standards of confidentiality the public will not trust them. Without such trust people may not seek therapy leading to poorer health care for the population. On this view, high standards of confidentiality are important because they lead to the best consequences.

The grounds on which you base the importance of confidentiality can affect judgements about how serious a breach is. For example, if a patient is unaware of a breach, and is not harmed by it, from a consequentialist perspective the breach may be trivial. From the perspective of respect for autonomy the breach could be serious.

The law, and professional guidelines, give much weight to therapist confidentiality, principally on consequentialist grounds, but confidentiality is not absolute.

The professional body for UK doctors gives useful guidance:

> Disclosure of [patients'] personal information without consent may be justified where failure to do so may expose the patient or others to risk of death or serious harm.... You should generally inform the patient before disclosing the information.
>
> (General Medical Council, 2004)

How might the principle of confidentiality be applied to specific situations?

When a patient tells you of a crime they have committed or may commit

There is in general no legal requirement to breach confidentiality simply because you become aware of criminal activity by a patient. The Department of Health (2003) Code of Practice states that staff are permitted to disclose personal information: 'to prevent and support the detection, investigation, and punishment of serious crime'. 'Serious crime' includes rape, murder, manslaughter, treason, kidnapping, and child abuse. Most crimes against property are probably not sufficiently serious to justify a breach. All guidelines give considerable room for professional judgement.

When a patient is in danger of telling you about a crime

Suppose you become aware that a patient may tell you about his involvement in potentially serious crimes. What should you do? There are three possible responses.

1. Wait to see whether your patient admits to crimes. If he does, you are then faced with the issue discussed above of whether to breach confidentiality.
2. Warn the patient that if he tells you about a serious crime you may be obliged to inform the police.
3. Probe, without warning the patient, in order to find out as much as possible about the crimes in order to inform the police: to play detective.

Course 2 maximally respects patient autonomy and places central importance on the value of trust.

Course 3 is perhaps consistent with a purely consequentialist approach but it turns your role from therapist to criminal investigator. This could be seen as an abuse of your role as therapist.

Behavioural experiments in public places

Most therapy is carried out behind closed doors. In CBT, it may be appropriate for a therapy session to take place in a public place, as when a therapist accompanies a patient in the course of a behavioural experiment. Therapists will need to be very careful in such settings to ensure that any confidential discussion cannot be overheard. But the very act of carrying out the experiment may enable members of the public, or an acquaintance of the patient who happens to be present, to discover confidential information. It is important to discuss these possibilities with your patient beforehand in order to work out how to minimize the risks, and to allow your patient to decide whether he/she is willing to take the risks.

Autonomy and the professional relationship

The relationship between therapist and patient is one of the cornerstones of therapy. It is an important component of effectiveness. It also has many ethical implications. The therapist can help motivate a patient to make changes; but providing motivation can become coercion. A therapeutic relationship is a personal relationship; but it can become too personal. A therapist may wish to explore the possibility of major changes to a patient's life; but can such changes be too major? It is valuable to reflect on the variations in patient-therapist relationships and on your own experiences of such relationships.

Four models of the doctor-patient relationship

Emanuel and Emanuel (1992) proposed four models of the doctor-patient relationship.

The paternalistic model

A good father does what is best for his child. He may override the child's wishes for the child's good. The paternalistic model sees the therapist as making the main decisions about health care, in the best interests of the patient, because the therapist is viewed as being in the best position to do this. The therapist, however, should act solely to promote what is best for the patient, and not what is best for the doctor or society.

This model may appear to be a far cry from the nature of the patient-therapist relationship in CBT but consider how often you believe you know what is best for your patient, and how much control you have over the direction of therapy. CBT prides itself on its scientific credentials of effectiveness. If firmly guiding a reluctant patient to face his/her phobia is effective is that what you should do? And if you do, how close is that to adopting the paternalistic model?

The consumer (informative) model

According to the consumer model the therapist's role is to provide the patient with the facts relevant to allow her to decide what she wants, and then to carry out that part of the management plan that requires his technical or clinical skills.

The consumer model is based on the view that patient autonomy is maximized by providing relevant information only and that any further discussion (other than clarification of the information) is undue influence. This model is difficult to apply in its extreme form to CBT because therapy requires more from the therapist than the provision of information, but its implication is that therapists should minimize persuasion: inform, don't persuade.

The interpretive model

According to the interpretive model therapists should help patients to make those decisions that are most in keeping with patients' values. This may involve using persuasion to try and prevent patients from making decisions not in keeping with their values. This model can be derived from a view of autonomy that sees helping people to make decisions consistent with their values as promoting autonomy.

The interpretive model provides patients with more support in reaching decisions than the consumer model. CBT involves helping patients clarify their core values and living in a manner consistent with these values. The interpretive model fits closely with the therapeutic relationship inherent to CBT.

The deliberative model

The deliberative model is similar to the interpretive model except in one respect: the therapist not only helps the patient to clarify his/her values, but may also challenge them. The therapist, on this view, should be prepared to try and persuade the patient to alter values the therapist believes are wrong, just as a teacher or friend might do. This model derives from a view that sees moral development as an element in promoting autonomy.

Values might be at stake when the doctor believes that a patient is over- or under-valuing aspects of health care that impinge on others, for example, if the patient is behaving in a way that has a negative impact on her children. This could arise, for example, with an obsessional patient who makes her children ritualize—not severe enough to invoke legal action—but of concern. The patient however may give relatively less consideration to her children's welfare than the therapist believes is right. According to the deliberative model, the therapist might raise this as a moral issue with a view to persuading the patient to give more weight to her children's interests.

Persuasion and coercion

When does legitimate persuasion become unacceptable coercion? This issue might arise, for example, when the therapist wants to persuade the patient to do something difficult as part of a behavioural experiment. There are two distinct reasons for persuading a patient. The first is because it is in his/her best interests. The second is on grounds of respecting autonomy because the persuasion aims to bring the patient's behaviour and decisions into line with his/her values. The first reason is consistent with the paternalistic model; the second with the interpretive model. These two reasons have different implications for how you should try and persuade. If on grounds of respecting autonomy the method of persuasion should itself respect autonomy—it should involve helping the patient clarify his/her own values. If on grounds of best interests then you may be justified in using effective means of persuasion that go beyond respecting autonomy.

Should you ask a patient to do something that you would not be prepared to do yourself?

In the treatment, for example, of obsessional disorders and phobias it may be helpful for patients to do something that the therapist would not be willing to do himself/herself. This might arise because the therapist shares a similar phobia (e.g. of spiders) or because the behaviour is relatively extreme (e.g. putting a hand into a toilet bowl). Is there an ethical rule: never ask a patient to do something that you would not (willingly) do yourself?

What principle would support such a rule? The rule might act as a valuable guide to what it is reasonable to ask of patients. But if a behavioural experiment has developed as a result of collaboration and is relevant in achieving the patient's goals then what is appropriate for the patient may not be something that the therapist would be willing to do. A therapist may, for example, have a fear of flying which does not interfere with his/her life, whereas the patient may have a job which demands foreign travel.

Advising to make major changes in a person's life: the precautionary principle

Sometimes the therapist may believe that a major change in a patient's life is desirable, such as leaving a long-standing partner. Should a therapist be as persuasive in encouraging a patient to leave a partner as he/she might on occasions be in encouraging a difficult behavioural experiment?

There are two reasons for being circumspect in these circumstances. First, another person, the partner, is strongly affected and the therapist has no professional relationship with this person. Second, if the therapist's judgement is wrong there is the potential for great harm to the patient. Fools step in where angels fear to tread, and perhaps a wise therapist uses the precautionary principle. This principle is that in circumstances where the outcome of an action is highly uncertain but includes the possibility of great harm, then the action should not be taken unless there are particularly strong reasons in favour of taking it.

Boundaries of the relationship

To what extent can the patient-therapist relationship be a personal as well as a professional relationship? Treatment in CBT sometimes involves the therapist being with a patient outside the normal setting of the consulting room, as for example, when visiting an earlier site of trauma or in accompanying a patient with phobic problems to a restaurant. This can result in a relationship that feels less professional and more like that of a friend. A patient may want to have a closer relationship with the therapist and perhaps invite him/her to dinner. Why shouldn't the therapist take up this invitation?

It is important that therapists understand that their relationship with a patient is, first and foremost, a professional one and that this has several implications.

1 The therapist has obligations that are both legal and professional including a duty of care to the patient.

2 The patient has come for help with a problem and the therapist has some expertise relevant to that problem.

3 The patient is paying, or being paid for; the therapist is receiving payment for the therapy.

4 The patient may be vulnerable and need to reveal more about himself/herself than he/she would do outside a professional relationship.

5 The purpose of the relationship is to help the patient and not the therapist. The therapist's needs should not affect the therapy or the relationship.

Thus, if the relationship develops so that the personal interests of the therapist become significant then the patient may be harmed because the patient's interests are no longer the sole focus. This does not mean that the therapist must be cold. Within a professional relationship people can have warm feelings for each other and behave in a sensitive and caring fashion. There are a number of specific implications of these considerations in the context of CBT?

- There should be no physical relationship (e.g. a sexual relationship) between therapist and patient. A therapist might physically touch a patient, for example, in comforting the patient in times of great distress. But even then the therapist must consider whether the patient might mistake the meaning of the contact, perhaps thinking it has a sexual component.
- When a therapy session takes place outside the consulting room, for example, in a restaurant, some normal social conversation is almost inevitable. Furthermore, there are no fundamental theoretical grounds, as there are in analytic forms of therapy, for disallowing aspects of the therapist's life to be discussed. The therapist, however, should ensure that the relationship remains a professional one.
- More generally the issue arises as to how much of himself/herself should the therapist reveal. Two guiding principles are: first that the therapist's sharing of his/her personal information should be done only with the purpose of helping the patient. It should not become a burden for the patient. Second, it should not lead to a level of intimacy that threatens the professional nature of the relationship.

Resource allocation

You and your time are scarce resources

Your time is limited. Economists use the concept of *opportunity costs*. The opportunity cost of an activity is the value of what is forgone, of what does not happen, because of carrying out that activity. There is an *opportunity cost* whenever you see a particular patient. This cost can be thought of as how else you might have spent that time. For example, you might have spent that time seeing another patient, or in research, or administration, or have gone home earlier. Your employer might think more in terms of money than time.

The ethical question is: how should you spend your time; or how should the organization spend its money? These are aspects of the broad issue of how (scarce) healthcare resources should be allocated. For individual therapists this question most obviously arises when asking which patients you should see and for how many sessions. Even therapists who are relatively constrained by employers are likely to have some freedom to make choices. You may choose to see one patient for only a few sessions in order to take on a new patient earlier. You may be involved in assessing new patients and determining who should, and who should not, be put on the waiting list for therapy. What are some of the principles that are relevant to making resource allocation decisions? I will discuss four principles.

Four principles of resource allocation

Principle 1: Maximizing welfare gain

One principle is to use resources to maximize overall welfare. This derives from utilitarian theories of ethics. On this view, the purpose of health care in general is to increase both the quantity and quality of life of patients. CBT is focused mainly on increasing the quality of life of patients.

One view of the welfare gain of a course of CBT is the increase in quality of life resulting from therapy multiplied by the time period for which the patient experiences such gain. This is similar, conceptually, to the integration of 'moment utilities' discussed above (see section 'Promoting patients' best interests'). Whatever the specific account of welfare, most successful therapy should result in an overall predicted welfare gain for the patient. Consider two patients A and B. Patient A has had 10 sessions of CBT and experienced as a result an overall welfare gain of x (in whatever units are appropriate). You believe, however, that A would benefit further from 5more sessions leading to an extra gain in welfare of y units. If, however, you stopped treating A after the 10 sessions and gave the extra 5 sessions to B, B would gain z units of welfare. According to the principle of maximizing welfare gain, if $y > z$ you should give those 5 sessions to A and if $z > y$ to B.

Principle 2: Treatment according to need: prioritizing the worst off

A quite separate principle is that of prioritizing the worst off. Consider patients C and D. If you have the resources to treat only one, who should it be? Patient C, let us suppose, has moderate quality of life (let us rate this arbitrarily at 0.4). Therapy will increase this quality to 0.8. Patient D has a lower quality of life of 0.2 and this will rise to 0.4 with therapy. Assuming that both patients would need roughly the same number of sessions, and both would enjoy the gain in quality of life for roughly the same length of time then, according to principle 1 (maximizing welfare gain) you should treat C. But it might be argued that D should have priority on the grounds that D is (before therapy) worse off than C: D *needs* therapy more. The principle should be: give highest priority to treating the worst off.

A conflict between principles 1 and 2 will not arise in all cases: sometimes the person who is worse off to begin with will also gain the most from treatment. But this will by no means always be the case. Should we use our time as CBT therapists to maximize the amount of gain in welfare or to help the worst off?

Principle 3: The Master Mind principle: I've started so I'll finish (a duty of care to complete a reasonable course of therapy)

Once you start therapy you have a duty of care towards the patient. That duty might be interpreted as requiring that you continue therapy until the patient has overcome the relevant problem, at least as far as that is reasonably possible. We would not normally advocate only half treating patients. According to principle 3, therapy that has been started should be continued to a point where it is reasonable to consider it completed, even if there are other potential patients who are more needy or who would gain more quality of life. The basis for such a principle lies in the idea of the patient-therapist relationship: that once you have formed such a relationship you have a duty to stick with the patient until a reasonable end point. This raises, of course, the question of what is a reasonable end point. This could be in terms of the actual level of functioning: that if the person's symptoms, or quality of life, are at an acceptable level the end point is reached, even if they might improve further. It could be in terms of closeness to the best end point that could be reached for that patient if there were no limit to therapy. It could be based on rate of change: that from now on the rate of improvement is very slow.

Principle 4: Help as many people as possible

According to this principle when resources are scarce we should aim to provide some help to as many people as possible rather than providing more help to some, and no help to others. To apply this principle we have to determine the level at which the help is so small as not to be worthwhile at all. This principle is likely to be most compelling when there are no good reasons to believe that some potential patients should be at higher priority than others, for example, that neither principle 1 nor 2 can be effectively applied.

Application of the principles

These principles can be applied to various situations. For example, when deciding which patients should go on the list for therapy some balance between principles 1 and 2 seems sensible. Clearly a patient, however severe his/her condition or however low his/her quality of life, should not be considered for CBT if such therapy is (almost certainly) ineffective. But how should one prioritize patients who are needy, and who are likely to gain a small amount of benefit from CBT? Should such patients be given higher or lower priority than patients who are likely to gain much from CBT but who are not so badly off in the first place. Many of the patients who can make best use of CBT are those who are not suffering with major problems.

There is no definitive answer and to some extent the answer has to be a personal judgement as to which way of spending your time is better. In choosing who is to be placed on the list for CBT it seems reasonable to use a mix of both principles 1 and 2: ability to benefit and severity of condition.

In deciding when to stop therapy with one patient in order to take on another, the principles suggest that three factual issues are of most relevance: how badly off is each patient; how much benefit is each likely to gain over the next sessions; and what is the likely maximum gain if given extensive CBT. Although these are difficult judgements to make they are necessary if the allocation of your resources is to be at all rational. But there is a further step. Having made the judgements about the facts, a decision must be made in the light of the ethical principle or principles that you believe right.

Key points

- Clinical practice involves ethical as well as technical and scientific skills. The ethical aspects of therapy will need to stand up to scrutiny, in a court if necessary, just as much as will the scientific and therapeutic aspects.
- Two key ethical principles for therapists are promoting patients' best interests and respecting their autonomy. On occasions, the interests of others may also be relevant.
- These various ethical principles can come into conflict in some clinical situations. Maintaining patient confidentiality, for example (an example of respecting autonomy) can occasionally put others at risk. In such situations, judgements will need to be made, taking professional guidelines into account.
- Conflicts also arise when patients are making decisions that the therapist believes are not in their best interests. How much persuasion should the

Key points *(continued)*

therapist use? Different models of the patient-therapist relationship give different answers to this, and other questions.

- Ethical issues are important not only when there are conflicts of principles but also in ensuring that standards are not lowered through lack of awareness. The maintenance of confidentiality when performing behavioural experiments with patients in public places is one example.
- Therapists' time is a scarce resource. How should it best be allocated? Which patients should be offered therapy and which should not, given that not everyone who could benefit can be treated? Several principles are relevant in answering these questions.

Further reading

Beauchamp, T.L. and Childress, J.F. (2008). *Principles of Biomedical Ethics*. Sixth edition. New York, NY: Oxford University Press.

This best selling textbook of medical ethics provides a systematic and detailed account of key general principles and their applications.

Campbell, A., Gillett, G. and Jones, G. (2005). *Medical Ethics*. Fourth edition. Melbourne: Oxford University Press.

Accessible and relatively small textbook written by a team of philosophers and doctors.

Hope, T. (2004). *Medical Ethics: A Very Short Introduction*. Oxford: Oxford University Press.

Intended as an introduction, each chapter makes an argument for a particular ethical position concerning an issue in medical ethics.

Hope, T., Savulescu, J. and Hendrick, J. (2007). *Medical Ethics and Law: The Core Curriculum*. Second edition. Edinburgh: Churchill Livingstone.

Another short textbook intended for doctors but many of the key legal aspects are relevant to all health professionals.

Singer, P. (ed.) (1991). *A Companion to Ethics*. Oxford: Blackwell.

An edited book with excellent philosophical accounts of different approaches to ethics including virtue, duty-based, and consequentialist approaches.

Two relevant professional codes of ethics are:

The British Psychological Society: Code of Ethics and Conduct (2006). Available at: http://www.bps.org.uk (accessed on 18 February 2010).

The General Medical Council: Good Medical Practice (2006). Available at: http://www.gmc-uk.org/guidance/ (accessed on 18 February 2010).

References

Department of Health (2003). Confidentiality: NHS Code of Practice. Available at: http://www.dh.gov.uk (accessed 14 January 2009).

Dworkin, G. (1988). *The Theory and Practice of Autonomy*. Cambridge: Cambridge University Press.

Emanuel, E.J. and Emanuel, L.L. (1992). Four models of the physician-patient relationship. *Journal of the American Medical Association*, **267**, 2221–2226.

General Medical Council (2004). Confidentiality: Protecting and Providing Information. Available at: http://www.gmc-uk.org (accessed 14 January 2009).

Hope, T., Savulescu, J. and Hendrick, J. (2007). *Medical Ethics and Law: The Core Curriculum*. Second edition. Edinburgh: Churchill Livingstone.

Kahneman, D. and Riis, J. (2005). Living, and thinking about it: two perspectives on life, in Huppert, F., Baylis, N. and Keverne, B. (eds.), *The Science of Well-being*. Oxford: Oxford University Press, pp. 285–304.

Mill, J.S. (1859). *On Liberty*. There are many modern editions, including Harmondsworth, Penguin Books (1982).

Padesky, C. (1993). *Socratic Questioning: Changing Minds or Guiding Discovery?* Keynote address to European Congress of Behavioural and Cognitive Therapies, London.

Plato (1977). The Apology. There are many translations with slightly different wordings (e.g. Euthyphro, Apology of Socrates and Crito, translated by J. Burnet, Oxford: Oxford University Press). This quotation is at 38.

Singer, P. (ed.) (1991). *A Companion to Ethics*. Oxford: Blackwell.

Young, R. (1986) *Personal Autonomy: Beyond Negative and Positive Liberty*. London: Croom Helm.

Chapter 5

Patient perspectives on receiving CBT

Written by Patients

Commentary by Martina Mueller

Introduction

We invited several patients to write about their experience of treatment, to share their insights into what it is like to have CBT. We asked them: what they found helpful, what not so helpful, and what advice they might give to CBT therapists on the basis of their experience. Contributing patients were drawn from a wide range of settings: primary care, more specialist hospital settings, research units, and prison in-reach teams. Some patients had sought treatment for one specific problem, while others had treatment for more wide ranging difficulties; some had sought CBT and/or other treatments before. We would not wish to claim that these accounts are drawn from a representative sample of patients: they were just people who responded to our call for contributions, most were treated in and around Oxford and we did not include anyone who dropped out of treatment or appeared to gain little benefit from their experience of CBT. Nevertheless, these accounts offer a rare opportunity to hear patients speak for themselves about what it is like to experience CBT.

Contributors responded in their own way and we have chosen to keep the accounts in the form they were offered. To protect patient confidentiality, we have used pseudonyms and removed or modified identifiable details unless we were asked to acknowledge the patient's real name. One of our contributors, Jess, is a mental health professional. Her account offers a detailed analysis of the experience of treatment from the perspective of a CBT practitioner as well as that of a patient. To reflect her professional perspective we have placed her contribution in Chapter 20 'Therapy for Therapists'. Although each contribution tells a different story, they all share one crucial message: *the experience of receiving treatment is very different from the experience of delivering it.* We consider what we can learn from these accounts later on in this chapter.

Patient experiences of CBT

Thomas: my experience of short-term CBT for paruresis

I am a man, in my mid-thirties. I work in a research environment and am trained in a scientific field. Since my teenage years I have had the condition avoidant paruresis (AP), the inability to urinate in the presence, real or perceived, of others. Related problems were present earlier than this, from as young as five or six, but I cannot recall any specific trigger, for example, a traumatic incident. This condition led to feeling of isolation and shame, severe limitations in my professional and personal life, principally relating to various forms of avoidant behaviour, with travel being particularly problematic, and has at times resulted in high levels of anxiety and sub-clinical depression.

I first decided to seek help in my early twenties, approaching a general practitioner (GP), but based on what I perceived as a very negative reaction from them I didn't pursue this, and therefore it did not lead to any treatment. This was the first time that I had talked to anyone about my problem.

Until a couple of years ago I sought no further help, and accepted my situation until pressures at work, relating to my unwillingness to travel, made my anxieties intolerable, and I contacted the counselling service provided through my workplace. The service offered only open-ended talking therapy, and I engaged in this for the best part of 2 years. At first I found it impossible to reveal the underlying cause of my anxieties, and talked in general terms about problems with travel. When, after a few months, I reached the point where I felt that it was unproductive to continue without the counsellor knowing the specific nature of my problems, so I made them known. While I found it beneficial to have someone to talk to about my problems, the therapy didn't lead to any improvement in my symptoms, and the feeling that the travel situation at work was escalating again led me to discuss my problems with the Occupational Health team at my workplace. They suggested that I talk to my GP, which led to a referral to specialist mental health services, which involved in the first instance an assessment, and then a recommendation for me to undergo a course of CBT.

The first session included a general description of the ways that anxiety problems relate to avoidant behaviour, physiological and thought processes, and the ways in which these feedback into the anxiety. Also, it was made clear that the treatment would not operate on the causes of the problem, such as past experiences and beliefs, and this contrasted with the previous talking therapy that I had experienced. The finite nature of the treatment was also mentioned, and although it was something I was generally aware of regarding CBT before the treatment started, I did have some reservations that what sounded like a relatively short course of treatment would be sufficient for me to make significant progress. This concern was based both on the length of time I had already been in therapy, and perhaps more importantly on the fact that I couldn't see how I would make the first step in tackling my problem. My only other concern was that my therapist didn't have detailed knowledge of my condition, which I judged from questions that I asked about how successful CBT was at treating it, and I did consider that this may have some impact on the success or otherwise of the treatment.

The remainder of the session then covered how the treatment outside the sessions with the therapist would progress. In these exercises, the aim for me was to put myself into the situation that I had been avoiding, and each time to make notes about various internal (e.g. anxiety) and external (e.g. environmental) factors. It was agreed that we would meet a week later, after I had attempted the exercises. It was emphasized that the point of the exercises was not about specific goals, but to make observations in situations which my avoidant behaviour had previously meant I had generally not entered into.

My first impressions of the CBT model were that in general terms it made sense to me. I was particularly receptive to the idea of making records, some objective, some subjective, of my experiences of putting myself into a variety of unfamiliar situations. Having made progress through talking therapy to the extent of being able to talk to people about my problem, and having been offered further help, I was determined to try to get the most out CBT.

I started my exercises at a local shopping centre. The aim at this stage was to attempt to urinate in a stall, and record information in each case. I made a number of attempts over the course of a few hours, gradually loading with more fluids, and on the third attempt, I was successful. From these initial exercises I had already learnt that other people were not taking an interest in what I was doing, and I was not the focus of anyone else's attention. This meant that a busier toilet might actually present a more favourable environment, an idea that previously had been counterintuitive to me. I also learnt that there was a correlation between urgency and success. My typical behaviour had been to use a toilet based on the likelihood of success (e.g. go at lunchtime at work when most people were elsewhere), rather than based on my urgency. The failures were useful data, as they made it clear that any number of previous failures did not necessarily preclude eventual success.

At the second session, it was again emphasized that the exercises were about getting data and building experience of situations that I had been avoiding for many years. We discussed my good initial progress, in particular how many of the assumptions that I held were being challenged. We agreed that I would continue with the exercises, and would next meet in 2weeks. Between the second and third sessions, I had some failures and some successes, and varied the places that I visited. A key success for me was voiding at a urinal with other people present, an act that I could not recollect doing, and perhaps had not done for up to 20 years. At the third session, we discussed continued practice and successes, how some situations (in particular at work) were still problematic, and we agreed to meet again in 4 weeks. At the fourth session, we again discussed progress, and agreed that future sessions should be less frequent, with the next scheduled 4 months later. At the fifth session we discussed progress, and some setbacks, but agreed that there was no requirement for further sessions. While not free of the problem, and with some situations still very challenging, I realized that by this stage the sessions were not introducing any new aspects into my recovery, which henceforth could be pursued independently of any formal treatment.

I had no practical problems with the CBT treatment that I received, as I could make the appointments on days that I worked from home, and practice the exercises at weekends. It was sometimes draining to do the exercises, since the weekends would usually be a time when I had a break from my problems, but this was not so difficult to accept once the benefits of the exercises became apparent, which in my case was from very early on in the treatment.

After discussing the first set of exercises that I had been set by my therapist, further exercises became self-directed, and decisions to increase the difficulty of the exercises, and introduce new elements were taken by me. The therapy sessions were then mostly left to cover the outcome of the exercises and progress being made. I believe that this mode of working suited me particularly well because of my experience of independent learning and research.

What the therapist brought to the treatment were insights about the problem, a methodology for tackling the problem, and ideas about how to challenge the assumptions that the problem fostered. I had not been able to provide any of these elements, but once they were available I felt that I was equipped with everything that I needed to make progress, and the rest would be down to time and practice.

Because the sessions quickly became less frequent, and the number of sessions was small, no major adjustment was required when the therapy ended, although I did have some concerns about being less disciplined and regressing. So far this has not been a problem, and my recovery continues.

I had a good experience with CBT, which I believe was down to having a skilled practitioner and willingness on my side.

Becky: multiple courses of CBT for anorexia nervosa

My initial encounter with a psychologist was when I was 15, a hurried appointment arranged after a crisis admission to hospital. The week before I had collapsed at school, and was subsequently diagnosed with anorexia nervosa. My parents told me I was lucky, as both family therapy and individual sessions were set up immediately, avoiding the usual long wait. I didn't feel lucky though, as despite being emaciated, depressed, and too weak to attend school, I didn't believe I had a problem. I was resentful of my parents trying to feed me, and met with the psychologist under duress. My therapist was a National Health Service (NHS) child psychologist, working in an outpatient unit at the local children's psychiatric hospital, and I saw him for about 18 months. Looking back, I can see that what he did with me was CBT, but I didn't know it at the time. Each week I arrived, was weighed, handed over my food diaries and then sat down for the requisite hour. I didn't want to be there. I was mature for my age and found the setting (a room filled with toys) and manner in which I was spoken to patronizing, and I never engaged with my therapist. Being terribly compliant, I completed all my homework tasks—but they were mostly works of fiction. I never told anyone how I felt or what I was thinking. One problem was that I was a quick thinker and could anticipate questions and give the appropriate answers. I spent most of each session saying what was expected, while planning in my head how to cut down at meals and fake weight gain. The matter was made worse by the content of sessions being reported to my parents, which led me to close off from them all completely. Unsurprisingly, I gained nothing from therapy besides a distrust of psychologists, and increased bitterness towards my family. The anorexia was still with me, and was stronger than ever.

Over my A-level studies, I saw two private psychologists for CBT, each of whom I saw for about 6 months. The problems were similar to those I had with my first therapist, and I was only held back from disaster by my parents controlling my diet and activities.

In my first term at medical school I suffered a major relapse of my anorexia, and after a massive fight with my parents decided to look for help. My GP referred me to a program offering 40 sessions of CBT to patients with eating disorders. I liked the psychologist who assessed me, and as someone who likes to feel in control, was reassured by being offered a very structured treatment schedule. Unfortunately, I was put with another therapist for treatment, whom I didn't connect with at all. I had to attend twice a week at first, which interfered with my university commitments and was rather excessive. The therapist was very underweight herself, and this made me too jealous to be able to take her advice. I didn't feel I could trust someone to help me overcome anorexia when they were in such a contradictory position themselves. The sessions were very structured—weigh, update, discussion topic as per schedule, set homework, close—which was a helpful framework. Although I didn't gain much out of the sessions due to my not trusting the therapist, I worked on the material at home and bought a CBT book to go through as well. By the end of the 40 sessions I had made no physical progress, but understood anorexia better and had started to make connections between my thoughts and actions. This period happened to coincide with the psychology part of my medical course, and I found having some insight into how therapy works very useful in applying it to myself. I had hoped that once the 40 sessions had finished I might be referred elsewhere, but that didn't happen, so I went back to coping on my own.

The fourth year of my medical degree was a time of change—friends doing other courses had graduated, I moved from the safety of the library into the clinical environment, and there were problems between my mother and sister at home. I retreated into anorexia more deeply, slipping downward until the medical school suggested I look for treatment. I was scared, wanting to change but was discouraged by my previous experiences. My GP referred me to the specialist adult eating disorders service. I waited about 6 weeks for the assessment, which was done by a female psychologist with whom I connected immediately. It was the first time I had met someone who seemed to want to help me, and persisted despite my initial resistance to change. She was able to think quickly and challenge my thoughts and feelings. Gradually I tested the waters, but over a few sessions started to trust her and to open up more. Soon I felt able to discuss all my concerns freely, something I still cannot do with friends or family. I found the explicit explanations of feelings → thoughts → behaviours very helpful, and the use of diagrams and food/feelings diaries constructive. Treatment was disrupted by two lengthy hospitalizations, but the continuity of having the same therapist as I moved from outpatient to inpatient and vice versa was invaluable. One particularly helpful aspect of my therapist was that she appeared (or at least pretended convincingly) to enjoy my company, and responded to my thoughts in a human way. The superficial empathic listening while avoiding counter-transference has always left me uncomfortable and suspicious. The next appointment was always made at the end of a session, which I found reassuring and helped with feeling in control of my life. No therapy can ever be perfect, and I would have preferred a more set agenda for each session, and more specific homework tasks. It hasn't been an easy journey, but after 4 years I have recovered sufficiently to complete my medical degree, improve relations with my family, and start work as a doctor.

In the course of my illness, I have been exposed to other forms of psychotherapy including dialectical behaviour therapy (DBT), group CBT, The Maudsley Method, Acceptance and Commitment Therapy (ACT), and elements of the 12-step program. Out of these, all but individual CBT and ACT were futile. I found CBT particularly helpful for changing specific destructive behaviours (e.g. avoiding cheese), and learning to recognize the thoughts that led to them (e.g. Mum says cheese is fattening). The difficult part of this is that when challenges were set—eating cheese at home—I had to try and do this alone, and often failed. One problem with all my treatment was that it was suggested that if I gained weight and ate normally the anorexic thoughts would go. This never happened, so I always relapsed. However, ACT has a specific book for anorexia which teaches techniques for accepting that the thoughts will remain, but managing recovery around this. Combining this book with CBT techniques was an essential for me to make progress.

My main advice to patients thinking about having CBT would be to make sure YOU are the one who is choosing to do so, and not to be forced into it by others. Accept from the start that time for appointments will be lost from other pursuits—this will reduce weekly anxiety. During the session make notes of your therapist's advice, and between appointments keep a list of problems that arise/topics to discuss to ensure you get maximum benefit from the experience. Finally, if you don't engage with your therapist after a few sessions (and you are genuinely ready for making life changes), see if you can swap to someone else.

Ironically, many psychological problems arise from relationship difficulties, and yet providing effective therapy is reliant upon building a strong relationship between patient and therapist. I think it is pointless for therapy to continue when it becomes obvious that either the patient is unwilling to fully engage, or that there is no connection between you. Usually the patient will not be forward enough to say this, so it is up to the therapist to suggest a switch to another psychologist, or an alternative treatment plan. My experience is that it is important to tailor your approach to the individual patient—what is their usual level of functioning? A patronizing or far too intellectual approach will be a big turn off. As a clinician myself, I would suggest that if things aren't going well, discuss the case with a colleague—they might have ideas that you hadn't thought of.

For me, the key to making progress with CBT was twofold; overcoming my denial of having anorexia, and then finding a therapist with whom I could place my trust and who didn't give up on me despite several major setbacks.

Bev: CBT for long-standing problems

Background

I have had mental health problems for the past 17 years. To date I have received three courses of CBT.

My experience of CBT

My initial course of CBT was given to me at the age of 14 by my consultant psychiatrist. I had been seeing her both as an inpatient and as an outpatient for several months but we had never discussed anything other than medication.

I was now presented with the daunting task of embarking on a treatment which I knew nothing about, with a very austere person whom I am convinced came straight out of a Dickens' novel! To talk about my most private and painful things. I was extremely anxious and scared as to what was expected of me; nothing about this treatment had been explained to me. Sitting in her office at our first session I knew we wouldn't be able to work together, but I suppressed those feelings and forged ahead anyway. I tried to answer her questions as honestly and fully as I could but, I soon felt she wasn't really listening to me. As her questions became ever more probing, I would do my best to avoid them: by now I really didn't like or trust her. She never gave me the chance to talk, to elaborate on a question, or to ask a question. After some time she decided to end our sessions as it wasn't working. I felt so relieved! This experience put me off seeking the therapy I needed for almost 13 years.

My second course of CBT began at the age of 27 with a consultant clinical psychologist, after being on a waiting list for 18 months. Before letting myself in for a repeat performance of last time, I read everything I could find about the subject. This time I had an assessment before treatment commenced. I used this opportunity to ask as many questions as I could so that I was able to understand the demands and limitations that it entailed. This time I was slightly apprehensive but not scared. At our initial session, I was pleased to discover that my therapist was very friendly, polite, and softly spoken. I knew then that we would get on and she would be able to keep me calm when things got difficult. This time there were no deep probing questions to begin with. Initially, we just talked and tried to work each other out. At this stage, I still had problems with trusting people, so we set boundaries and an agenda, so that we both knew what was expected of each other. For the first few sessions we didn't focus on 'the problem'. We talked around it and got to know each other. This period for me was invaluable as it gave me the opportunity to learn to trust again; to assure myself that my therapist was not going to 'freak out' at something I said; and that she was going to be there for the long haul. As sessions went by I felt increasingly more able to say things that had been eating me up for many years. Each week I was set homework, which usually consisted of practicing something I had learned in therapy or keeping records of symptoms to be discussed at the next session. I never liked going to therapy sessions but I did appreciate the opportunity to talk. My therapy lasted 2 years before I was able to 'go it alone'.

My last course of CBT began just as the previous one was ending. This was to work on a different problem. They overlapped for a while which was really demanding. Again I saw another brilliant consultant psychologist who was also easy to get on with. After years of trying, I finally found myself in a place where I could say *anything* and not be judged. At last I started work on the most difficult aspects of my life. Gradually, over time, the pain diminished and I could look forward to a more contented life, after being so ill for so many years.

To conclude

I personally feel that finding the right therapist is crucial. At no stage in treatment was I ever given a choice of whom I saw. Over the years I have seen many therapists for different reasons and different treatments, some were good, some less so, and one was less than professional. In my opinion, a bad therapist can do much damage to an already fragile person. Trying to find a balance between keeping a professional relationship and giving something of yourself is very difficult on both sides. I could not have worked with someone without rigid and safe boundaries but I also needed some human warmth for reassurance. Four years of intensive treatment is a very big commitment. There were times when I felt like giving up, because it was easier than facing the painful issues. I was quite a hard patient to work with because I needed so much reassurance. However, I found the strength from somewhere to see it through and have managed to come out of the other side a much more stable, contented, and more able-to-cope individual. I do have one regret, which is not allowing myself to face one specific aspect of necessary treatment. Having not done this, treatment will never be as complete as it could have been. I just wish I had that opportunity again. I have learnt so much about myself, my behaviour, and how to cope more positively with life's problems.

Recommendations to new therapists

- First impressions count!
- Be honest and reliable. If you promise to do something, make sure you actually do it.
- Know when to give a patient time to tackle something and when they are avoiding it—and therefore know when to give encouragement.
- Allow other forms of communication, not just the verbal, for example, email and writing. This is valuable to test things between sessions and get clarification.
- Give lots of reassurance, because facing ingrained problems can be frightening.
- **GOOD LUCK!**

Cathy: Intensive CBT for post-traumatic stress disorder within a research context

Many years ago I suffered a serious road traffic accident with injuries and some subsequent amnesia but recovered well, despite neglect and little compassion from my parents. More recently an accident at work triggered distressing symptoms including memories of the first accident which intruded on daily life to the extent that I felt unable to work, and did not understand what was happening to me. An Occupational Health doctor diagnosed post-traumatic stress disorder (PTSD) and recommended treatment. This proved difficult to access on the NHS but my GP knew of an ongoing CBT trial locally and I was allocated to intensive treatment within less than 3 months. This I felt was significant to me in terms of how I engaged with the therapy in that the symptoms did not have time to worsen or become entrenched; a problem-solver by nature, not being able to work through these symptoms myself was very distressing; also the intensive delivery of the therapy, 18 hours over 1 week with several follow-ups over the next year allowed me to examine minutely the nature of what was happening to me.

I knew nothing of CBT except that it is a well-regarded and researched therapy, I was more than happy to take part in the trial and wanted it to begin as soon as possible as life was so difficult at that time. I can say that I was desperate for insight into these symptoms which seemed to have appeared out of the blue and so I was willing to be open-minded about CBT, the therapist, the venue. In the end, this flexibility paid off as it turned out to be a package of treatment which put me firmly back in control of my life.

My therapist explained that I had to be willing to bring everything out into the open by looking at contributory events in detail using a variety of methods. She likened the upcoming therapy to a scene at a station with me looking at a moving train, examining each carriage as a part of the trauma which had caused my post-traumatic stress and then letting it go: turning my back and so avoiding parts of the scene would only perpetuate the symptoms of fear and anxiety; thorough examination and processing would put everything where it belonged, in the past.

Supported by my therapist, I relived the two traumas as far as I remembered, recording the events on a tape then with guidance, I looked for any positive parts of the story to help me feel safer and not so threatened: I found this especially effective in dampening anxiety symptoms as it proved that indeed I had been looked after at the time by most people involved. I dealt with more difficult memories by initiating a conversation with people about forgotten parts of that time in order to fill in the gaps in my memory: this helped change my perception of events and change the memory from neglectful to relatively caring and has helped train my brain to have more positive feelings about the bad times. Unhelpful thoughts would prolong the problems.

By examining these events, we were then able to pinpoint physical triggers in everyday life which might exacerbate symptoms of fear and anxiety. Initially, we went out to look for triggers to unwanted memories together, to examine the reality of them and I practiced this daily so that they became less of a burden and my perception of threats became mitigated. Eventually after some weeks, we were able to revisit the scene of the first accident and relive it: although challenging this enabled me to understand exactly what had had happened to me and put it in perspective together with the old memories. Later we visited the second accident site.

We talked a great deal about how the styles of behaviour around me as a child might have influenced my personal sense of value as an adult. I have had to learn that I need to look after myself and ensure that my own needs are voiced and met; we practiced this by putting a wish list in place for things I wanted to do to help me move on and ways in which I wished to be treated. I was also taught a technique called the Assertive Defence of the Self which means being able to state one's own views clearly in order to achieve positive outcomes in dealings with other people. This has enabled me to improve my self-image and confidence and gives me a valuable interpersonal tool to use in any situation where I feel that I am not being heard. Another valuable technique is to look at how my childhood core beliefs might have influenced my perception of the second accident. It was possible for me to see that some of the ways in which I had been treated as a child, for example, with a lack of nurturing and care, may have contributed to me not paying enough attention to my own needs. Ensuring that I am better heard by myself and others has meant a far greater sense of well-being, both physical and emotional.

During the therapy I was not working so I was able and willing to devote lots of time to it. This involved much practicing of the techniques as well as listening to the reliving tapes made during sessions. I kept a diary of my progress which has been very helpful in highlighting unhelpful hotspots. I found that devoting some time daily to CBT to be effective in keeping things moving; just thinking about issues sometimes was enough to keep ideas alive for when problems crop up. The relationship with the therapist is crucial; trust is paramount and at the beginning the therapist is leading the way in helping the client to feel safe enough to explore painful issues but the aim of therapy must be to enable the clients to take control of their life gradually using the tools being taught. It is an exhausting process to go through, being kind to oneself is essential and even more important allow other people to be kind too. CBT can be overwhelming: only so much can be dealt with at a time. One of the most helpful things I was told at the outset was that everything that was happening to me was a normal response to abnormal events and that CBT would help me get better in time; my therapist gave me some sheets outlining the symptoms of PTSD which I referred to frequently in order to recognize the illness as real and know there is a way to put it firmly in the past where it belongs so that I could move on with my life.

For the client

- Be prepared for the unexpected, positive as well as negative.
- Devote time to the therapy while it is ongoing to maximize benefit.
- Be very kind to yourself, therapy is a taxing time.
- CBT is not a magic cure; the strategies are for the client to learn, practice, and use as/when necessary in order to keep moving forward.
- Keep a diary as a witness to your progress.

For the therapist

- Clients may be oversensitive; the therapy environment is best kept neutral but comfortable.
- Therapy is very hard work, particularly if delivered in an intensive format: breaks and drinks are helpful.
- A reference sheet or key points/homework is very useful for between sessions to keep clients on task and to keep support going at a distance.
- An email address/phone number for contact helped me feel not alone at the end in case a query came up.

Lewis: CBT for depression and low self-esteem in a prison setting

When I started my treatment I had long-standing beliefs that I wasn't worth anything. I had such a low opinion of myself I believed I was there just for others. I believed I should have done and been better, I shouldn't burden others with my problems, and that if something good were to happen to me it would be taken away. I was suffering from depression and low self-esteem.

I found it hard to talk about my life to start with. I listened and talked over my problems and things that affected me and the way I saw myself and how I believed others saw me. Over the weeks of talking I opened up as my therapist made me feel relaxed, I began to challenge my beliefs by looking at alternatives. For example, rather than thinking that if something good happens it will be taken away, an alternative would be to think that nothing lasts forever and that changes can be opportunities. I was slowly able to look around me and find positives in my day-to-day life. People I had only thought of as workmates turned out to be true friends willing to help me, who made me believe that I'm worth something.

Before, I had often freaked out when things would go out of control, I'd go into panic mode. Through keeping a daily diary and so taking a step back I learned to cope with whatever happen and calm stressful situations down. I found the more open I was with people and talked about things the better I became, I had gone from believing that I should bottle everything up to a position of talking over problems with my friends and asking for help when I needed it.

My sessions were on a one-to-one basis, my therapist made me feel relaxed and at ease. I felt that I could talk about anything, I wasn't being judged, it felt like someone wanted to listen to me and help me. My treatment lasted for 10 sessions of about 2 hours at a time. I did homework which we then talked about the following week. We wrote down the positives from my life and we talked about my achievements, skills, and strengths and listed them. Over time, I was able to build up a list of the good things which helps you to believe in yourself, you begin to believe that you are not rubbish, you are worthy. I also made columns of my beliefs on one side and on the opposite a list of 'more realistic' alternatives, this helps you to change the way to see yourself and how others may see you.

Advice for patients

I think you need to go into CBT with your mind open and put your trust in your therapist. You need to be proactive and try to look at a bigger picture and how others might see you. Try to look for positives rather than the negatives.

Advice for therapists

I think the therapist must be able to make you feel totally relaxed and allow you to be confident in them, so you can put your trust in them. The therapist needs to listen to you and not to judge you. I can honestly say that CBT has helped me. I still do a daily diary and I have found life so much easier because I understand myself better.

Tulip: CBT for a driving phobia

In 2002, I started to experience panic attacks when driving the car. This was disturbing as I had retired in 2000 and had, previously, been used to driving over 30,000 miles a year without a problem. The attacks developed fairly slowly, as follows:

1 One major panic attack on an A road in July 2002 when I felt dizzy, faint, and hot. I thought that I had absolutely no control and was a danger on the road and would inevitably crash the car.
2 I began to suffer 'the jitters' two or three times a month during 2002–2003.
3 I developed a phobia about driving on very straight roads during 2004–2006.
4 I stopped driving on straight roads in 2007.
5 Could not face driving of any kind at the end of 2007 and so stopped driving altogether.

During this period, I consulted a doctor, psychologist, and hypnotist, but this failed to halt the trend.

In April 2008, a friend intimated that I might be able to get help at the local hospital. I was at the end of my tether, but decided to make contact as a 'last chance'. I arranged a discussion with a CBT therapist at local hospital and this gave me a glimmer of hope. What was really helpful was the confidence my therapist had in CBT to treat my problem. I did not feel as confident, but as this was my last shot, I had to give it a go. We agreed a series of appointments, which progressed as follows:

1 My therapist came to my home and managed to get me to sit in the car. I was then persuaded to drive while she followed, on a short, easy journey. This was the first time I had driven a car in approximately 9 months.
2 I was persuaded to get back in the car and drive for 1 hour a day on 'comfortable' roads. I did this with difficulty for a couple of weeks.
3 I was persuaded to 'stretch' myself on roads I considered to be more of a problem and I did this, once again for an hour a day for a couple of weeks.
4 Then I had a small breakthrough. I was asked to criticize my driving performance and had to admit that I decelerated when cars approached, and probably held on to the steering wheel too firmly (sheer terror!). My therapist signalled that this was 'no good' and insisted that I concentrate on improvement in these areas. This I did, but with great difficulty over the next week.
5 After time, I was then persuaded to drive on A roads and a motorway (shock horror), once again for an hour per day every day. This I managed to do with difficulty.

6 At this point I had a major breakthrough. I had explained to my therapist that although I was now driving the car, I was so terrified, particularly on fast roads that I could not move out of the slow lane. Once again, the signal coming was that this was 'no good'. I remember this discussion really well, as I left it that I would try to drive 'normally', but I had absolutely no confidence that I would be able to do this.

7 I will never forget the next day. I was terrified as I approached the slip road, horrified at the prospect of overtaking, suddenly, with the words 'no good' ringing in my ears, I found myself accelerating past slower vehicles, just like the old days.

8 After a couple of weeks of practising 1 hour every day, I found myself driving, maybe not as well as ever, but certainly good enough for a man of 71 years, on all roads, without a major problem.

I have certainly learned from my therapy to remain positive when the odd feeling of insecurity occurs. For me, specifically, this was to relax and accelerate away from the perceived problem.

If I were a therapist, I would:

1 Be really confident and make sure the patient is persuaded to share the confidence that CBT works.

2 When progress is being made, find out from the patient what is 'not happening'. For me and my treatment, this was the breakthrough—viz: relax, accelerate normally, and do not slow down without reason.

3 Push the patient, with forceful persuasion, to progress past the really difficult times.

4 Keep the appointments closely linked, maybe weekly, and look for regular improvements.

5 Maybe signal a maximum of appointments to achieve a result.

In conclusion, I am enormously grateful for the treatment I received. It was the best few quid I have ever spent!

Jenny: CBT for recurrent severe depression

Over the last 30 years I have suffered from many episodes of severe depression. Throughout this time I have been prescribed numerous drugs, had counselling, and been given electroconvulsive therapy (ECT). Although these treatments may have offered some short-term relief, none of them helped me to achieve a long-term recovery.

A few years ago, while I was in hospital under 'section', I was told about a new initiative by the local trust, to offer CBT in conjunction with the local university. I had never heard of CBT, but I was desperate, and willing to do anything that may help me to return to some kind of life. When I was first assessed for CBT I was told that I was lucky to be offered it. I was struck with how that reinforced all my beliefs about being worthless. It seemed as though CBT and other 'talking therapies' were only for the privileged.

After 4 months in hospital I was discharged and began to try and rebuild my life. CBT became a hugely important part of that recovery. I had one-to-one CBT for several months, and then joined a group for Mindfulness-Based CBT.

CBT was a struggle. I was being asked to change the habits and behaviours of a life time. Not something that is easy to do when you are in a good place, desperately hard when you are in as bleak a place as I was. Gradually, the work with my therapist began to make some sense and the skills and techniques became incorporated into my thinking, at a 'conscious' and at an 'automatic' level. This awareness of my thoughts and behaviour allowed me to see choices that had not existed before and to begin to make changes.

I found the whole process of CBT incredibly difficult; I frequently worried that I was 'getting it wrong', that the therapist thought I was wasting his time, etc. Gradually, the exercises and practice helped me to realize the 'automatic' nature of these thoughts and to challenge them. Some of the things that I found helpful were:

- Flexibility is the approach to help me to maximize the benefits of each session. This was crucial due to my varying levels of concentration and memory.
- A clear structure for the sessions. It can be easy for sessions to dissolve into a general counselling type of session which is not the best use of the time.
- I found that it was really helpful for me to understand what the homework was trying to help me to achieve in order to maintain the commitment needed.
- The use of a variety of techniques—particularly when I felt 'stuck' at different points in the course of treatment—was helpful in moving my learning forward and enabling me to find a variety of ways to carry out homework tasks.
- The constant repetition of the need to 'just do it' even when it did not seem to be achieving anything.
- Providing reassurance that there was no overall 'right' way to 'do' CBT.
- A sense of humour.

CBT has enabled me to develop an understanding of my depression, to recognize what is happening, to provide insight into triggers, and most importantly, has helped to prevent recurrence. The skills I have gained have been long-lasting and I use them all the time. I am often unaware that I am using them now because they have become such a natural part of my life, replacing the unhealthy thinking and behaviours associated with my depression. My skills have developed and changed according to my needs, and in many ways that is the real strength of CBT, unlike medication it offers an ongoing benefit, which can be used repeatedly, without side effects, it can be adapted to suit the individual and it is very cost-effective!

One of the most important things that CBT offers is ownership—ownership of your illness, your treatment, and your recovery. Medication cannot do that. Medication is given to me, something administered by those with power and knowledge, by people who will make me better. Although medication has an important place in the treatment of depression, I feel that for long-term or recurrent depression it can only ever be a temporary solution. Medication is too often seen as the only answer, offered as an apparently quick and simple solution to a complex condition. It does not assist you in moving forward, but maintains a position of dependency and illness. Depression makes you powerless and for many years the treatments offered have exacerbated that powerlessness. Medication can take away power, control, and responsibility. What psychological therapies can offer is a way of taking back some of the control which is lost through depression. CBT turns the whole issue of power and strength on its head. It offers the chance to become the expert, the knowledgeable, the owner of recovery and well-being. CBT has given me the insight into my condition that enables me to ask for help before I have another crisis. Although I may not have completely broken the cycle of depression, I now feel confident that if the black cloud ever descends on me again I will recover.

CBT has helped me to discover inner strengths and resources that I can use to prevent depression recurring. It has enabled me to begin to trust myself. It has given me and my family hope for the future, and the opportunity to contribute positively to life. After nearly 30 years I no longer take any medication for depression. I am mentally stronger and healthier than I have ever been. I could not have achieved this without CBT.

What can we learn from these contributions?

These patient accounts gave us much to reflect on. We highlight some of the important messages below that stood out for us and consider what implications this might have for how we practice CBT.

The therapeutic relationship is important

The importance of a good therapeutic alliance has long been acknowledged by all forms of psychotherapy, including CBT (Castonguay *et al.*, 2006). Thus, it comes as no surprise to see the importance of the relationship echoed by many of our contributors. When first entering treatment almost all contributors to this chapter appeared to have asked themselves:

- Does my therapist understand me?
- Does my therapist feel warmly towards me?
- Does my therapist appear to be knowledgeable and competent?
- Can I be open and honest about my problems and my struggles with CBT without fear of negative judgement?

In that sense, the assessment is very much a bilateral process where therapist and patient ask essentially the same question: 'Can I work with this person'. As therapists we need to remain mindful that first impressions count: our patients will construe our words and attitudes in certain ways and they will assess us on the basis of what we do and say. This is highlighted by Jenny's and Cathy's observations.

> Jenny: When I was first assessed for CBT I was told that I was lucky to be offered it. I was struck with how that reinforced all my beliefs about being worthless.

> Cathy: The relationship with the therapist is crucial; trust is paramount and at the beginning the therapist is leading the way in helping the client to feel safe enough to explore painful issues but the aim of therapy must be to enable the client to take control of their life gradually using the tools being taught.

More subtle elements of communication can also be important. Becky struggles to work on her anorexia because:

> [My therapist] was very underweight herself, and this made me too jealous to be able to take her advice. I didn't feel I could trust someone to help me overcome anorexia when they were in such a contradictory position themselves.

Bev's comment reminds us that authenticity and genuineness matter (and may be much more easily noticeable than we think!):

> To find a balance between keeping a professional relationship and giving something of yourself is very difficult on both sides. I could not have worked with someone without rigid and safe boundaries but I also needed some human warmth for reassurance.

And Becky tells us:

> ... superficial empathic listening whilst avoiding counter-transference has always left me uncomfortable and suspicious.

We need to be very careful not to overestimate our capacity to establish and maintain a good therapeutic alliance. We need to remain attentive to unvoiced signals from our patients that something doesn't feel quite right, and address these openly and with care. Different aspects of the therapeutic alliance matter to patients to different degrees depending on the nature of their difficulties and past experiences. For example, Middle and Kennerley's (2001) research on patients' preferences within the therapeutic relationship suggests that overt 'Rogerian' qualities are particularly valued by those with traumatic interpersonal experiences, while evidence of therapist skills and knowledge is valued more highly by patients with relatively uncomplicated histories and presenting problems.

The therapy tasks and procedures matter, too

The contributors' experience of treatment appear to underline Bordin's (1976) idea that the quality of the alliance is a product of the extent to which the patient feels understood and respected, but also the extent to which the patient and therapist can work collaboratively on therapeutic tasks and goals, highlighting the interdependence of the technical aspects of CBT and the relationship. Thomas reflects that:

> I was particularly receptive to the idea of making records, some objective, some subjective, of my experiences of putting myself into a variety of unfamiliar situations.

Becky reports similar findings:

> I found the explicit explanations of feelings → thoughts → behaviours very helpful, and the use of diagrams and food/feelings diaries constructive.

Several contributors acknowledged the importance of learning and using new, or perhaps, rediscovered skills.

Jenny:

> CBT turns the whole issue of power and strength on its head. It offers the chance to become the expert, the knowledgeable, the owner of recovery and well being. CBT has given me the insight into my condition that enables me to ask for help before I have another crisis.

Cathy:

> CBT is not a magic cure; the strategies are for the client to learn, practise and use as/when necessary in order to keep moving forward.

Jess (Chapter 20):

> The educational component of therapy was one of the things that I valued the most.

The structure of CBT is important

Although novice CBT therapist can sometimes feel a little uncomfortable with structuring treatment, Jenny and Jess' comments reflect how agenda setting not only helps to focus treatment but also promotes collaborative working.

Jenny:

> ...a clear structure for the sessions. It can be easy for sessions to dissolve into a general counselling type of session which is not the best use of the time.

Jess (Chapter 20):

> I found that agenda-setting reduced my anxiety about sitting in the sessions as I wasn't on edge all session wondering what the therapist was going to bring up. It fostered a true sense of collaboration and transparency.

CBT isn't a spectator sport

To engage in CBT is to become an active agent in change. It takes time and energy to understand what is maintaining a problem and to try out strategies to see if they can aid recovery or facilitate progress. As Jenny tells us:

> One of the most important things that CBT offers is ownership—ownership of your illness, your treatment, and your recovery. Medication cannot do that. Medication is given to you, something administered by those with power and knowledge, by people who will make me better.

> And: CBT has helped me to discover inner strengths and resources that I can use to prevent depression recurring.

Jess (Chapter 20) comments:

> I really liked having homework! It helped me feel like I was doing everything I could between sessions to help myself. It also helped me feel less alone with the difficulties I was struggling with. There were often things I couldn't comprehend at all in therapy that a homework task would help me process between sessions.

Furthermore, CBT has a strong action direction, recognizing that doing things differently is an important and effective way of changing how we think and feel. It thus requires patients to engage actively with the tasks of therapy and many contributors highlight how powerful (if exhausting) it is to change what you do or how you do it, both in and outside the therapy room.

Cathy:

> I was able and willing to devote as much time as I could to it. This involved much practising of the techniques as well as listening to the re-living tapes made during sessions. I kept a diary of my progress which has been very helpful in highlighting unhelpful hotspots which need to be addressed as time has gone on. I found that devoting some time daily to CBT to be effective in keeping things moving.

Thomas:

> We agreed that I would continue with the exercises ... between the second and third sessions, I had some failures and some successes, and varied the places that I visited. A key success for me was voiding at a urinal with other people present, an act that I could not recollect doing, and perhaps had not done for up to twenty years.

Tulip:

> I will never forget the next day. I was terrified as I approached the slip road, horrified at the prospect of overtaking, suddenly, with the words "no good" ringing in my ears, I found myself accelerating past slower vehicles, just like the old days.

Lewis:

> Through keeping a daily diary and so taking a step back I learned to cope with whatever happen and calm stressful situations down. I found the more open I was with people and talked about things the better I became, I had gone from believing that I should bottle everything up to a position of talking over problems with my friends and asking for help when I needed it.

Confidence and optimism are infectious

CBT has a positive, problem-solving stance which can counteract the hopelessness which frequently accompanies mental health problems and undermines a patient's capacity to deal with difficulties constructively. Many contributors highlighted how important it is to have confidence in the possibility of change and to remain hopeful in the face of setbacks and difficulties.

Tulip tells us:

> What was really helpful was the confidence my therapist had in CBT to treat my problem.

Or as Jess puts it:

> Keep hopeful, it's contagious!

Finally, one of our contributors chose to reflect on therapy in the form of a poem which again captures the message that satisfactory therapy requires a balanced approach which attends to the therapeutic relationship and teaching self-help skills.

D. Barrett: 'In therapy'

Waiting expectantly for you to start

Spilling the beans

Revealing things that have torn you apart

Tentative steps

Feeling your way

Exploring the events

That blacken you day

Painful sometimes

Like raking hot coals
What do you need to achieve?
What are your goals?
Discussing in detail
The shadows of life
Sometimes can wound
Like turning a knife
And yet suddenly
A chink of light seems to appear
You want to reach out, hold it
To draw it near
Someone who listens
Adds no burden or blame
Doesn't laugh at your feelings
Doesn't fill you with shame
Slowly unravelling the tangled web
Feelings of anxiety beginning to ebb
Calmness descends
Like a comforting hand
Acceptance and knowledge sharing the same land
Learning to stop the round-about
From going full spin
Controlling the turmoil
You can find yourself in
Using the brakes
The tools you've learned
To finally find the peace
You have so rightfully earned

References

Bordin, E.S. (1976). The generalizability of the psychoanalytic concept of the working alliance. *Psychotherapy: Theory, Research, Practice, Training*, **16**, 252–260.

Castonguay, C.G., Constantiona, M.J. and Grosse Holtforth, M.G. (2006). The Working Alliance: Where are we and where should we go? *Psychotherapy: Theory, Research, Practice, Training*, **43**, 198–205.

Middle, C. and Kennerley, H. (2001). A grounded theory analysis of the therapeutic relationship with clients sexually abused as children and non-abused clients. *Clinical Psychology and Psychotherapy*, **8**, 198–205.

Chapter 6

Low-intensity CBT

Dave Richards

The low-intensity CBT context

From the very beginnings of cognitive behavioural therapy (CBT), practitioners and researchers have striven for a world where CBT treatments are available to all those who could benefit from them. It is almost impossible to recall a time when this was not a major driver behind the development of CBT. Pioneers such as Isaac Marks laboured to make therapeutic information available in as many different and accessible forms as possible. Marks published one of the first and most widely translated CBT self-help books, Living with Fear (Marks, 1978). With colleagues he also initiated the uniquely pluralistic nature of CBT in the United Kingdom by founding the multidisciplinary British Association of Behavioural and Cognitive Psychotherapies (BABCP: www.babcp.com) and by the then-revolutionary expedient of training nurses to deliver these empirically supported psychological techniques. In the twenty-first century, if you want to work in CBT, you must engage with the results of this legacy. We may have come a long way since those early days, our methods may have changed, and our thinking may have developed, but the idea of what we now call 'low-intensity' treatment persists in the CBT movement's consciousness. Low-intensity treatment must be a major component of any CBT service.

Why is low-intensity working important?

We may often picture CBT as a complex and in-depth process, requiring intense study and practice by patient and therapist alike. However, in the United Kingdom from 2008 onward, the multi-million pound Improving Access to Psychological Therapies programme will specifically train at least 40% of its CBT therapists to deliver exclusively low-intensity versions of CBT. Therefore, as a consequence of the higher volumes treated by low-intensity therapists, the *majority* of patients in these services are likely to be receiving low-intensity forms of treatment. Clearly it is absolutely essential that all CBT practitioners, high- and low-intensity specialists alike, have a sound understanding of what low-intensity CBT is all about. This chapter will tell you about the knowledge, skills, and attitudes you will need to function effectively in this low-intensity environment.

Introduction

Picture this scene. We are working for a psychological therapies service in an average Primary Care Trust in the United Kingdom with around 300,000 potential patients over 16 years of age. What we know about help-seeking, coupled with the epidemiology of anxiety and depression, would suggest that up to 7,000 patients per year may come forward for help. In actual fact, current experience suggests that around 4,000 patients will be referred by their general practitioner (GP), themselves, or other agencies such as workplace or work assistance organizations. We have not got off lightly, however. Assessing and treating 4,000 patients effectively is a big task.

If we work in a traditional high-intensity orientated CBT service we have a number of options: we could employ a workforce equivalent to the PCT's total annual budget; we could put up artificial barriers in front of patients such as requiring them to 'opt-in'; we could close the waiting list.

There is another way.

Challenge number 1: let's change our attitudes

- Large referral numbers are not the PCT's problem, the GPs' problem, or the patients' problem. They are our problem.
- Patients are the best managers of their own mental health; after all they have far more years of experience of doing so than we have.
- Giving every patient we see an in-depth, lengthy, and highly intensive treatment programme is neglectful of our public health responsibilities.
- We are not selling patients short if we give them the least burdensome treatment option necessary for their recovery.
- Telephone treatment is not second rated. Patients like talking to therapists this way. Until they try it, most therapists hate it. But whose treatment is it anyway?
- It is OK to talk about medication and definitely OK to help patients make the best use of it. A lot of patients, including many CBT therapists who experience depression, swear by it.

In other words, we have got to remember that the majority of people are perfectly equipped to run their own lives. When they hit emotional problems they often lack only two things: (1) information to help them understand and address these problems; (2) support while they do this (Rogers *et al.*, 1999). There is a lot of distress out there and we have just as much of a responsibility to people who are in the queue for our services as to those in our consulting room. Working in a modern CBT environment might mean learning to be comfortable with not dotting every 'i' and crossing every 't'. That is the patient's job.

Challenge number 2: get out of the CBT knowledge silo

There is a whole literature out there waiting for the CBT community to discover. Many other mental health specialists know about it, why don't we? For example, in terms of the number of patients in clinical trials, the total size of the evidence base for a system of care called 'collaborative care' (Bower *et al.*, 2006; Gilbody *et al.*, 2006) vastly overwhelms that for CBT. Why don't most of us know about it?

Another system is called 'stepped care'. What do you know about it? Contrary to received wisdom, stepped care was not invented by the UK National Institute for Health and Clinical Excellence (NICE) for their depression guidelines (NICE, 2009). Furthermore, stepped care is not a treatment, nor is it a system unique to mental health; it is not a system of rationing, and it definitely does not have NICE's five steps. We will not achieve stepped care just by providing self-help or computerized treatments. Stepping or allocation, triage or review—these are all factors which will have major impact on system performance. Is it not time we thought a bit more constructively about stepped care and considered how to apply its principles?

Challenge number 3: think creatively about new ways of working and new workers

Many of us have spent years in professional training and have then taken more time learning CBT, undertaking continuing professional development and receiving in-depth supervision. This has had two effects. Firstly, we can become desperate to apply every new technique we have learned from attending workshops delivered by renowned international specialists. Secondly, we can be very proud of our skills and protective of the effort we have expended in getting them. Most therapists believe that this powerful combination of experience and training is an essential part of being an effective CBT practitioner. The BABCP supports this view by making it extremely tough to accredit as a therapist. They and most therapists believe that this protects patients receiving CBT.

Let us question these beliefs. How much do they reflect the desire to protect patients rather than the desire to protect CBT? Are these beliefs really as magnanimous as one might imagine, or are they about power and control, remuneration, and professional prestige? Although all professional bodies aim to regulate and protect patients from charlatans and abuse, most, for example, the British

Medical Association, evolve into powerful advocates of professional groups, gate-keeping entry to their respective 'guilds'. Is our situation any different?

In fact, CBT-specific techniques are not the whole story. To quote an early pioneer of clinical behaviour therapy, '...the importance of the relationship between patient and therapist [is] the single factor which seems most relevant to the outcome of behaviour therapy'. (Meyer and Gelder, 1963, p. 26) ... Meyer tartly adding, 'You will get further with a patient with a good therapeutic relationship and a lousy technique, than you will with good techniques and a lousy relationship' (quoted in Bruch and Bond, 1998, p. 141). Although the therapeutic relationship in CBT has been variously dismissed as merely the 'context' in which specific techniques are applied (Beck et al., 1979, p. 45) or 'like the anaesthesia that allows for a surgical procedure to be performed' (Goldfried, 2004, p. 98), other CBT researchers have suggested that there may be an association between the therapy relationship and clinical outcomes, independent of the relationship between outcome and specific CBT techniques (Waddington, 2002; Ilardi and Craighead, 1994; Safran and Segal, 1996).

These 'common factors'—the alliance building and communication skills so essential for any psychological therapy—can be taught. We now know that it is possible to train completely inexperienced workers rapidly in both common therapeutic factors and specific CBT techniques. Marks and colleagues first demonstrated that it was possible to train nurses—a group of workers previously thought to be beyond the pale when it came to delivering psychological therapies. Medical students were also shown to deliver outcomes equivalent to experienced therapists. A combination of clinical simulation and supervised practice, allied to modelling by experienced workers and careful supervision, forms the bedrock of the national UK curriculum for low-intensity psychological therapists (Department of Health, 2008; Richards and Whyte, 2009). Our ability to deliver such training means we can now recruit and train a vastly more diverse group of CBT workers from communities and groups who have not previously accessed such training. Our services can begin to look like the communities we serve, can employ people who share the values of those communities, and can begin to connect with the concerns of the many different groups that make up our society (Richards, 2007). And we can do this quickly and efficiently.

The above discourse has asked you to think about your knowledge and attitudes. Before we move on to identifying skills for working in a CBT environment that includes low-intensity working, what follows is a brief section on the evidence for low-intensity CBT, collaborative care, and stepped care. Given the brief nature of this chapter it can only be a taster and you are advised to follow the references for further detail.

Low-intensity working

The term 'low-intensity' working has evolved from previous descriptions such as 'self-help' or 'brief therapy', terms which it has tended to subsume. Some commentators have questioned whether low-intensity CBT is essentially a smaller 'dose' of CBT, whether it is something different, or whether it is not really CBT at all. These reservations centre on the 'What is therapy?' debate, which is not the subject of this chapter. However, alternative means of accessing psychological information and support (Rogers *et al.*, 1999) have been part of the CBT consciousness since its inception and are just as much therapy as the traditional face-to-face system.

Low-intensity treatment is characterized by:

- Fewer sessions
- More emphasis on self-management
- The structured and central use of written material as a core strategy, rather than merely an adjunct to therapy
- Variation in administration methods, such as delivery via the telephone or computer

These factors can be illustrated by the largest field trial of low-intensity methods so far (in Doncaster, UK), where workers provided guided self-help in an average of just over five contacts per patient, 75% of which were delivered using the telephone. Results were benchmarked against relevant randomized controlled trials and reports from routine clinical practice, and found to be broadly equivalent. The effect sizes for patients completing treatment were very large, with recovery/remission rates around 75% (Richards and Suckling, 2009).

In terms of the evidence for guided self-help, in randomized controlled trials the controlled clinical effect size for low-intensity CBT for depression is very similar to high-intensity CBT (0.8) (Gellatly *et al.*, 2007) but more varied and generally lower for anxiety disorders (range 0.18–1.02) (Hirai and Clum, 2006), although low-intensity CBT for generalized anxiety has a large effect (0.92).

Collaborative care

Collaborative care is a 'systems level' quality improvement approach consisting of a multi-professional approach to patient care, a structured patient management plan, scheduled patient follow-ups, and enhanced interprofessional communication (Gunn *et al.*, 2006). As a quality improvement intervention, collaborative care does not *add* additional therapeutic ingredients but *optimises* the delivery of existing treatments—pharmacological and/or psychological.

In collaborative care systems, mental health workers ensure that patients remain in contact with mental health care services and that they get the maximum benefit from their chosen treatment. To do this, workers often assertively keep in contact with patients using the telephone to ensure that patients do not lose contact with services and 'drop through the net'.

To illustrate collaborative care in action we can take the example of a depressed patient, 'Frank'. In a traditional service model Frank may be prescribed antidepressants by his GP and if lucky referred to counselling. After a wait of some weeks, Frank is sent an appointment letter which he neglects to open. After receiving a second letter, warning him that he must respond within two weeks or his referral will be cancelled, Frank arranges an appointment. At the appointment, the counsellor arranges to see him for six sessions of Rogerian non-directive counselling in the general practice surgery, requiring Frank to take time off work to attend each week. After two sessions he drops out. After three months Frank discontinues his antidepressant medication. Six months later he is still depressed and Frank is told he has 'treatment resistant depression' which requires specialist psychotherapy. He is prescribed a different antidepressant and put on the psychology department's 18 month waiting list.

In a collaborative care service model things would be very different:

Frank is still prescribed antidepressants but instead of counselling he is referred to a case manager. The case manager telephones Frank to arrange an appointment. Although the case manager does not get an initial reply, she continues to call Frank until he answers. Frank is offered a face-to-face appointment followed by as many telephone follow-up calls as he wishes, with the option of further face-to-face appointments if he so desires. At the first appointment the case manager gathers information on Frank's medicines and his attitude to taking them, and gives Frank written information on antidepressants, depression and low-intensity CBT. Together they make a shared decision on a pharmacological and psychological treatment plan. The case manager shares this information with her supervisor and, with Frank's agreement, provides the GP with a short summary of the treatment plan. The case manager telephones Frank weekly to support him in undertaking a programme of behavioural activation. After a few weeks, Frank is feeling somewhat better and expresses to his GP a desire to come off his medication, which the GP agrees to. In discussion with the case manager, however, Frank learns that the chances of relapse are increased significantly unless he remains on antidepressants for six months post-recovery. Although he is disappointed at this news, he agrees to keep taking them. The case manager discusses this in supervision and talks to the GP about renewing the prescription. Four months later Frank is scoring well below threshold on routine measures of depression and is feeling subjectively much better. The final session with the case manager is focused on relapse prevention, and Frank writes a plan to continue his beneficial activity programme, identify trigger situations and symptoms of depression, and initiate actions if his depression begins to return.

Frank's first case scenario is illustrative of traditional systems where only about 40–50% of depressed patients referred to a mental health specialist attend an initial appointment, with a median of a further two follow-up appointments attended. Indeed, just like Frank, many patients who do see a mental health professional do not receive evidence-based psychological treatment. The contrasting story highlights how collaborative care is multi-professional, evidence-based, and assertive. Frank is supported by the case manager, his GP, and a specialist. The treatment he receives is effective and focused on Frank's long-term recovery. Because of this support he is concordant with pharmacological treatment, receives an evidence-based psychological treatment, recovers, and is prepared for the possibility of relapse. He does not attract the inappropriately pessimistic label of 'treatment-resistant depression'.

The evidence for collaborative care is very strong, consisting of over 12,000 patients in 36 studies. Although a recent systematic review (Bower *et al.*, 2006) found that the combined effect size for collaborative care in these studies was relatively modest (<0.3), the review found that this was because of the very varied nature of collaborative care. The review was able to identify the components of this complex system which predicted improved patient outcomes. We found that the effectiveness of collaborative care could be optimized by employing mental health workers with specific (albeit not necessarily extensive) mental health training and who also received regular expert supervision. Recent UK trials which utilized these effective ingredients achieved larger effect sizes (0.67) as a consequence (Richards *et al.*, 2008) and formed the underpinning evidence base for the Doncaster low-intensity clinical delivery method (Richards and Suckling, 2008).

Stepped care

Stepped care has two fundamental principles:

1 Treatments delivered should always be the 'least restrictive', in that the burden on patients should be as low as possible whilst achieving a positive clinical outcome. This principle is usually interpreted as the delivery of a low-intensity treatment such as guided self-help, unless other high-intensity treatments are indicated.

2 Stepped care should be self-correcting. This refers to the systematic scheduled review of patient outcomes to assist in clinical decision-making, using validated outcome tools such as symptom schedules.

Despite the fact that stepped care is a widespread health service principle and runs through many (although not all) international guidelines for depression and anxiety disorders (e.g. Andrews and Tolkein II Team, 2006; NICE, 2009; 2009), specific evidence for it is relatively sparse. Stepped care is often combined with collaborative care in clinical trials and so it can be difficult to extract specific evidence. Although based on the common sense proposition that it is as harmful to over-treat as under-treat common mental health disorders, NICE guidelines provide little evidence to support the implementation of stepped care. However, there are indications that some ways of organizing care which might be described as 'stepped' can increase the usual recovery rate compared to standard treatment in depression.

Stepped care is absolutely critical to low-intensity working and modern CBT practice. CBT is uniquely positioned to take advantage of a system of care that asks for a menu of treatments which increase in intensity. Unlike most other psychological therapies which regard therapeutic change to be *uniquely* a product of the relationship between the therapist and the patient, CBT regards its specific empirically supported factors as also being a major driver of change. As such, its techniques can be designed to be mainly patient-enacted or therapist-supported.

An example of stepped care in action can be seen in the stories of Frank's wife Marisa and her friend Fatima. They were friends from the school run and both found that when their children became old enough to walk home they lost confidence and began to experience panic and agoraphobia. Initially, when they went to their GP, they were given a referral to the local psychology department, where 18 month waits for treatment were the norm. However, after six months they both received a letter saying that their GP practice was involved in a pilot 'IAPT' service. They both went for an interview with a 'Psychological Wellbeing Practitioner' who outlined a treatment programme based on graded exposure to their feared situations. Each time the practitioner had an appointment with them, they were asked to fill in a set of rating scales. After six appointments, Fatima's ratings were coming down and she was entering previously avoided situations with minimal anxiety. Marisa, however, was not doing so well. Her treatment programme was not very effective and her ratings remained high. After discussing this with the practitioner, Marisa was 'stepped up' to a cognitive-behaviour therapist who was able to help her understand and challenge the way she interpreted her panic symptoms. After a further seven sessions she too was entering previously avoided situations with minimal anxiety.

Marisa and Fatima's stories show how in stepped care an initially effective and low-burden treatment is applied first. Graded exposure is effective for many people with agoraphobia, including Fatima. However, Marisa needed some high-intensity work and this need was identified through the use of routine outcome measures. In a traditional system, both would have been referred to the cognitive-behaviour therapist, which in Fatima's case would have been an example of overtreatment. Although it might be argued that Marisa had an experience of 'treatment failure' the integration of low- and high-intensity CBT in the stepped care service meant that Marisa, who had already been 'socialized' to the CBT model, could make rapid progress with high-intensity CBT. In the traditional scenario, both would have had a considerable wait for treatment, caused by both the scarcity of cognitive-behaviour therapists and the numbers of patients overtreated.

Major challenges for low-intensity working

From the above sections of this chapter, it should be clear that low-intensity working presents considerable challenges to mental health workers. These challenges can be summarized as issues of managing volume, clinical decision-making, the coaching role, and high volume supervision. The rest of this chapter will address these issues.

Managing volume

The expectations placed upon modern mental health services have been raised significantly through lobbying and political action by those, such as Richard Layard, who regard the lack of access to effective psychological alternatives to medicines as contributing significantly to a major waste of human potential. Most of this expectation falls on the shoulders of low-intensity workers, who must treat greater volumes of patients than their high-intensity colleagues. Typically, low-intensity workers will have 50–70 active patients on their caseloads, at least twice as many as their high-intensity colleagues. Although one can argue that the stress of treating half as many patients intensively is as great as twice as many patients treated in low-intensity working, there are unique challenges in high volume working.

Clinical record keeping, whether paper or computer based, is a necessary aspect of clinical governance and patient protection. Large caseloads will generate more paperwork. In order to survive, workers need to develop succinct and accurate record keeping styles and need to be supported by systems which are efficient and reduce the need for multiple records on the same patient being made. Good information technology is an essential tool for survival.

Forgetting specific patient details is a danger when large numbers of patients are seen regularly. Low-intensity workers need to take tips from other health workers like GPs who also see large volumes of patients. Memory aids are regularly used, such as small family genograms or other unique details, independent of the person's difficulties. Workers need to convert each 'patient' into a 'personality' in some way. Access to such details needs to be available before each new contact and will enable workers to more easily recall specific patient details.

Imposing arbitrary session limits can be a confused organizational response to the pressure of volume. Originally prevalent in practice-based counselling, the idea that mental health care in primary care should be rationed to a specific number of sessions, irrespective of patient response, still persists. Although low-intensity working generally means fewer sessions, it is nonsense to stop half way through a course of low-intensity treatment where a patient is beginning to respond. Low-intensity workers can find this terribly frustrating and must argue against such systems. The best survival strategy is to work with stepped care scheduled review systems using routine outcome data to demonstrate progress, or lack of it.

Follow-ups can be neglected as volume builds. When a patient does not attend, or misses a telephone contact, therapists have a tendency to see the missed appointment as an opportunity to catch up on other things. In a low-intensity service, particularly those working through telephone contact, this time can be used to make calls to other patients. The original patient may be overlooked. Indeed, in a high volume situation it is very easy to allow patients to 'drop through the net' and never be followed up. To avoid this, low-intensity workers require extremely good organizational backup. This is almost certainly best delivered by computer systems such as those developed for the IAPT (Improving Access to Psychological Therapies) programme from US case management software (e.g. www.pc-mis.co.uk or other bespoke systems) which automatically alert workers to situations where patients have not been followed up for their next appointment.

Clinical decision-making

Low-intensity working operates in the context of stepped care. There are at least two points in stepped care systems where clinical decisions have to be made. Firstly, the 'stratification decision point', after an initial assessment, directs a patient to low- or high-intensity treatment. Secondly, the 'stepping decision point', after a period of low-intensity treatment, is the point at which the decision is made to cease treatment or step a patient up to high-intensity treatment. Many low-intensity workers will be making decisions at both points, supported through supervision.

Furthermore, evidence-based low-intensity treatments include a wide range such as large group psycho-education, bibliotherapy, guided self-help, and low-intensity versions of established CBT treatments such as behavioural activation. Low-intensity workers, therefore, not only have to decide whether low-intensity treatments are appropriate but also *which* of them to recommend, as well as when to persist and when to recommend stepping up to a more intensive treatment approach. Two survival strategies can be employed here. Firstly, explicit clinical decision algorithms can be utilized, which assist workers to balance important factors such as severity, chronicity, disability, patient preference, and likely response to treatment. Secondly, the use of routine outcome measures, collected at every session, will ensure that stepping-up decisions are informed by empirical evidence. Once again, intelligent information technology is an invaluable survival tool.

A real-life example of how low-intensity workers might use these factors to make shared clinical judgements with their patients is illustrated in Table 6.1, taken from an actual UK stepped care service. In this example of depression, following an initial pathway allocation based on symptom severity, the decision moderators are problem duration, the experience and effect of past treatment, and the impact of the problem on a patient's life. Low-intensity workers can use this set of decision guides to assist them in present treatment options and information to patients for joint decision-making.

Becoming a coach not a therapist

The essence of low-intensity working is learning to act as a 'coach' rather than a therapist. The role is just like an athletics coach, or a personal fitness trainer. If people go to the gym or play sports, fitness trainers don't do the actual physical work of getting them fit. That is up to the individual. However, the trainer will help devise a fitness plan, monitor a person's progress and keep encouraging them when the going gets tough. A low-intensity worker will act in the same way. Although some of these coaching behaviours are similar to traditional CBT practice, low-intensity working coaching behaviours are made very explicit, and the nature of the coaching relationship is made clear from the outset.

Coaching is a supportive position. Taking on such a role explicitly acknowledges that the patient is going to do the required work towards wellness. As a coach, a low-intensity worker has a role as an educator and supporter, helping motivate the patient but always acknowledging that the real work is being undertaken by the patient.

Coaching also involves setting clear targets. The similarities with high-intensity CBT are closer here and a low-intensity coach will be regularly reappraising the targets and revisiting them.

Coaches often devise treatment according to a coaching manual, and this idea can help differentiate between traditional therapy and low-intensity treatment. In low-intensity treatment the main focus of the treatment is often on a manual or other material (sometimes computerized), whereas in high-intensity work the materials are usually adjuncts to the work of therapist, not the main focus.

One thing is very clear. A fitness manual on its own is unlikely to work. Supportive work from a coach will reap greater rewards, through encouraging

Table 6.1 Example of a low-intensity treatment decision algorithm for depression.

Pathway	**A**	**B**	**C**
Severity (PHQ)	**<10**	**10–14**	**15+**
Default intervention	No more than one more appointment: • Information • Predict recovery • Seek help again if condition worsens • Signpost if required	A small number of contacts only, to be reviewed in supervision after four sessions: • Information • Depression Recovery Programme • Possible CCBT • Medication management • Signpost if required	Multiple contacts reviewed regularly in supervision: • Information • Depression Recovery Programme • Possible CCBT • Medication management • Signpost if required
Duration and past treatment	>1 month duration or previous unsuccessful treatment consider: • Pathway B	<1 month duration consider: • Pathway A Previous unsuccessful low-intensity treatment consider: • Pathway C or high-intensity treatment	<1 month duration consider: • Pathway B Previously unsuccessful low-intensity treatment consider: • High-intensity therapy
Impact	No or minimal disruption to work, home, social, personal, familial life Moderate disruption consider: • Pathway B Major disruption consider: • Pathway C	Moderate disruption to work, home, social, personal, familial life Major disruption consider: • Pathway C	Major disruption to work, home, social, personal, familial life:

Abbreviation: CCBT, computerized cognitive behavioural therapy.

closer adherence to the fitness plan. The same is true in psychological therapy, where the evidence is that non-guided self-help is clinically ineffective (Gellatly *et al.*, 2007). Low-intensity CBT workers have to learn to work through a self-help treatment plan, usually written down and largely patient-directed. This can cause difficulties as workers may want to take over, and work through the therapeutic contact rather than through the materials. A survival strategy here is to keep the materials as the focus of the session, whether face to face or on the telephone, physically ensuring that the materials take up a central position in the space between the worker and the patient. Good quality materials, used as a constant reference point, help maintain the focus on the written 'fitness plan' and ensure that low-intensity working is very different from more usual counselling or discursive approaches.

In the United Kingdom, there is now a well-established education programme for workers delivering low-intensity CBT. The curriculum for this programme is published on the IAPT website (www.iapt.nhs.uk) with comprehensive educator and student support materials also available on the same website (Richards and Whyte, 2009). The curriculum supports the coach model and stresses the importance of both 'common' and 'technique specific' therapeutic factors, putting great emphasis on patient-centred clinical skills development. Although most of the specific techniques are CBT-based, the common techniques are those used in any psychological therapy to develop an effective therapeutic alliance. Students learn patient-centred information gathering, information giving, and shared decision-making via a mixture of expert modelling, clinical simulation role–plays, and supervised real-life practice. One survival strategy for anyone undertaking low-intensity treatment using the coaching role would be to download the teaching material and watch the accompanying DVDs or, even better, enrol on such a course.

Supervision

Although supervision is widely regarded as essential for therapist development and clinical governance, we now have evidence that supervision actually *predicts* increased patient outcomes. In other words, if clinicians receive effective supervision, their patients will improve more than if they only receive supervision in an *ad hoc* manner. This evidence comes from the collaborative care literature and refers to the supervision of low-intensity workers in depression (Bower *et al.*, 2006). The model of supervision which gives this result is one where the supervisee does not have a choice as to the content of supervision—a major contrast with the usual CBT model, where the supervisee decides which cases to bring to supervision. The final challenge of low-intensity working, therefore, is to organize supervision to reflect this finding.

In the most effective low-intensity supervision model, decisions to discuss patients are made according to pre-set algorithms. These algorithms could include rules whereby a worker and supervisor should discuss:

- All their new patients
- Those with high levels of morbidity on routine outcome measures

- Patients who are above a certain level of risk
- All patients after a specific duration in treatment
- Any patient who has missed an appointment

(Richards and Whyte, 2009, pp. 104–106)

We can alter these rules according to the needs of different patients and services, but the key element is that *all* patients who meet the criteria should be discussed.

In a high volume, low-intensity service there is a significant risk that patients can 'drop through the net'. As well as its clinical governance function, the form of supervision described above is designed to ensure this does not happen. One of the most useful survival strategies is to use the IT systems referred to earlier to automate the process of identifying patients requiring supervision. An electronic patient management system such as PC-MIS (Patient Case Management Information System) uses automated supervision alerts to notify supervisor and supervisee that certain patients require discussion. These patients remain on both supervisor and supervisee screens until the supervisor confirms that supervision has taken place and records this in the patient's notes. Other similar patient management systems are also available.

An example of supervision conducted this way would be the case of Alice, Fatima and Marisa's case manager. Alice has 56 patients on her caseload and sees her supervisor, Mary, weekly. PC-MIS automatically helps them to decide which patients need discussion. Both Fatima and Marisa were included in the automatic alert as 'new patients'. Alice presented a brief summary of Fatima and Marisa including their basic demographic characteristics, their problem summary statement, their risk status, their scores on PHQ9, GAD7, phobia scales and the treatment plans that Alice had agreed with them. Mary agreed with the plans. The next time these two patients were discussed was after a further four weeks, when PC-MIS flagged them up as patients who were scheduled for a supervision review. At this appointment, Mary looked at the outcome sessional measures and agreed with Alice that Fatima was progressing well and should continue with low-intensity treatment. Reviewing the graphical presentation on PC-MIS of Marisa's outcome measures it was clear that Marisa was not improving. After a discussion, Mary recommended that Alice suggest to Marisa that she be referred on to one of the team's cognitive-behaviour therapists for some high-intensity CBT. This helped Alice plan her next session with Marisa. They then moved on to discuss another 13 patients scheduled for supervision.

Here we have another lesson about adaptation for low-intensity CBT working. In traditional supervision systems Alice may not have brought Marisa (or Fatima) for supervision, meaning that Mary would not have had an overall view of Alice's caseload and individual decision-making. Marisa's stepped care treatment programme was rendered efficient and effective through this supervision system. Supervision is, therefore, as high volume as the organizational setup. It is essential for improved clinical outcomes, and works best when initiated by automatic flags or alerts.

Key points

- In the future, the majority of patients undertaking psychological therapy for common mental health problems are likely to receive low-intensity CBT.
- We must revise our attitudes to patients, to treatments, and to therapists in order to meet this challenge.
- Low-intensity therapy differs significantly in philosophy and delivery from standard CBT.
- Stepped care has two principles: firstly, that of initial allocation to the least restrictive treatment possible; and secondly that of systematic scheduled review with the degree of stepping and stratification dramatically altering system performance.
- Routine outcome measures taken at each clinical contact are essential to clinical management in stepped care systems.
- Supervision, when managed in an automated and scheduled manner, predicts increased patient outcomes.
- Novice workers can be effectively trained to deliver low-intensity CBT via national training programme curricula.

Further reading

Lovell, K. and Richards, D. (2008). *A Recovery Programme for Depression.* London: Rethink.

Richards, D.A. and Whyte, M. (2009). *Reach Out: National Programme Educator Materials to Support the Delivery of Training for Practitioners Delivering Low-intensity Interventions* 2nd edition. London: Rethink.

Roth, A. and Pilling, S. (2007). *The Competences Required to Deliver Effective Cognitive and Behavioural Therapy for People with Depression and with Anxiety Disorders.* London: Department of Health.

Westbrook, D., Kennerley, H. and Kirk, J. (2007). *An Introduction to Cognitive Behaviour Therapy: Skills and Applications.* Michigan: Sage.

References

Andrews, G. and Tolkein II Team (2006). *A Needs-Based, Costed Stepped-Care Model for Mental Health Services.* CRUFAD: University of New South Wales.

Beck, A., Rush, A., Shaw, B. and Emery, G. (1979). *Cognitive Therapy of Depression.* New York, NY: Guilford Press.

Bower, P., Gilbody, S., Richards, D.A., Fletcher, J. and Sutton, A. (2006). Collaborative care for depression in primary care. Making sense of a complex intervention: systematic review and meta regression. *British Journal of Psychiatry*, **189**, 484–493.

Bruch, M. and Bond, F. (1998). *Beyond Diagnosis: Case formulation. Approaches in CBT.* London: John Wiley & Sons.

Department of Health (2008). *Improving Access to Psychological Therapies: Implementation Plan: Curriculum for Low-intensity Therapies Workers.* London: DH/Mental Health Programme/Improving Access to Psychological Therapies.

Gellatly, J., Bower, P., Hennessy, S., Richards, D., Gilbody, S. and Lovell, K. (2007). What makes self-help interventions effective in the management of depressive symptoms? Meta-analysis and meta-regression. *Psychological Medicine*, **37**, 1217–1228.

Gilbody, S., Bower, P., Fletcher, J., Richards, D.A. and Sutton, A. (2006). Collaborative care for depression: a systematic review and cumulative meta-analysis. *Archives of Internal Medicine*, **166**, 2314–2321.

Goldfried, M. (2004). Integrating integratively oriented brief psychotherapy. *Journal of Psychotherapy Integration*, **14**, 93–105.

Gunn, L., Diggens, J., Hegarty, K. and Blashki, G. (2006). A systematic review of complex system interventions designed to increase recovery from depression in primary care. *BMC Health Services Research*, **6**, 88.

Hirai, M. and Clum, G. (2006). A meta-analytic study of self-help interventions for anxiety problems. *Behavior Therapy*, **37**(2), 99–111.

Ilardi, S.S. and Craighead, W.E. (1994). The role of nonspecific factors in cognitive-behavior therapy for depression. *Clinical Psychology: Science and Practice*, **1**, 138–156.

Marks, I.M. (1978). *Living With Fear.* New York, NY: McGraw-Hill.

Meyer, V. and Gelder, M.G. (1963). Behaviour therapy and phobic disorders. *British Journal of Psychiatry*, **109**, 19–28.

National Institute for Clinical Excellence (NICE) (2007). *Anxiety (amended): Management of Anxiety (panic disorder, with or without agoraphobia, and generalised anxiety disorder) in Adults in Primary, Secondary and Community Care.* London: National Institute for Health and Clinical Excellence.

National Institute for Health and Clinical Excellence (NICE) (2009). *Depression: the treatment and management of depression in adults (update).* London: National Institute for Health and Clinical Excellence.

Richards, D. (2007). Reforming psychological therapies—a recipe for happiness? *Openmind*, **145**, May/June, 18–20.

Richards, D.A., Lovell, K., Gilbody, S., Gask, L., Torgerson, D., Barkham, M., Bower, P., Bland, J.M., Lankshear, A., Simpson, A., Fletcher, J., Escott, D., Hennessy, S. and Richardson, R. (2008). Collaborative care for depression in UK primary care: a randomised controlled trial. *Psychological Medicine*, **38**, 279–288.

Richards, D. and Suckling, R. (2008). Improving access to psychological therapy: the Doncaster demonstration site organisational model. *Clinical Psychology Forum*, **181**, 9–16.

Richards, D.A. and Suckling, R. (2009). Improving Access to Psychological Therapies (IAPT): Phase IV Prospective Cohort Study. *British Journal of Clinical Psychology*, **48,** 377–396.

Richards, D.A. and Whyte, M. (2009). *Reach Out: National Programme Educator Materials to Support the Delivery of Training for Practitioners Delivering Low-intensity Interventions 2nd edition.* London: Rethink.

Rogers, A., Flowers, J. and Pencheon, D. (1999). Improving access needs a whole systems approach. *British Medical Journal*, **319**, 866–867.

Safran, J.D. and Segal, Z.V. (1996). *Interpersonal Process in Cognitive Therapy*. Northvale: Jason Aronson Inc.

Waddington, L. (2002). The therapy relationship in cognitive therapy: a review. *Behavioural and Cognitive Psychotherapy*, **30**, 179–191.

Chapter 7

Brief CBT in GP surgeries and community settings

Louise Hankinson and Rebecca Mitchell

Introduction

There is a large body of evidence supporting the effectiveness of cognitive behavioural therapy (CBT) delivered according to research trial standards, often prescribing 12–20 sessions for most common disorders (e.g. Clark *et al.*, 1994; Clark *et al.*, 1998; DeRubeis *et al.*, 2005). However, the reality of working in many services is that they have to work within a briefer therapy remit, due to pressures to reduce costs and waiting times by achieving results in less time. This is particularly true in primary care and community-based services, where the main issues are often high demand, overstretched resources, and long waiting times.

Evidence to support a brief CBT model is now growing. Recent guidance from the National Institute for Health and Clinical Excellence (NICE) mentions the use of brief CBT, in particular with some anxiety disorders (NICE, 2004a) and mild to moderate depression (NICE, 2004b). The Government's Improving Access to Psychological Therapies (IAPT) programme was launched to address the gap between supply and demand, and advocates a stepped-care model. It has brought increased funding to train more cognitive behavioural therapists, and is supporting the development of new ways of working, so that CBT can be available to more people, in accessible, non-stigmatizing settings (see Chapter 6). It is therefore a time of great change, excitement, and innovation, and there are many opportunities for those with CBT training.

Models of service delivery within an IAPT framework will differ but all follow the same steps:

- Step 1 is provided in primary care by general practitioners (GPs) and other practice staff and involves monitoring, support, and the use of psychoactive medication.
- Step 2 is where low-intensity CBT is provided by trained staff. This can include bibliotherapy, guided self-help, group CBT, and computerized CBT (see Chapter 6).

- Step 3 involves trained staff delivering high-intensity CBT in one-to-one therapy of up to 20 sessions. Self-referral is an option in many services to access help at Steps 2 and 3.
- Step 4 is available for people with moderate to severe psychological problems and is provided by Community Mental Health Teams and specialist psychological therapies services. Referral is via a GP or other professional worker.

Although many services have an upper session limit of around 20 sessions, it is likely that the pressure to see patients for fewer sessions while still achieving positive clinical outcomes will spread across all levels of service delivery. It is our belief therefore that if you can learn to do CBT briefly, and do it well, the rewards, both personal and professional, are many.

For the purposes of this chapter we define brief CBT as 6–8 sessions of formulation-driven therapy, which may include work on schemas and core beliefs—in other words therapy that, although brief, still adheres to standard CBT principles. When CBT is delivered in this way, careful consideration has to be given to the selection of patients, and to assessment, formulation, and intervention, in order to achieve the best possible outcome. In this chapter we will aim to address some of the clinical, personal, and practical challenges of working within a brief therapy model in community settings.

Direct work

Before you start

The current publicity regarding CBT may lead both patients and referrers to have unrealistic expectations as to what can be achieved with a 'bit of CBT'! Some patients may have had a few sessions with a low-intensity worker at Step 2, and be reluctant to enter into more CBT at Step 3, thinking they've already 'been there and done that'. Others may come expecting a cure, having read about CBT and its large evidence base, yet knowing little about what is actually involved. Some may not have heard anything at all about CBT, and be reluctant to attend because of fear of the unknown.

Here are some ideas about how you might manage these issues before the start of therapy:

- Talk to referrers about what you can offer. Stay realistic—therapy is not always about a cure, but about helping patients understand their difficulties, and facilitating their discovery and use of strategies to tackle these. Emphasize the collaborative nature of CBT and the fact that brief therapy is the *start* of a process of change that should continue beyond the end of therapy.

- Send out leaflets to patients prior to assessment, to explain CBT, what it can and cannot offer, what will be expected from them, and how many sessions they can expect to receive.
- Patient motivation is another factor to consider—'the brief psychotherapy patient or client is expected to act rather than suffer, and to become an involved participant in the therapeutic process' (Wells and Phelps, 1990). Ask referrers to talk to patients prior to referral about their expectations, ensuring they are prepared to put in the necessary work and are ready for therapy at this time, both in a practical and emotional sense.

Assessment in brief CBT

Effective screening of referrals is important in any service, but what can aid your assessment of suitability for brief CBT?

- In your introduction to the patient, state that the purpose of the assessment is to find out if there is a match between what they want and what you can offer. This can help focus both your minds on the task in hand.
- Look for evidence that the patient might be able to make use of brief CBT:
  - Is the patient ready? A patient keen to make changes, or one who has come via Step 2, might be better suited to brief work than one who arrives confused as to why he is there and cynical as to how much he might gain from therapy. Similarly, one who appears quite passive and only attending because his GP persuaded him may not be ready.
  - Can the patient identify with the cognitive behavioural model straightaway—does it help her start to make sense of her difficulties? Can she talk about her thoughts and feelings?
  - Are there signs of overdependence on other services, for example, excessive visits to his GP? If so, he may be looking for a similar relationship with you, and this would need to be directly addressed.
  - What stresses are there in her life at the moment? If she is being made homeless, has split up from her partner, has a sick child, or is under a lot of stress at work, she may not have the capacity to make full use of limited sessions at the current time. It may be appropriate to see the patient, but shift the focus of the work, or put therapy on hold and review in a few months. Alternatively, you could consider a referral to Step 2 where there may be access to less intensive but supportive therapy.
- Look beyond the diagnosis/label:
  - A diagnosis can be helpful but we would advise against making decisions on this basis alone. Referrals for panic are not always straightforward,

whereas referrals relating to obsessive compulsive disorder (OCD), or even childhood trauma, may present in a way that permits some effective brief work.

- Therapy is not always about offering the patient a cure. Ask yourself if there is an aspect of this patient's problem that might respond to brief CBT, and whether this can be worked on without increasing the patient's vulnerability.
- Having said this, be mindful of patients presenting with a history of self-harm, addiction, and difficulty forming trusting relationships, or those labeled as having a personality disorder. It is unlikely that you will be able to offer the support or time that they need, and therefore it may be best to refer on to an alternative service, for example, at Step 4.

◆ Make the most of the assessment session. You cannot afford to spend two or three sessions taking a detailed history, listing every problem, qualification, job, relationship, etc. In order to make the assessment as efficient as possible it is often necessary to limit the history taking to a summary. Here are a few examples of the sorts of questions that can be helpful in this:
  - Can you tell me briefly about any events in your past that you consider relevant to your difficulties?
  - Could you briefly sum up your childhood and teenage years for me?
  - Are there any people or times in your life that have been particularly important to you, either negatively or positively?

◆ Support your assessment with one or more standardized questionnaire(s). Examine responses on individual items as well as looking at total scores, and feedback scores to patients.

◆ Start to formulate:
  - In brief work there is less time to review and reformulate, and therefore more need for an accurate and helpful early working formulation that helps make sense of the patient's difficulties and allows you to see clear targets and goals. Use a white board or pencil-drawn diagram whenever possible, and give the patient a copy to take away.
  - Don't be in such a hurry that you present a 'ready-made' formulation to the patient that does not fit for them. Use a 'wondering aloud', non-dogmatic tone, which should allow you to check out the accuracy of the formulation and allow the patient to correct aspects of it.

◆ Set some goals and homework, right from the beginning:
  - Treatment options will be discussed at the end of the assessment session and, if therapy is to be offered within the service, the goals can be agreed.

- It may also be necessary to define what will *not* be targeted, especially in the case of a focused piece of work with a patient with complex problems.
- Some recommendations for self-help can be made (including reading), particularly if the patient will have to wait for therapy to begin. It is not possible to offer a comprehensive review or list of self-help literature here, and it is likely that your service will provide a list of recommended self-help literature for you to refer to. In our practice, we regularly use books and workbooks from the Overcoming series (www.overcoming.co.uk) and also the Oxford Cognitive Therapy Centre booklets (www.octc.co.uk).
- Don't be afraid of setting homework after the assessment, where appropriate. For example, the patient may immediately identify a lack of activity as a problem, and be able to set some goals for behavioural change. We have also given out thought records or information about challenging negative automatic thoughts to patients who are clearly ready to get started. However, gauge what the patient is capable of taking on board at this stage, so that you don't overwhelm someone who isn't ready.

A woman with long-standing depression associated strongly with the CBT model when it was presented to her towards the end of the assessment session. She was able to fit her real life experiences with the model, and identify vicious cycles. She described it as a "revelation" when we talked about thoughts being open to challenge and that they are "just thoughts not facts". As a result we discussed what she could do to help herself whilst she waited for therapy to commence. I talked her through a handout describing unhelpful thinking patterns (e.g. "all or nothing thinking", "mind-reading" and "negative filter") and how she could start recording her negative thoughts, which she was already well able to identify. She was keen to start generating alternative perspectives by examining the evidence. We were able to introduce this early on because she was highly motivated, ready to make changes and because the cognitive model had validity. In addition, because the referrer was knowledgeable about the service, he had been able to make a good judgement about her suitability for a brief CBT service.

Therapy

We shall now consider some of the core concepts of CBT and how they sometimes require modification in brief work.

The therapeutic alliance

In brief therapy, you have to be able to communicate empathy and understand fairly rapidly, and also quickly establish a good and trusting relationship with your patient. Where there is less time to work on the alliance, or to mend a relationship that becomes disrupted, some of the following may help:

- Self-disclosure can help to illustrate the model, show that you are human (we all make thinking errors and avoid things we fear), and show that there might be other ways of dealing with situations that your patient has not considered. This is *not* about telling the patient that you also had trouble sleeping last night! It is about sharing something that helps the patient feel understood.
- Using adequately disguised illustrative examples from other patients can reduce stigma and help patients feel they are not alone in their problems. This enhances empathy, which in turn can strengthen the alliance.
- Humour, when used appropriately and with warmth, can facilitate a good alliance.
- Pay attention to the alliance from the start. You may want to be explicit in the therapy contract about how problems in the alliance should be dealt with. It is helpful if both you and the patient feel able to raise any problems in the alliance in a gentle but direct way, perhaps with reference to issues highlighted in the formulation.

  A patient did not attend a session, which was unusual—in fact she usually arrived early for appointments. She responded to a routine letter and the problem was discussed at the next session. It transpired that she had not been able to complete the homework task due to her anxiety and was worried that this would provoke criticism. We were able to relate this back to her perfectionist tendencies, identified in the formulation. It was extremely helpful to be able to reflect on this and use it to challenge her ideas about criticism and her unhelpful tendency to avoid situations where she might be criticised. She was able to see how this long-standing tendency was counter-productive and that the "failure" to complete her homework was something that could be overcome.

The CBT toolbox

A sound knowledge of CBT, both in terms of the theory and the techniques involved, is vital when carrying out brief work. If you know a full range of techniques for intervening at all levels with cognitive, behavioural, and physical symptoms then you can ensure that the correct strategies are aimed at the correct problems, reducing the amount of time needed while maintaining effectiveness.

- Stay aware of the core competences (Roth and Pilling, 2007) and focus your clinical supervision and continuing professional development on those areas that are weakest.
- Strong CBT skills and theoretical knowledge ensure that sessions are planned and structured in an optimal way, again making maximum use of the limited time available. The use of an agenda is a key component. It enables the

therapist to focus on agreed goals effectively and to ensure homework tasks are looked at, enhancing the patient's motivation to continue these tasks.

- Use guided discovery whenever possible, as it enhances learning. As clinicians we have experience of how powerful a tool this can be when done effectively, but we also appreciate how working briefly can put pressure on the therapist to steer patients more directly towards a new understanding. Consider the following:
  - It is important to be sensitive enough to gauge things appropriately so that therapy does not become too didactic.
  - Be wary of making assumptions about the patient's experience and meaning. Don't assume you know what their anxious thoughts or bodily sensations are on the basis of a recent situation. Let them tell you.
  - There may be times when you enter 'teaching mode' and this can be very appropriate; for example, when you are explaining the importance of a behavioural experiment, outlining the basics of effective problem-solving, or stressing the links between mood and activity levels.
  - Ask the patient to summarize key points back to you at the end of the session to ensure they have not been left behind.
- The use of stories or metaphors can also be helpful in illustrating complex ideas in a simplified and memorable way.

A man with OCD was struggling to stop asking his wife for reassurance. In order to remind him how this reassurance seeking was one of the things maintaining his anxiety, we discussed a gardening metaphor. Being a keen gardener he was able to see that reassurance seeking was like weeding without pulling out the root of the weed. It kills off the weed (or anxious thought) for a certain amount of time, but it hasn't really removed it and it grows back pretty quickly. He later said that this was a turning point in helping him understand how to deal with his worries about causing harm to others.

Core beliefs

In some circumstances it is possible to commence work on core beliefs in brief therapy, although it may not be possible to complete the work. You must be equipped with a good knowledge of methods such as continuum techniques, evidence logs, (Padesky, 1994) and constructing a new bottom line (Fennell, 1999). The Prejudice Model is also very helpful (Padesky, 1990).

A woman in her late 40s, who scored in the very severe range for depression and anxiety, almost shook with anxiety at assessment, and avoided all eye contact. Whilst she was continuing to work, she was struggling to do much else. Her 19 year old daughter had a number of issues, and was very dependent on her mother for support. The patient was often being called at all hours and was expected to drop everything to go and help. She had a very supportive partner, whom she was pushing away and refusing to commit to. She saw herself as 100% bad.

We spent two sessions drawing up a formulation, and then used continua and a positive data notebook to challenge her core belief. She came back a week later and smiled for the first time since we met. During the following three sessions she continued to record three positives every day, and would read these out aloud to herself. She went from being 1% good, to 20% good, to 35% good, and went out with friends from work for the first time in years. She also accepted support from her partner and managed to say "No" to one of her daughter's unreasonable requests.

Patient's strengths

Look out for positives and resilience in your patients, as in the above example, where a supportive partner and the patient's ability to maintain a stable job demonstrated areas of strength that could be built on in therapy. Padesky and Mooney's (2002) 4-step model for building resilience can be a very helpful tool for this.

Don't just talk about it—do it!

As therapists we have all had the experience of sitting there thinking of some great behavioural task which will enhance learning and move therapy forward, and yet we can't bring ourselves to suggest it or carry it out. Bennett-Levy *et al.* (2004) is full of helpful ideas, and graded desensitization programmes abound, but it can still feel difficult to push forward with such plans. Therefore:

- If you have some ideas about behavioural experiments, share them with the patient and see if together you can come up with a realistic plan.
- Use your imagination—even if the first idea for an experiment needs modifying, that initial creativity may get the ball rolling.
- If you're aware you're avoiding doing something (e.g. taking a client onto a bus, carrying out a survey, putting your hand down the loo!), don't wait until it's too late. Take it to supervision, and look into what might be getting in the way. It may be a practical issue, or it may relate to your own fears or beliefs (see below, in 'Your beliefs'), which can be addressed.
- You may help patients to start programmes of graded exposure by accompanying them on trips outside the consulting room. If you do, then make it clear that these are the early steps and that they have to move towards enlisting the support of someone else, or doing it autonomously.

Staying focused

As a therapist you have to remain focused and motivated. At a recent training event, the majority of CBT therapists present admitted to sometimes 'zoning out' during a session, or to sometimes allowing the patient to go 'off track' a little. Therapists know how frustrating, or disheartening it can be when a patient comes to a session not having thought about their homework. It is possible the patient may also feel like this following a session when we haven't challenged them, therefore:

- You can minimize wasted time by sticking to an agreed agenda and looking after yourself to ensure you are not too tired, or hungry, to concentrate (see Chapter 3).
- Don't overdo the clinical work. Is your service putting too much pressure on you to do too much or see too many clients? Can you reschedule your clinics to offer some more breaks, and time to prepare?

Your beliefs

Working in a brief CBT service can put pressure on the therapist. Not only are there the relentless referrals, and often no team to share the allocation, there is also that pressure to deliver something significant within a limited time frame. Common beliefs we hear in supervising others are 'If only I could see them for longer…', or 'I haven't done enough for them…', or 'Their needs are more important than mine…' (see Chapter 1 for more on therapist beliefs).

More helpful beliefs might be 'CBT is not just about a cure, it's about offering insight, and teaching strategies to help people break unhelpful patterns of thought and behaviour', or 'I am working with the patient on one problem out of many—this can still be helpful and may be enough to lead to change in other areas'. It is also helpful to remind yourself that responsibility for change is shared by both the therapist and the patient. You can also:

- Make it clear from the start how many sessions are on offer, and stick to it. You might want to refer back down to Step 2 for some maintenance work, if that fits with your service model.
- Agree with patients what will happen if they do not attend a session. You might be tempted not to count them, as one missed out of 6 is a far greater reduction than missing one out of 12. Decide what your policy is going to be with regards to this issue, and stick to it—then try and 'let go' of the frustration caused by a missed session.
- Avoid the assumption that brief CBT is easy just because there's less of it. Your training may have equipped you specifically to work briefly, in which case working in this way will be your *forte.* If you are moving from a more traditional model into a briefer one, be mindful:
    - Sometimes brief therapy is easier as there are patients with less chronic and severe problems, whose interpersonal style facilitates therapy.

However, there is little that can prepare you for the high throughput of patients, with possible expectations to see 6 or more patients in a day, every day. You may feel a pressure to get things 'right', without going down *any* dead ends: this is, of course, unrealistic. Use supervision to explore any pressures you might be feeling in terms of caseload or patient progress.

- Consider your personal style and ability to cope with the hopes of clients who may need more than you can offer, or with referrers, who clearly expect more.
- Consider how you will manage those patients who disclose traumatic histories or other complex needs to you, when you know you have the skills to help, but who you have to refer on elsewhere or end with because of service constraints. Take these issues to supervision.

Ending

With limited sessions, it is possible therapy may end when the patient is still experiencing some difficulty. To help facilitate a positive ending:

- Ensure that patients' expectations of therapy are realistic from the beginning, and work with them in the final sessions on a very structured blueprint for the future management of their difficulties.
- Guide patients towards further self-help materials, and consider offering future contact with the service (e.g. a follow-up review, or the prospect of re-referral for top-up sessions).
- We have often found it helpful to think with patients about a person they can recruit from their network, to help support them in implementing their blueprint and continuing to apply CBT in their everyday lives.
- Consider leaving patient files open for an agreed period (e.g. 3 months), during which time the patient can make contact and request to be seen without having to be re-referred. This can allow the patient to feel 'contained', and it reminds them they are still working on something. In our experience, patients rarely make contact during this time to ask to be seen. If you use this method, ensure you have a good administrative system in place to flag up files for closing at the end of the agreed period.

And a word about admin...

Given the high proportion of time spent in clinical contact and the variable levels of administrative support in GP surgeries and other such settings, it is important to learn strategies for keeping on top of admin. Here are a few hints that have helped us:

- Develop the skill of keeping session notes during the session, while maintaining as much eye contact as possible—this aids memory and avoids the necessity of spending time writing up notes after the session.
- Save templates of reports and letters on the computer system to aid report writing.
- Keep letters and reports brief: learn to summarize a history in a couple of sentences (e.g. X became vulnerable to depression as a result of criticism at home and bullying at school).
- Try to keep up-to-date with administrative tasks, as it takes much less time to write a brief report or fill out a registration form while the patient is still fresh in your mind.
- Be organized—have printouts of handouts and diagrams filed in such a way that they can be accessed quickly. If handing out CDs or booklets, ensure that you have well stocked supplies.

Requests for consultancy and advice

Often you may be the only mental health professional or therapist in your setting, and as a result may receive requests to share skills and provide a broader service: for example, liaison, consultancy, supervision, and training. In Chapters 10 and 16 you can read in more detail about working through others and supervision. We shall now focus on some of the issues that can arise when sharing your skills through consultancy and advice.

- The types of issue you may be able to advise on are referral routes, other available services, or the best therapeutic option for a patient with mental health problems. Make sure you know about other services at the steps below and above yours, so that you can give accurate information.
- You can also facilitate colleagues' understanding of different problems using a CBT framework, and advise them how to manage specific situations.

  Whilst in the kitchen at a GP surgery I was asked for advice about a patient who frequently presented to many of the GPs in the practice. Having agreed that we both had 10 minutes to talk further, we re-located to an office to protect confidentiality. I asked the GP to summarize his concerns or difficulties in dealing with this patient and was able to hypothesize that the patient may have health anxiety to a fairly severe degree. Whilst in agreement, the GP stated that a referral for a CBT assessment had been discussed with this patient but she did not consent as she was convinced her problems had an entirely physical basis and were not being taken seriously by the doctors. I provided the GP with a booklet about health anxiety and the CBT formulation. I also gave advice on dealing with the patient's requests for unnecessary tests and her regular reassurance-seeking. We agreed he would more clearly state to the patient that further tests or examinations were likely to be unhelpful; instead he would offer alternative explanations for the patient's symptoms. The GP was going to ensure that all staff in the practice dealt with the patient consistently and we discussed what could be done to help reception staff manage this highly anxious patient.

- It's important that you are not pushed into answering questions without sufficient information, time to think, knowledge, or expertise. If you don't know something it is both professional and ethical to say that you don't know and that you will try to find out, or that you need some time to think further about it.
- Be prepared for more unusual, or personal requests for advice, some of which you may need to discuss in supervision, before agreeing to advise.

A GP asked if I "had a moment for a chat." We entered into a discussion about the difficulties arising from the fact that this GP had a patient who was also a personal friend. The GP wanted to know how psychologists or therapists would deal with this situation. I advised that we would seek an alternative therapist for a patient who was also a personal friend, because of the complications that arise from such a blurring of boundaries. The GP said she felt incredibly relieved and that she'd always felt it wasn't an effective way to help her friend (who had complex needs), but there had always been an expectation, from her friend and from colleagues, that she should be the named GP. We brainstormed some ways in which she could broach this subject with her friend.

Working across multiple settings

It is often a feature of providing CBT in a primary care or community setting that you may have no single office base. In addition, you may be required to work across two or more settings in a single day and multiple settings in a working week. This can be extremely stressful and it is entirely appropriate to bring any concerns you have to supervision, or to the attention of your line manager. These concerns may centre around the demands of traveling between multiple sites without a base, or may involve specific issues with a certain setting. We outline below some of the challenges that have arisen in our own work in primary care:

- We have been required to offer therapy in rooms equipped with beds, dentist chairs, surgical devices, or virtually no space! We have also turned up for clinics where there has not been a room available at all. It is best to be mentally prepared for all eventualities and sometimes the use of humour, when appropriate, can help smooth over an awkward situation. Communicate clearly with the settings you work in about your requirements and the reasons for them. If the setting has not accommodated mental health therapists before, do not assume they know not to interrupt you or that a session usually lasts for around 50 minutes. It may be necessary to follow up any conversations with a letter to the manager of the facility listing your requirements.

- Access to a computer and printer is often necessary for record keeping, writing letters and reports, and printing patient handouts. You may also need paper, envelopes, and secure storage facilities for patient files. You will need support from your line manager if there is uncertainty about who should pay for and provide such facilities.
- Insufficient time to travel between sites is one of the most common stressors in this type of work. Try to set up your working week to minimize travel as much as possible. If you are going to be late then phone ahead so that reception staff can inform your patients.
- Drawing boundaries around your work in any particular setting is crucial so that you don't attempt to fit in more than is actually possible in the time. In high-intensity therapy it is usual to see a maximum of 3 patients in a half-day. You may also find that you cannot keep up with all the administrative demands if all your patients attend, so you may need to ring-fence time for these tasks.
- We have found it essential to carry CBT resources around with us, but one of the easiest ways to do this is to save patient handouts (e.g. thought records, information sheets, and free website links) on a memory stick or similar device. There is usually a facility for printing out what you need in the consulting room, or a nearby office.
- If you spend a little time and effort getting to know the administrative and clinical staff in a setting, that can enhance cooperation and make your working life more pleasant.
- In order to deal with isolation it is crucial that you maintain a professional identity and keep abreast of developments in the field. You can:
  - Make contact with fellow therapists/mental health professionals via websites.
  - Set up peer supervision groups if possible, or establish other informal links.
  - Subscribe to professional or academic organizations such as the British Association of Behavioural and Cognitive Psychotherapists (BABCP) or British Psychological Society (BPS). Make sure you allow time to read

papers on-line or in journals you subscribe to, as it is a requirement of many organizations that you maintain a professional development log. Most employers should support you in this.

- Attend conferences to stay in touch with your core training, and with other CBT therapists (see Chapter 15).

Key points

- Communicate well with referrers and patients about the scope and limitations of brief CBT.
- The assessment should be focused on the current problem(s) and ascertaining suitability for brief CBT. Aim to share an initial formulation and give advice on strategies at the end of the assessment session so that therapy can start even before the first treatment session.
- It takes skill and practice to hone standard CBT skills to a brief model. Therapy may be a little more didactic and will certainly be more focused—but get going as soon as possible with tasks, such as behavioural experiments, that will bring about cognitive change. *Don't just talk about it—do it!*
- Contain anxieties about ending by sticking to the agreed number of sessions and developing a good blueprint, so that hope and change continue after therapy has ended.
- When offering consultancy or advice, do not feel pressured into giving an instant answer. If you lack the knowledge or experience it is best to say that you don't know, but that you will try to find out and report back.

Further reading

Bond, F.W. and Dryden, W. (eds.) (2002). *Handbook of Brief Cognitive Behaviour Therapy.* Chichester: John Wiley & Sons.

The 'Overcoming' Series website. Available at: www.overcoming.co.uk (accessed 26 February 2010).

The Oxford Cognitive Therapy Centre website. Available at: www.octc.co.uk (accessed 26 February 2010).

References

Bennett-Levy, J., Butler, G., Fennell, M., Hackmann, A., Mueller, M. and Westbrook, D. (eds.) (2004). *Oxford Guide to Behavioural Experiments.* New York, NY: Oxford University Press.

Clark, D.M., Salkovskis, P.M., Hackmann, A., Middleton, H., Anastasiades, P. and Gelder, M.G. (1994). A comparison of cognitive therapy, applied relaxation and Imipramine in the treatment of panic disorder. *British Journal of Psychiatry*, **164**, 759–769.

Clark, D.M., Salkovskis, P.M., Hackmann, A., Wells, A., Fennell, M., Ludgate, J., Ahmad, S., Richards, H.C. and Gelder, M.G. (1998). Two psychological treatments for hypochondriasis: a randomised controlled trial. *British Journal of Psychiatry*, **173**, 218–225.

DeRubeis, R.J., Hollon, S.D., Amsterdam, J.D., Shelton, R.C., Young, P.R., Salomon, R.M., O'Reardon, J.P., Lovett, M.L., Gladis, M.M., Brown, L.L. and Gallop, R. (2005). Cognitive therapy vs medications in the treatment of moderate to severe depression. *Archives of General Psychiatry*, **62**, 409–416.

Fennell, M.F. (1999). *Overcoming Low Self-esteem: A Self-help Guide to Using Cognitive-Behavioural Techniques.* London: Constable and Robinson.

National Institute for Health and Clinical Excellence (2004a). *Anxiety: Management of Anxiety (panic disorder, with or without agoraphobia, and generalised anxiety disorder) in Adults in Primary, Secondary and Community Care.* Available at: http://guidance.nice.org.uk/CG22/guidance/pdf/English (accessed 20 January 2009).

National Institute for Health and Clinical Excellence (2004b). *Depression: Management of Depression in Primary and Secondary Care.* Available at: http://guidance.nice.org.uk/CG23/guidance/pdf/English (accessed 20 January 2009).

Padesky, C.A. (1990). Schema as self-prejudice. *International Cognitive Therapy Newsletter*, **5/6**, 16–17.

Padesky, C.A. (1994). Schema change processes in cognitive therapy. *Clinical Psychology and Psychotherapy*, **1**(5), 267–278.

Padesky, C.A. and Mooney, K. (2002). *Two-day Workshop: Cognitive Therapy to Build Resilience: A 4-step Model.* 14–15 May 2007. London.

Roth, A.D. and Pilling, S. (2007). *The Competences Required to Deliver Effective Cognitive and Behavioural Therapy for People with Depression and with Anxiety Disorders.* Available at: http://www.ucl.ac.uk/clinical-psychology/CORE/CBT_Competences/CBT_Competence_List.pdf (accessed 20 January 2009).

Wells, R.A. and Phelps, P.A. (1990). The brief psychotherapies: a selective overview, in Wells, R.A. and Giannetti, V.J. (eds.), *Handbook of the Brief Psychotherapies.* New York, NY: Plenum Press.

Chapter 8

CBT in groups

Joanne Ryder

You are feeling the pressure of referrals. You do not want to reject them but nor do you want to build up a long waiting list. As some of your referrals are for similar difficulties, your thoughts turn to group therapy. However, this consideration is accompanied by many questions: Have you the skill to manage a group? Will you be able to decide who is suitable? What is the evidence that group intervention is effective? What will you do if it all gets out of hand?

Introduction

The provision of therapy within a group setting has long been established within the psychodynamic tradition. Over the past 30 years, group cognitive behavioural therapy (GCBT) has become an increasingly popular means of delivering cognitive behavioural therapy (CBT) to people presenting with similar problems at the same time. As increasing pressure is placed on providers of psychological services to ensure that people are seen promptly, together with the fact that the demand for psychological therapy (and in particular CBT) tends to exceed its supply, then the provision of GCBT is one of the obvious ways to square this circle. GCBT has the potential to enable clinicians to meet the demand for providing CBT to more patients in a timely fashion, especially if they can be confident that the treatment is both clinically and cost-effective.

This chapter will help you decide if GCBT is relevant for you and, if it is, how to get the most out of it. It will guide you through some of the important considerations that you will need to address when developing and running GCBT, and will discuss some of the obstacles and difficulties that you might encounter along the way, providing you with possible solutions to these.

GCBT has been developed using the same principles on which individual CBT is based. As a result, it mirrors the therapy structure within individual CBT, and incorporates many recognizable features of individual CBT, such as the use of agenda setting, the establishment of a collaborative relationship, formulation, goal setting, socialization, cognitive and behaviour interventions, the evaluation of dysfunctional assumptions and beliefs, homework tasks and blueprinting. Its applicability to presenting problems is also comparable to that for individual CBT. There is evidence that suggests GCBT can be provided for a number of disorders such as depression (Scott and Stradling, 1990) and anxiety (White, 1995), as well as for psychosis (Bechdolf *et al.*, 2004) and bipolar affective disorder (Patelis-Siotis *et al.*, 2001).

There are many reasons you may choose to run a group. Apart from factors associated with the clinical and cost-effectiveness of groups, it is incredibly rewarding to be the facilitator of a group that has enabled a number of members to undergo a life-changing experience. In my experience, the main advantages of GCBT are:

- It can normalize group members' experiences.
- It allows members to support one another in doing tasks (e.g. behavioural experiments, which might be particularly useful in social anxiety).
- It enables members to learn through others' cognitions (e.g. when recognizing and challenging cognitive distortions, people can often identify in others what they cannot see in themselves).

The disadvantages of GCBT are:

- It provides the therapist with only a very limited ability to tailor sessions to the idiosyncratic beliefs and behaviour systems of the individual.
- Patient outcome is dependent upon the dynamics of the group, not just on the patient's own motivation to change.

In some cases, GCBT has proven to be as clinically effective as individual CBT (see Morrison, 2001 for a fuller review of the literature). However, the evidence relating to the cost-effectiveness of GCBT is inconclusive. Where GCBT has been deemed to be cost-effective, this assessment has been based largely on it being clinically effective, and therefore by extension cost-effective because of the number of patients involved in each group. Tucker and Oei (2007) evaluated the existing research on the cost-effectiveness of GCBT, and concluded that the apparent findings of cost-effectiveness (see Scott and Stradling, 1990 for depression) might be based on inadequate or incomplete estimates of the costs associated with GCBT. Costs of GCBT that are often overlooked include the additional preparation time for the facilitators, and the extra costs incurred by participants as a result of the reduced flexibility in the timing and location of the group when compared with individual therapy. Therefore, the assessment of the cost-effectiveness of GCBT is dependent on the appropriate measurement of *all* the costs (see Tucker and Oei, 2007), and this is what you will have to bear in mind.

Getting started

There are several key factors to consider before embarking on a GCBT programme:

- Is there a clinical justification for running the group?
- How does running a group fit within the service in which you work?
- What is the purpose of the group, and who is the group for?
- Does your workplace have the necessary resources to enable you to develop this programme?
- Do you have the necessary skills to do it?
- Do you need a co-therapist?
- Do you have the time?

  Have you allowed yourself enough time to both prepare and run the group? You need to include any administrative work before and after the group, such as correspondence to the referrer and note-keeping. Often this aspect of running groups is underestimated.
- Where, when, and how will the group take place?
- How do you intend to measure the effectiveness of the group?

  This is particularly important when required to justify the resources allocated to run the group.
- What supervision is available to you while the group is running?

Selecting the type of group

There are already a number of established group protocol programmes (that have evolved out of individual CBT) for specific disorders (see Bieling *et al.*, 2006, for an overview). However, my experience suggests that some of these programmes should be modified. For instance, the length of session and the material that you present will depend on either the patient group with whom you are working or the requirements of your service. If you are offering GCBT in a primary care setting that is targeted at people suffering with mild to moderate depression, you might consider offering a reduced length of treatment when compared to GBCT for moderate to severely depressed people.

You may also consider offering GCBT in a briefer format if it is designed to be purely psychoeducational. You will find that some groups evolve, so that what might have started as a purely psychoeducational group becomes something that is less didactic, where group members are encouraged to speak openly about their difficulties. This process can present you with one of the clear advantages associated with GCBT: by encouraging more group discussion (which can be promoted through the use of exercises, such as ones that are designed to identify or to test negative automatic thoughts), you can assist in normalizing the group's experiences. In addition, patients can often identify from others' experiences what is not obvious to themselves. On the other hand, encouraging group discussion of individual experiences has the potential for the session to degenerate into a general discussion, or can result in the session becoming dominated by one or two group members who are able to identify with each others' experiences (see section 'Group process').

Format

The format of the group will be dependent on your own work setting. Variants of GCBT have been developed for different purposes, for example, large scale psychoeducational groups versus small scale targeted groups, and closed groups versus rotating open groups that might be more suited to an inpatient setting.

Group size

The size of the group you will run depends on the group's objectives and availability of therapists. Group size would typically lie between 10 and 25 in most settings, but can be as large as 50. As the size of your group increases, so does the spread in presenting difficulties. You could offer a very small group if it would be more cost-effective for you to see 2-plus patients in the same amount of time as seeing one patient. For instance, if you have recently assessed a small number of patients presenting with similar difficulties, and you feel that they would work well together, then offering a group programme for 2-plus people would be sensible. There is the additional benefit that patients will be able to share their experiences with one another and operate as co-therapists. Large groups of 30 or more patients are more challenging, and will require you to have gained experience as a large group facilitator. Also, a larger group might need more than two facilitators to manage difficulties that arise among the group members and to properly observe the group. As the group you run becomes larger, so it will tend to become more didactic (see White, 1995), with limited opportunity for fuller patient participation.

Closed groups

This is where all the participants join the group at the same time and follow the same group programme. This format tends to run for between 8 and 14 sessions and would usually be weekly, although it could be more frequent if you are working with inpatients. Within primary care, GCBT is often aimed at symptom management, and might therefore be somewhat shorter. Each group session tends to last for between 1½–2 hours. If you aim for a 2-hour session, you will have greater flexibility and more discussion in the group, but you might want to schedule a short break.

Open-ended groups

The alternative to a closed format is the open-ended, rotating format, where participants join the group at any point during the programme. Sessions are often held more frequently than in the closed format, and are likely to have a more psychoeducational bias, or have a skills focus. This format is frequently used in an inpatient setting since patient admissions are often relatively brief. However, this format can hinder group processes, such as those identified by Tuckman (1965).

An associated issue you will need to consider is whether the group is to be predominantly experiential or didactic. For more didactic GCBT, you might state this in a leaflet distributed prior to the programme starting, and also remind participants in the first session, that:

> *This is a skills based course—we will be learning new skills to help manage X. It is not intended to be group therapy. No one will be expected to talk about themselves, or their own particular difficulties, in front of the whole group. We will, however, be asking you to think of relevant examples from your current situation, and to use these as examples in the exercises.*

Facilitator(s)

The size and nature of the group you run will influence how many facilitators are required. For smaller groups, often only one facilitator will be required, if you are working with a highly distressed patient group you may still want to consider having another person on hand to manage distressed patients. This additional facilitator can be less experienced or qualified, but should be able to contain a patient's distress. You will need to define their role clearly to the group at the outset. A second facilitator is also useful so that both group process and content can be attended to at any one time, whatever the group size. Where two facilitators are required, it is again possible that, depending on the group format and patient group, the second facilitator will be less qualified or experienced than the leader of the group.

As the leader of the group you need to be clear about the role and expectations of the second facilitator. Should you choose to have a co-facilitator, outline their role before, during, and after the group, so that you are both clear about your responsibilities. The role of the main facilitator is to keep the group on track, and will include tasks such as:

- Structuring the format of the group
- Maintaining clinical records
- Corresponding with the referrer
- Fielding telephone calls between sessions
- Following up any patients who have been distressed
- Addressing any risk issues that have become apparent

If you are working within a secondary care setting, you might want to avoid being the care coordinator for patients in groups, although this needs to be negotiated with the referrer prior to the patient's inclusion in the group. You might also want to consider whether to include a patient who has been seen by a facilitator for individual therapy, as they may have expectations of the facilitator that cannot be satisfied and other group members might feel disadvantaged.

Selecting patients for GCBT

All groups should have inclusion and exclusion criteria. It is important that you pay careful attention to these criteria as selection of patients can make or break a group.

Inclusion criteria

Your inclusion criteria will depend on the type of group you plan to run, and might include a primary diagnosis based on the focus of the group, for example, depression. It is important that individuals are motivated to engage in GCBT, are socially able enough to benefit from the group, and will not undermine its functioning. It is also beneficial if they are able to learn cooperatively and vicariously. Otherwise, they will be unable to take full advantage of being in the group, and might also adversely affect the dynamics of the group. Your criteria for inclusion might mean that you will want to exclude someone who is:

- Actively suicidal
- Engaging in self-harming behaviour
- Misusing substances
- Actively psychotic

These are very general guidelines. You will need to modify them when working with a more complex patient group. If this is the case, you should have contingency plans in place if a situation occurs that will detract from the running of the group. For instance:

- If you are running a group for substance misuse and a member arrives intoxicated.
- Someone becomes threatening to a group member or facilitator.
- A patient's self-harming behaviour increases when you are running a group for people with personality disorders.
- A patient's presenting problem worsens so that they can no longer function well in a group.

It is crucial that you adhere to your inclusion criteria to reduce the likelihood of such situations occurring. Being flexible and accommodating is not necessarily in the best interests of potential patients. For example, if you allow a person who is severely depressed to attend GCBT for people presenting with mild to moderate depression, they might become despondent about not improving as quickly as other group members, and drop out as a result. Conversely, others within the group might be discouraged from continuing as they will view their difficulties as insignificant in comparison.

Patient characteristics

If the focus of your group is concerned with the management of problems across diagnoses (as might be the case for a group offered within an inpatient setting, or for a group of survivors of childhood trauma), then it is more likely you will include a wider range of patients. You will need to take into account such characteristics as the gender, age, and ethnicity of potential group members. For example, you will need to consider how well a single male would fit in a group of females. You will also have to pay close attention to language (particularly where English is not a person's first language). Such patients may find it difficult to involve themselves fully in the group, unable to ask questions or seek clarification because they feel that they are slowing the group down. Conversely, other group members will become frustrated if they perceive they are waiting for others.

Similar difficulties may arise where patients have a specific learning difficulty, although sometimes you will be able to resolve or accommodate them quite quickly.

For example, a member of a group struggled to complete her homework tasks until the facilitator was able to identify that she had dyslexia. On discovering this, the woman was provided with a dictaphone, enabling her to record her homework tasks and so participate fully in the group.

Screening

Screening potential patients for suitability for the group can be time consuming, and therefore you need to decide in advance how this will be done, and how much time you are prepared to devote to it. You should screen referrals for GCBT even if the patient has been assessed and considered suitable for CBT. You might offer a brief telephone screening, where you can explain the nature and purpose of the group, and address any concerns the patient may have about the group. For more complex patients such as those with chronic depression or a history of childhood sexual abuse (CSA), your screening will need to be face to face and more detailed. Such screening also allows you to determine the patients' expectations of the group, and how they will fit in with it. When people are referred without a CBT assessment, I would recommend that you assess their suitability for CBT and attending the group at the same time. You will need to consider the patients' psychological mindedness, which includes their ability to engage in therapy, together with how they will fit in with, and enhance, the group.

In general, you should try to avoid including someone who is likely to undermine the cohesiveness of the group, and in turn undermine the whole process. You will therefore need to be prepared to convey sensitively to patients who you do not wish to include in the group that it is unlikely to meet their current needs. This can be easier to do if you have considered in advance the alternatives open to these patients, and you are therefore able to explain to them that these alternatives are more suited to their needs. For a general discussion on selecting patients for CBT, see Chapter 1.

Information leaflet

It is useful to provide a referrer's leaflet and a patient leaflet explaining the GCBT. The former serves to educate potential referrers about the group, by defining who would be suitable. You need to be clear about what the group can, and can not, offer. A typical leaflet is shown in the Appendix 8.1. You may also wish to include a referral form that elicits the basic information that you will need before being able to consider accepting the referral for the group.

A patient leaflet is also a useful resource when you recruit to a group. Your leaflet should state:

- The purpose of the group.
- Who the group is suitable for.
- Some basic, useful information such as where the group will be held and who will be the facilitator(s), with contact numbers.
- The expectations of the group.

It is particularly important that you outline your expectations of group members since people's reluctance to attend a group is often due to the perception that 'they need to reveal all'. By dispelling this myth about GCBT at an early stage, you will find it much easier to encourage people to attend.

Group process

As the facilitator, you will not only need CBT skills, such as those used in individual therapy, but you will also have to manage the group process and dynamics. You therefore need to be able to use the available time effectively, to manage dominant group members while continuing to pay attention to others in the group, and to stay on track and cover the agenda for that particular group session. Your interpersonal style is an important factor to consider, just as it is in individual therapy. Your ability to form a collaborative therapeutic alliance is essential, as is your ability to use the group process to foster learning (see Chapters 16 and 17 on training and on supervision).

In many ways, you will need to perform a juggling act that balances the needs of the group while at the same time imparting CBT techniques. Yalom (1995) has identified 12 therapeutic factors that are present to a greater or lesser extent in a group, and are also dependent on the developmental stage of the group. He suggests that the factors needing close attention are: interpersonal interaction, catharsis, self-understanding, and group cohesion (for a fuller review, see Yalom, 1995, and also Burlingame *et al.*, 2004). Furthermore, Tuckman (1965) has also identified a number of stages through which groups proceed, including:

- Forming (engagement and affiliation),
- Storming (control, status, competition, and individual differentiation),
- Norming and performing (productive working phase accompanied by engagement and cohesion), and
- Adjourning (the ending of the group).

In general, paying close attention to these will help you build group cohesion, enhancing your ability to work effectively within a group setting. However, there is a view that group cohesion can be destructive to the group or the group's function (see Whitaker and Lieberman, 1964). For example, a high degree of support from other patients in the group may allow an individual patient to maintain his/her avoidance behaviours.

The group should be as interactive as possible, in order to encourage active participation by all the group members. You need to ensure each group member receives approximately the same amount of time and individual attention. Just as in individual CBT, you will be using Socratic method to elicit information, although in GCBT you will also be making use of group examples to illustrate the particular perspective or CBT skill that you are trying to impart. If the group is more experiential, allowing group members to share their experiences can encourage other group members to share strategies that are particularly focused on problem-solving. This approach will help you to shift the perspective of group members.

In my experience, there is often one group member who attempts to dominate. This may range from them wanting simply to tell their story so that they feel that they are understood by the group, to monopolizing the sessions by continually restating their own difficulties with little regard to others in the group, to interrupting other group members and regarding other group members' difficulties as being less relevant or significant. You should also be aware of the difficulties of the silent member, the patient who is tearful, the 'complainer', and the disengaged. You can use yourself, your co-therapist, *and* group members as a resource to overcome such difficulties.

John was a quieter member of the group. We used experiences from other patients to encourage John to engage in group discussion. Although initially reluctant to talk, John formed a strong alliance with other group members, which gave him the confidence to become more involved.

Aysha was initially tearful, to the extent that she would leave the group during a session and it was useful to have a co-facilitator who could attend more closely to her emotions when she left the group. As the facilitator, you must attend to individual affective change, but also balance this with the needs of other group members: to validate one person's emotional response, but then quickly refocus on the whole group.

Mary would seek reassurance from the facilitator about the homework task, much to the frustration of her fellow group members. She then extended her reassurance seeking to other group exercises. Referring her back to the written homework instructions or group task instructions did not stop her reassurance seeking, until a frustrated group member directly challenged her, saying "I've noticed it does not matter what X and Y say to reassure you about the task. It is taking time away from what we need to do here." Mary verbalised her need to "always get it right". The group was then able to help Mary evaluate her thought and experiment by doing something differently.

It is important that you work through the group process (in the here and now) in order to develop group cohesion. This means paying close attention not only to the verbal but also to the non-verbal behaviour of group members, and drawing upon the use of management and containment strategies.

Corrine had a number of social problems that influenced her low mood. Following assessment, she was referred to a Psycho-educational Managing Depression group. It quickly became apparent that Corrine would try to monopolise the group, recounting her past and present difficulties. At times she felt vulnerable after leaving the group because she felt she had been too open. The group leader appreciated that she needed to be skilful in the use of containment strategies. At the start of each session, she included a reminder about how the group best uses its time, and the importance of everybody who wants to talk getting a chance, and feeling they are listened to by the other group members. A general reminder of the ground rules discussed at the outset also proved useful. Whist this was the strategy used in the initial sessions, the facilitator spoke to Corrine individually to acknowledge her contribution to the group, but also to discuss the appropriateness of her contributions bearing in mind the psycho-educational aim of the group. Following the group, Corrine was referred for individual therapy.

Jane was always the first to answer questions and monopolise time. Other group members found her domineering and she had little regard for other group members. The facilitators recognised this pattern and quickly opened discussion to other members by reminding her that she had had her time and it was important that others should have a chance to talk. Another strategy that was used was to note that this was interesting but the group would have to move on because of a lack of time.

There may also be some group members who challenge you or the therapy. It is important that you do not engage with their arguments, but instead validate their difficulties and emphasise the role of personal responsibility and choice.

Leroy would frequently become confrontational towards the facilitator during group exercises. His frustrations were always acknowledged and considered by the group. Leroy was encouraged to focus on his thoughts and emotions about being involved in group exercises and in the group in general. This allowed him to communicate his anxiety about being in the group and "making a fool of himself". Once the facilitator had identified this, Leroy was able, with the group's help, to evaluate and test his thoughts.

It does not matter how well you screen people for inclusion in a group, there will be occasions when it becomes apparent that some members become unsuitable over time, perhaps as a result of deteriorating mental health. You need to be prepared to acknowledge this with the individual and the group, suggest that they discontinue the group, and propose an alternative therapy option that better meets their current psychological needs. You should try to do this with them individually, and then inform the group at the next session.

Jaideep was initially well motivated to attend a group for patients with bipolar affective disorder. However, after several sessions, his behaviour during the group became inappropriate, and it was apparent that he was cycling into a manic episode. After a discussion with the patient, the facilitator decided that he should no longer attend the group, and he was referred back to his care coordinator. When the group was informed that Jaideep would no longer be attending, the facilitator ensured that they were aware of the circumstances, and assured that these had nothing to do with him attending the group.

Other considerations

Location of the group

It is easy to overlook the importance, or potential impact, of the location of the group. In my experience, providing the group in a location that is away from a mental health setting, such as in a local community hall, leads to an increase in group attendance. The location of the group is often referred to by participants as being a factor that they regard as important. Holding the group away from a medical setting can be perceived as less stigmatizing and formal, particularly for those who have previously had less formal contact with mental health services. However, if you decide to run a group away from your usual place of work, remember to consider transport links, parking difficulties, and factor in additional costs, such as room hire.

Group rules

Assuming that you are running a closed group, the first session should include your expectations of group members and the 'group rules'. These rules will cover a number of issues.

- Confidentiality. It is important that participants understand that they should only share with others what they are happy to share, that discussions are private, that everyone should be respectful of confidential issues.
- Respect. They should listen to and respect others as they would wish to be listened to and respected, and should look for the value in what other people say.
- Attendance. You might want to stress that patients should arrive on time, and that they should try to contact the facilitator when unable to attend.
- What to do in a crisis. Make sure that patients have appropriate contact numbers, and if self-harm is a possible risk, then patients should have prevention plans (see Kennerley *et al.*, 1998).
- Troubleshooting. It is easy to overlook seemingly minor issues that can be significant for some participants. One example of this is 'what shall we do if we meet someone we know from the group?' This issue can cause a lot of debate, with responses ranging from 'I would say hello' to 'I would ignore them'. If group members choose to meet outside the group and offer each other support, you need to ensure that this does not affect the cohesiveness of the group. This illustrates the inherent complexities of working within groups.

When running an open group, you will need to provide a brief review of the above rules at the start of each session. However, it is always beneficial if you provide the patients with a written overview outlining the rules.

Record keeping

You will need to follow the protocol of the service in which you work and consider what information you will need to inform your session to session work. As a minimum, you should document attendance and any difficulties or safety issues that have arisen, and the appropriate action that you have taken. You may also find it useful to document what the particular session has covered, for example, an introduction to identifying negative automatic thoughts.

Evaluating the group

Just as with individual therapy, it is good practice to evaluate routinely your clinical outcome. It is also likely that the Service in which you work will require you to show that the group has been effective. You will therefore need to consider what outcome measures to use, and the frequency of their use. This may range from start, end, and follow-up of the group, to every session (although remember that this will impose an additional administrative task). Session-by-session evaluations can range from formal psychometrics to simple visual analogue scales—you need to consider what information you need and what it is reasonable to ask of your patients. You should also consider the use of a patient satisfaction questionnaire to enable you to identify those aspects of treatment that were successful, and those that might need to be re-evaluated for subsequent groups.

Supervision

You will need to decide whether you arrange clinical supervision separately in respect of your GCBT, or whether you can include this in your existing supervision arrangements. If there is more than one facilitator, it is important to have briefing sessions prior to the group, as well as debriefing sessions after the group. Your debriefing may focus on any difficulties that have arisen in the session, and ways to manage these should they arise again.

It is normally the case that no two groups are alike. Sometimes what went well in one group may pose a problem in another, and this is often due to the dynamics of the group, rather than the CBT intervention itself. Just as in individual therapy, so the process will need examining. Again, you can do this in a debriefing session with the co-facilitator should there be one. If an issue recurs, you may choose to discuss this in your personal clinical supervision, as it may be a reflection of a particular aspect of your leadership style, such as being inflexible or unstructured.

Issues associated with GCBT

Attendance

It is important that you attempt to maximize attendance, as this is likely to benefit all group members. A lot depends upon you as the facilitator. Above all, you must be well prepared at all times, which might even include providing refreshments at break time.

If you are running a closed group, consider when you would exclude a person from attending further sessions if their attendance is ad hoc or they have missed the first 2 or 3 sessions where you are socializing patients into the model and formulating difficulties. It becomes more difficult to do this as time progresses, so as the group facilitator you will need to consider the needs of the larger group. If you are forced to engage in catch-up with members who have missed sessions, then this will take time away from the rest of the group and may lead to tensions in the group. Also, if a patient misses a significant number of sessions, you might want to provide some guidance about what they should do to catch up.

Where possible, always include the individual and group members in any discussion on whether to exclude people from the group as a result of non-attendance. If it is a planned absence, then you might suggest some reading or homework that keeps the individual on track. If time permits, ask the patient to come to the group a few minutes early so that you can cover the previous week's programme with him/her. You might consider recording a session for a patient unable to attend, but remember you will need to obtain written consent from all the patients attending. When people do not attend the group and have made no contact with you, then you might choose to write to them, inviting them to the next session, or telephone them and try and encourage them to attend the next session. It is important that you keep the group updated with who is attending and not attending in any week, as consistent attendance provides a safe environment for disclosure by group members who have begun to trust the other group members and the group facilitator. This approach will be more difficult in a very large group setting, and will not be feasible in an open group.

Lateness

Lateness is probably best addressed with the individual at the end of the session. Try and help the person solve the problem of getting to the group on time rather than point out the negative impact of their lateness on themselves and the group in general. If another group member raises the fact that some members have arrived late, you may want to check whether others have concerns about this and put it on the agenda for discussion. However, be careful that any resulting discussion does not descend into an attempt to shame or vilify individual members of the group.

Homework

As with all CBT, homework is an important part of the therapy and you must pay close attention to members who do not do the homework. Your agenda setting should always include a review of homework. If you find that individuals have been unable to complete the task, try to determine why. You need to consider whether the task was not explained in sufficient detail, or whether a lack of time is the issue. If it is the latter, try problem-solving with the individual, and open the discussion up to the group to offer alternative solutions. Be mindful of time keeping, but paying close attention to the homework review sends a clear message to all group members that homework is an important task, is part of the group task, and should not be overlooked. Material from assignments can also be usefully explored in the session, providing examples for all group members.

There are many ways that you can review homework within a group setting, and you will need to find a way that works well for you and the group, especially if there are more than around 12 in the group. There are advantages and disadvantages of reviewing the homework individually. Although it is a good way of ensuring that all group members have completed it, it takes time, during which some group members might disengage. I find that reviewing homework in pairs (or small groups), with specific questions to answer and then asking for feedback, works well. This is a format I use when the group is over 12. Alternatively, you can ask for homework to be handed directly to the facilitator. This can then be reviewed and returned to members. Although this approach imposes an additional burden on you, it allows you to see that the task has been completed, and completed in the way you were expecting. When setting homework, provide written instructions about the task or encourage group members to write the instructions down. In this way, there is less room for confusion and the homework task is more likely to be completed.

Feedback

One of the challenges for you is to facilitate feedback from others in a helpful way. Always try to finish the group on time, while allowing for time for brief individual feedback just as you would in individual CBT. The sorts of things you might want to include are 'what will you take away from the group today', 'what went well', and 'what, if anything, did you not like'. Where individuals have struggled in the group session, for example, due to a significant affective change or disengagement, you might want to approach these individuals on their own to identify, and deal with, any potential issues that have arisen. You can use prepared forms if you want to ask for more formal feedback. These need not be onerous: they can simply ask questions such as:

- What did you find helpful about the group meeting?

- What did you find difficult or unhelpful?
- What suggestions do you have for improving the sessions?
- On a scale of 1–10, how did you feel at the end of the session?

Clearly you will tailor the questions to meet your needs.

Ending

Just as in individual therapy, it is important that you address termination issues and any associated anxiety that this brings. Allow time to discuss such issues, as well as time to develop a blueprint of therapy. You may choose to have an individual blueprint, or a group blueprint that covers similar questions to an individual blueprint. It is also useful to give individuals a resource file that includes everything that has been covered during the group, as people often misplace information that they have been given during the course of the sessions. If you have scheduled a group follow-up, then arrange this. Alternatively, if group members are to have individual follow-up, then discuss and arrange this too. Depending on the setting in which you work, you may discharge patients straight back to the referrer without follow-up. If you do offer individual follow-up, remember to allocate time for this. You could do this over the telephone, or in the form of brief face-to-face appointments. Questions that you will need to consider carefully include: what is the purpose of the follow-up, how will you decide whether a group member should be offered further one-to-one CBT, and are they likely to benefit from this?

Key points

If you are thinking about setting up a CBT group you will need to:

- Provide a clinical justification for running your group.
- Demonstrate how running the group fits with your Service needs.
- Determine if you have the resources available to run the group, as well as the time and skills that are required.
- Decide on the type and size of group that you plan to run, and how you will evaluate clinical outcome.
- Develop inclusion criteria, and screen potential patients.
- Provide an information leaflet for referrers and patients.
- Manage the group process while imparting CBT skills.
- Ensure your clinical supervision arrangements include your group work.
- End the group while allowing space to discuss termination issues as well as blueprinting.

Further reading

Bieling, P., McCabe, R. and ad Antony, M. (2006). *Cognitive Behavioural Therapy in Groups*. New York, NY: Guildford Press.

Morrison, N. (2001). Group cognitive therapy: treatment choice or sub-optimal option? *Behavioural and Cognitive Psychotherapy*, **29**, 311–332.

Safran, J.D. and Segal, Z.V. (1990). *Interpersonal Process in Cognitive Therapy*. New York, NY: Basic Books.

Tucker, M. and Oei, T. (2007). Is group more cost effective than individual CBT? The evidence is not solid yet. *Behavioural and Cognitive Psychotherapy*, **35**, 77–91.

Yalom, I. (1995). *The Theory and Practice of Group Psychotherapy*. New York, NY: Basic Books.

References

Bechdolf, A., Knost, B., Kuntermann, C., Schiller, S., Klosterkotter, J., Hambrecht, M. and Pukrop, R. (2004). A randomized comparison of group cognitive-behavioural therapy and group psychoeducation in patients with schizophrenia. *Acta Psychiatrica Scandinavica*, **110**, 21–28.

Burlingame, G., MacKenzie, K. and Strauss, B. (2004). Small group treatment: evidence for effectiveness and mechanisms of change, in Lambert, M., Bergin, A. and Garfield, S. (eds.), *Bergin and Garfield's Handbook of Psychotherapy and Behaviour Change*. New York, NY: Wiley.

Kennerley, H., Whitehead, L., Butler, G. and Norris, R. (1998). *Recovering from Childhood Sexual Abuse: Therapy Workbook*. Oxuniprint for OCTC.

Patelis-Siotis, I., Young, L., Robb, J., Marriott, M., Bieling, P., Cox, L. and Joffe, R. (2001). Group cognitive behavioral therapy for bipolar disorder: a feasibility and effectiveness study. *Journal of Affective Disorders*, **65**, 145–153.

Scott, M.J. and Stradling, S. (1990). Group cognitive therapy for depression produces clinically significant change in community-based settings. *Behavioural Psychotherapy*, **18**, 1–19.

Tuckman, B. (1965). Developmental sequences in small groups. *Psychological Bulletin*, **63**, 384–399.

Whitaker, D. and Lieberman, M. (1964). *Psychotherapy Through the Group Process*. New York, NY: Atherton Press.

White, J. (1995). Stresspac: a controlled trial of a self-help package for anxiety. *Behavioural and Cognitive Psychotherapy*, **23**, 89–108.

Appendix 8.1–Example patient leaflet for a psychoeducational group

Managing depression course

This leaflet will answer some of your questions about the course.

What is depression?

We all have times when we feel low in mood, however for most people this usually only lasts for a day or two. However, for some, low mood can become more severe and difficult to shake off. When low mood persists in this way, it is referred to as 'clinical depression'. Depression is common, it is estimated that as many as 1 in 6 people will experience clinical depression at some point in their lives. Below are some of the common signs and symptoms you may experience if you are depressed:

- **Emotions or feelings**
  - Feeling sad, numb, guilty, upset, despairing, or angry
  - Crying a lot, or feeling unable to cry
  - Anxiety and fear
  - Loss of interest and enjoyment
  - Feeling alone, isolated, and withdrawn
- **Physical or bodily signs**
  - Tiredness or exhaustion
  - Restlessness
  - Changes in sleep—waking early or interrupted sleep
  - Changes in appetite, eating, and weight
  - Poor memory and concentration
  - Worsening of chronic conditions
- **Thoughts**
  - Having upsetting and gloomy thoughts, generally expecting the worst
  - Thinking that everything is hopeless
  - Thinking that you hate yourself

  - Losing confidence in your ability
  - Difficulty in making decisions
  - Thoughts of death and suicide
- **Changes in behaviour**
  - Finding it difficult to be with people
  - Reduced activities
  - Self neglect

Treatment, be it medication and/or psychological treatment, can help to speed recovery from depression and reduce the chances of becoming depressed again.

What is the managing depression course?

It is an 8-week course (plus a follow-up session) for people interested in learning skills and techniques to help manage their depression. The course is for people who wish to understand what happens when we feel depressed and ways to feel better by approaching problems one step at a time. These skills and techniques are based on a psychological treatment called cognitive behavioural therapy (CBT). The main topics will be:

- Becoming more active and finding satisfying activities
- Distracting oneself from unhelpful thoughts
- Questioning unhelpful thoughts
- Solving day-to-day problems

The main aim of the course is to help you become your own therapist so that you will feel more confident at the end of the course to manage depression.

What will be expected of me on the course?

The course will be in the style of an evening class rather than a therapy group. This means that we will not be sitting in a circle talking about our problems. There is no expectation that you will disclose personal information about yourself, in fact self-disclosure will be discouraged. If personal information is disclosed then all participants on the course will be expected to keep this information **confidential**. During the first session group leaders will talk about depression in detail. Later on in the course you will be taught techniques and expected to practice them outside of the course.

There is a self-help booklet to accompany the course, called *Managing Depression* written by David Westbrook. It is recommended that you read this booklet in preparation for the course. If you do not have a copy of this you can request one from the group leaders: it is free of charge.

Who will attend?

The course is for adults who are interested in learning more about managing depression. We anticipate that there will be between 20–25 men and women attending.

Who will lead the course?

The group will be run by Ali Smith (CBT therapist and social worker) and Robert Jones (CBT therapist and community psychiatric nurse). Both are employed by County NHS Trust and can be contacted on the following number:

0111 222333

Where will it be held?

The course will be held at Town Centre Building, on the first floor. There is parking available and the number 3 and 4 buses stop outside the Town Centre Building.

When will it start?

The course will run for 8 consecutive weeks on Wednesdays from 6.00 pm to 8.00 pm. It will begin on 1st of July (refreshments will be available at all classes).

What to do next?

If you think this course will be helpful, then ask your GP or care worker to refer you to the course (if you have not been referred already). You will be then sent a letter outlining how you can contact a course leader prior to the course if needed to answer any queries. We will also ask you to complete some questionnaires before and after the group to monitor your progress.

Chapter 9

Systemic aspects of CBT

Claudia Koch, Anne Stewart, and Ailsa Stuart

Why think about systems?

You have been meeting with your patient for several sessions of CBT. However, progress is limited. Your patient tells you that his family is unsupportive, a neighbour has been unpleasant to him and he has been upset by media reports highlighting the dangerousness of people with mental health problems; he has also found it hard to cope with a recent change of therapist. You feel stuck and wonder what you might do to move forward.

Cognitive behavioural approaches have always considered the 'wider system' and its role in development and maintenance of problems (Beck *et al.*, 1979). However, cognitive behavioural therapy (CBT) has developed *primarily* as an individual therapy, focusing on the internal states and behaviour of the patient. When working individually you might feel stuck due to the impact of wider systemic factors, such as the patient's family, the community, the political context, or your own working environment. Indeed, individually based therapies have been criticized on a number of accounts, for example, the failure to resolve relational problems (Emanuels-Zuurven and Emmelkamp, 1996) and the finding that inpatients, treated individually, tend to relapse when returning to certain home environments (Kuipers, 2006). Emmelkamp and Foa (1983) argue that one reason for treatment failure in CBT is the incomplete assessment of social factors. Addressing the wider systems may be useful, if not inevitable, when you work therapeutically. A distinction can be made between systemic psychotherapy, carried out by qualified family therapists, and systemic practice, that is, the use of systemic ideas and approaches in the wider sense, including the system external to the family as well as the family itself (Vetere and Dallos, 2003). This chapter will focus on systemic practice.

Background

Theoretical perspectives

Many forms of therapy can be viewed as integrative in that they continuously evolve and assimilate new ideas. Over the past 60 years, both behavioural and family approaches have undergone considerable development; more recently there has been an increased interest in the integration across what have traditionally been viewed as 'pure-form therapies' (Norcross, 2005).

Drawing specifically on CBT and systemic ideas, Bandura and Goldman (1995) argue that the two approaches are based on different theoretical assumptions which they do not attempt to combine. However, they focus on common factors, such as belief systems and problem-solving patterns and propose that systemic ideas can help a CBT therapist and their adult patients (usually seen individually) understand and overcome difficulties when attempting to change. Examples include looking at the social costs associated with change or the influences of intergenerational patterns on cognitive schemas.

Noting that depression and family problems frequently co-occur, Uebelacker *et al.* (2008), on the other hand, propose an integrative formulation of intra- and interpersonal factors. This involves focusing on the reciprocal relationship between an individual's and the family's thoughts, feelings, and behaviour and a consideration of external stressors. Similarly, Burbach and Stanbridge (1998) describe an integrated family intervention model drawing on CBT and systemic ideas within a psychosis service. This includes psychoeducation, and homework tasks, as well as focusing on the wider context, using systemic interventions.

Regarding children and adolescents, Dummett (2006) describes the use of systemic CBT formulations. This enables greater understanding of the family and environmental context, leading to interventions that take these influences into account. Furthermore, Dattilio (2005) has described a style of family therapy known as cognitive behavioural family therapy (CBFT) which incorporates cognitive behavioural techniques within systemic family therapy. In CBFT, family schemas are identified and restructured in order to resolve family relationship difficulties.

A helpful model addressing both individual experience and the environment is the Life Cycle Model (Carter and McGoldrick, 2005) which locates the individual within various system levels, ranging from the immediate and extended family to the community and larger society. It acknowledges the impact of the wider context, including work, religion, politics, and economics, for example. The model highlights potential stressors, such as family patterns and beliefs, community changes, and societal prejudices on the one hand, and developmental, unpredictable, and historical events on the other.

For the purpose of this chapter we will focus on how ideas and practices from systemic therapies, including the Life Cycle Model, can be incorporated into CBT approaches.

Evidence base

Family interventions are now established as an effective approach for a number of disorders in adults, adolescents, and children (Carr, 2009). This is reflected in the NICE guidelines, that is, the National Institute for Health and Clinical Excellence, an independent organization providing national guidance on the promotion of good health. The guidelines specifically recommend making family interventions available for people with eating disorders (NICE, 2004a), depression (NICE, 2004b), post-traumatic stress disorder (PTSD; NICE, 2005), bi-polar disorder (NICE, 2006a), obsessive compulsive disorder (OCD; NICE, 2006b), schizophrenia (NICE, 2009a), attention deficit hyperactivity disorder (ADHD; NICE, 2009b), borderline personality disorder (BPD; NICE, 2009c), and antisocial personality disorder (NICE, 2009d). Moreover, the National Service Framework (NSF) for adults of working age and for children and adolescents recommends involving carers in treatment (Department of Health, 1999 and 2004).

Family interventions have had successful outcomes when carried out in conjunction with multi-systemic approaches, that is, including individual input as well as the wider system, such as schools and peer groups (Carr, 2009). With regard to cognitive behavioural approaches, Barrett *et al.* (2001) found that adding a family component to individual CBT can increase efficacy, although it is still not clear which families benefit most from this approach. A number of studies have looked at predictors of outcome in CBT with young people. These include treatment alliance (Chu *et al.*, 2004), negative thought change (Kaufman *et al.*, 2005), and skill acquisition and exposure (Kendall, 1994), all of which can potentially be influenced by family involvement. In addition, Cartwright-Hatton *et al.* (2005) found that working with parental beliefs can enhance parenting.

Regarding adults of working age, the effectiveness of family approaches is not conclusive, as the literature tends to confuse Family Management, based on CBT approaches, and Family Therapy, based on systemic ideas, as well as distinctions within these. Furthermore, most research is mainly based on diagnostic categories and individualistic medical models rather than qualitative models and those including family functioning in their outcome criteria. Bearing these limitations in mind, well-articulated family-based interventions have been shown to be effective for a range of problems. The majority of evidence is based on CBT or psychoeducational frameworks (Carr, 2009), but some research indicates that Family Management and Family Therapy approaches appear to be equally effective (Baucom *et al.*, 1998).

Current position and future developments

CBT has increasingly been applied to a wider range of populations yet little has been published on how systemic and CBT models might be integrated, and most of this is focused on children and adolescents. How to include systems within CBT, and the evaluation of such models remain important issues for future research.

Practical considerations

When and how to use systemic ideas

Clearly, it is good practice for you to take into account systemic factors when working with an individual and to meet with significant others as appropriate. However, you may find that there are times when it is helpful to incorporate *a systemic perspective* more specifically within CBT. You can achieve this in several ways:

- At referral and assessment take a systemic perspective (who the referral is from, who it is addressed to; what the expectations are for all professionals involved and the patient; and what are the living and working circumstances of the patient).
- Offer psychoeducation to the wider system (carers/family/co-workers/teachers, etc.).
- Use the family/partner to support the CBT: family/partner-assisted CBT (the family/partner/others provide support to the CBT).
- Actively incorporate the family/partner within CBT:
  - Family/couple CBT (the family/partner is incorporated within the CBT)
  - Working cognitively with parents of young children
  - Cognitive behavioural family therapy
- Work with the wider system, for example, school or the workplace.
- Work with the individual using a systemic focus (this may include systemic formulations and interventions).
- Carry out parallel family therapy with significant others.

Throughout this chapter, the following two case histories will be used to illustrate the above ways of working:

Malcolm, a 31 year old white British stockbroker, was referred by his GP for depression. As a teenager he suffered a road traffic accident resulting in chronic back pain necessitating the use of a wheel chair. He was frequently off work due to back pain and/or depression. His Pakistani wife wanted children, but he was reluctant, feeling he would be a bad father. He had received bereavement

counselling following the death of his grandfather the previous year. However, he felt that nothing had changed.
Anna, aged 15, was referred for treatment of health anxiety which had made it difficult for her to leave the home. In particular, she was worried about developing cancer, which had recently caused the death of two children living nearby. She had received individual CBT sessions with some response. However, in developing her formulation, it became evident that her parents were reinforcing some of her maladaptive behaviour, such as checking her body for signs of cancer.

Referral and assessment

Prior to the assessment, consider where the referral has come from, who it is to and what the expectations are. This will enable you to begin to take into account the wider context impacting on the problem. Your subsequent comprehensive CBT assessment should include enquiry regarding the family and wider system, both for child and adult patients. This can help you clarify the origin of key beliefs and the difficulties the patient may be experiencing in making changes. You can also explore the potential role of others in the system, such as partners, friends, or work colleagues in helping the patient. Considering the contextual and systemic aspects to the problem can be empowering for individuals who may blame themselves for their problems. With young people the family will usually be present; having significant others present with adults can also be helpful, although not always possible, for instance due to distance or personal preference of the patient.

A useful tool in assessing family factors is the genogram or a pictorial representation of key relationships (McGoldrick *et al.*, 2008). This can help you clarify relationships and family patterns and highlight where these are contributing to the patient's difficulties. Use of a genogram also ensures the wider family context is explored by asking about extended family, social networks, and cultural background as well as drawing out more detailed information about the patient's family of origin. This technique will highlight the systemic influences and the extent to which the wider system may need to be involved. The written genogram provides a useful record which can be referred to throughout therapy. Genograms for Malcom and Anna are shown in Figs. 9.1 and 9.2, respectively.

An important function of the assessment is to identify with the patient to what extent systemic factors could be incorporated within the treatment. For example, you might ask about family relationships, school/work environment, or cultural/racial issues. This may be a challenge for CBT therapists who have not been formally trained in family-based approaches. Some basic reading and/or basic training courses in family-based approaches may be useful in augmenting your knowledge (Dallos and Draper, 2000).

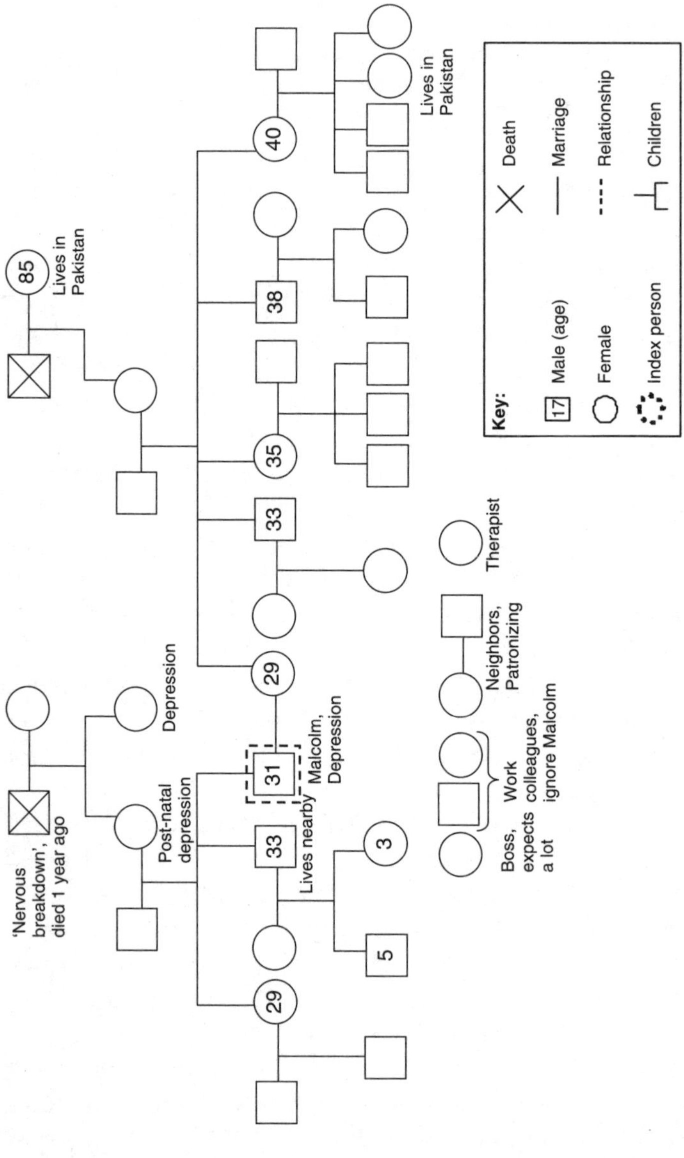

Fig. 9.1 Malcolm's genogram.

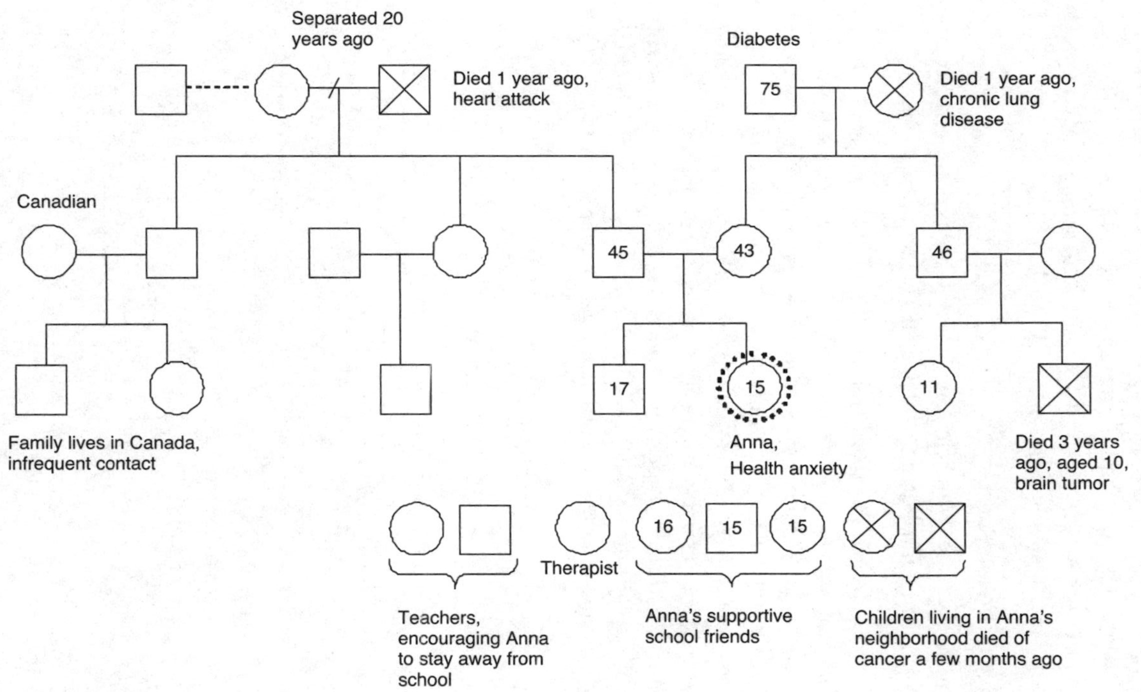

Fig. 9.2 Anna's genogram.

Formulation

During the initial assessment you may find it helpful to draw up a rudimentary formulation which indicates the key factors that are helping to maintain the problem. As therapy progresses you can produce a more comprehensive formulation, incorporating systemic factors as discussed later.

Figure 9.3 illustrates how the basic CBT formulation can incorporate wider systemic factors (indicated in bold).

Family patterns, beliefs, behaviour

A comprehensive assessment can help you identify patterns or belief systems in the family which have contributed to the patient's beliefs or behaviour.

Malcolm's grandfather, aunt and mother all suffered from mental health problems. This contributed to the family's belief that mental illness was immutable and genetic. In addition, over generations the men in the family tended to work, often in manual jobs, whilst the women took on the role looking after the household and children. This led to a belief in the family that men should be strong and fit and it is the role of males to provide financially.

Anna's parents had strong beliefs about the world being unsafe, leading to a need to overprotect their children. This arose from their own background; her father had experienced his parents marriage breaking up and had always

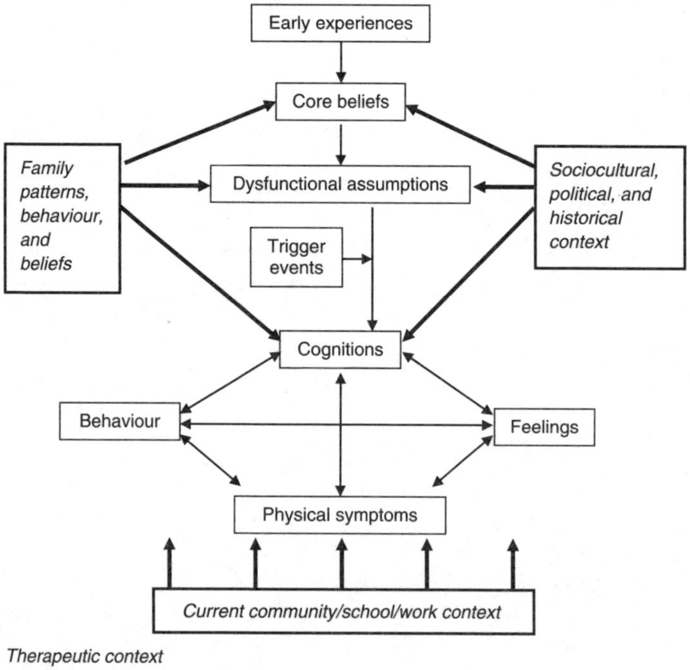

Fig. 9.3 Systemic CBT formulation.

felt unsupported and anxious as a child; her mother had experienced long term physical illness in her own mother and grew up believing that there is a strong vulnerability to illness in their family. Parental anxieties were reinforced by the family history of their favourite nephew dying of a brain tumour.

Sociocultural, political, and historical context

It can be important for you to identify sociocultural, political, and historical factors impacting on the patient.

Malcolm's family beliefs regarding mental and physical health were reinforced by attitudes in his work place, reflecting wider Western cultural beliefs that having mental and physical health problems is a sign of weakness. Malcolm reported that disabled toilets were difficult to access in some department stores. He also talked about feeling stigmatised about his lack of children following media reports that there are not enough young people to support the ageing population.

Current community/school/work context

The current context may also exert a strong influence. For example, the behaviour of peers, school teachers, employers, or other significant people in your patients' lives may impact on their cognitions and emotions.

Malcolm felt shunned or patronised by some of his neighbours and work colleagues when he used his wheelchair. His boss expected him to work long hours and maintain a high standard.

Anna was getting behind with school work which made it more difficult for her to go back to school. Some of her teachers, in wanting to support Anna, recommended that she take time off. Her school friends were anxious about her. However, they continued to keep some contact which was a positive influence in helping her progress.

Drawing up a formulation incorporating these different contexts and influences can be helpful for you in understanding the problems and deciding on the focus of treatment. Contextual influences may be hard to change in the short-term. However, your patient's perspective on them can be challenged and shaped in a helpful way which in turn can impact on the context.

Although a comprehensive standard formulation has been described above, not all these areas may be relevant. You may consider a briefer formulation, which makes sense to the patient, incorporates factors that impact on the problem, and provides a basis for intervention.

Malcolm: An initial formulation was discussed with Malcolm which was later expanded, highlighting how his early experiences, as well as wider contextual factors had contributed towards the development and maintenance of his depression. This enabled Malcolm to acknowledge that he did not experience

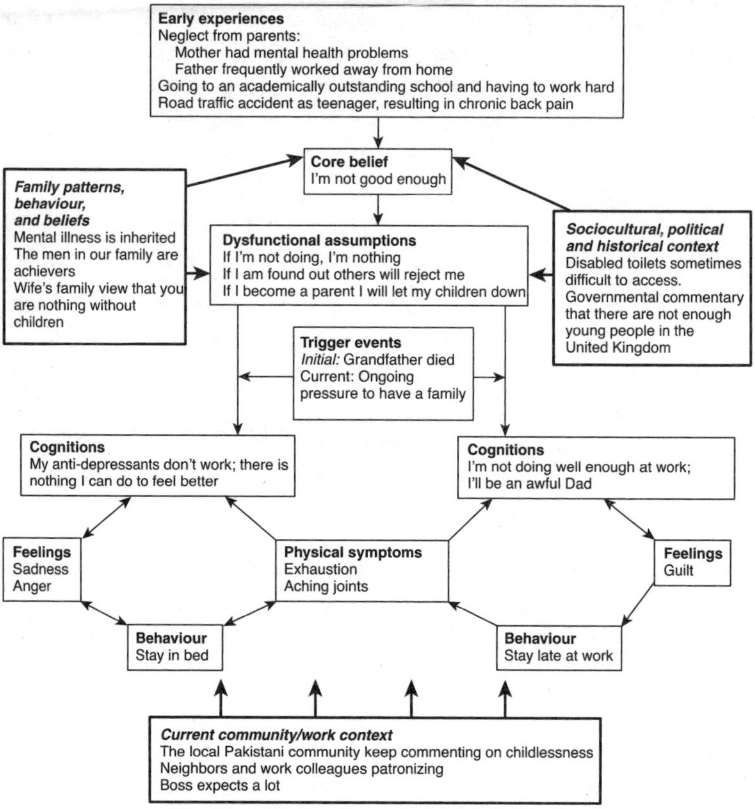

Therapeutic context: *Referred for CBT—problem located within the individual reinforcing negative beliefs about depression. Therapist is a different gender and same race.*

Fig. 9.4 Malcolm's formulation.

difficulties because he was inherently flawed, but because various external factors were impacting on his life, thus relieving some of his guilt and anger. (See Fig. 9.4)

Anna: An initial formulation drawn up individually was presented within a family session and expanded. Discussing the formulation together clarified the impact of her parents' anxiety on the maintenance of her problems. In particular, they were able to see how their anxiety about Anna's illness and frequent reassurance helped to maintain the problem. (See Fig. 9.5)

Developing positive reformulations from a systemic perspective

Having developed the formulation, it may become apparent to you how the family/wider systems can be incorporated in the intervention. As treatment proceeds you may consider redrawing the systemic formulation adding in positive elements which may indicate how changes in the wider system can influence the problem positively. Positive reformulations are particularly

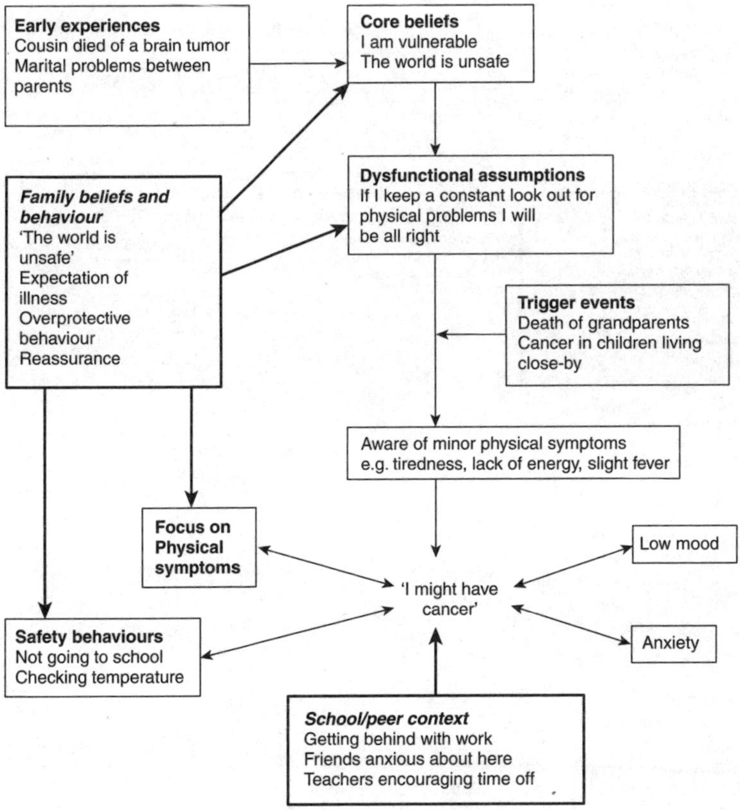

Therapeutic context. *Initially seen in psychiatric clinic. Therapist is same gender and race as Anna.*

Fig. 9.5 Anna's formulation.

pertinent to systemic CBT as they reinforce the notion that the family and wider system can be an active ingredient of change.

If it is inappropriate to involve relevant others directly, you may still find it useful to create a systemic reformulation with the individuals to enable them to see how their family can be a resource to them.

Anna: In redrawing the formulation, the family were able to see how the changes they were making were contributing positively to the changes in Anna. (See Fig. 9.6)

Interventions

Psychoeducation with family/partner/others

When a person attends for CBT there are often other family members who are concerned or perplexed about their relative's problems. Meeting with the family or significant others can provide you with a helpful opportunity for education regarding the nature of the problems.

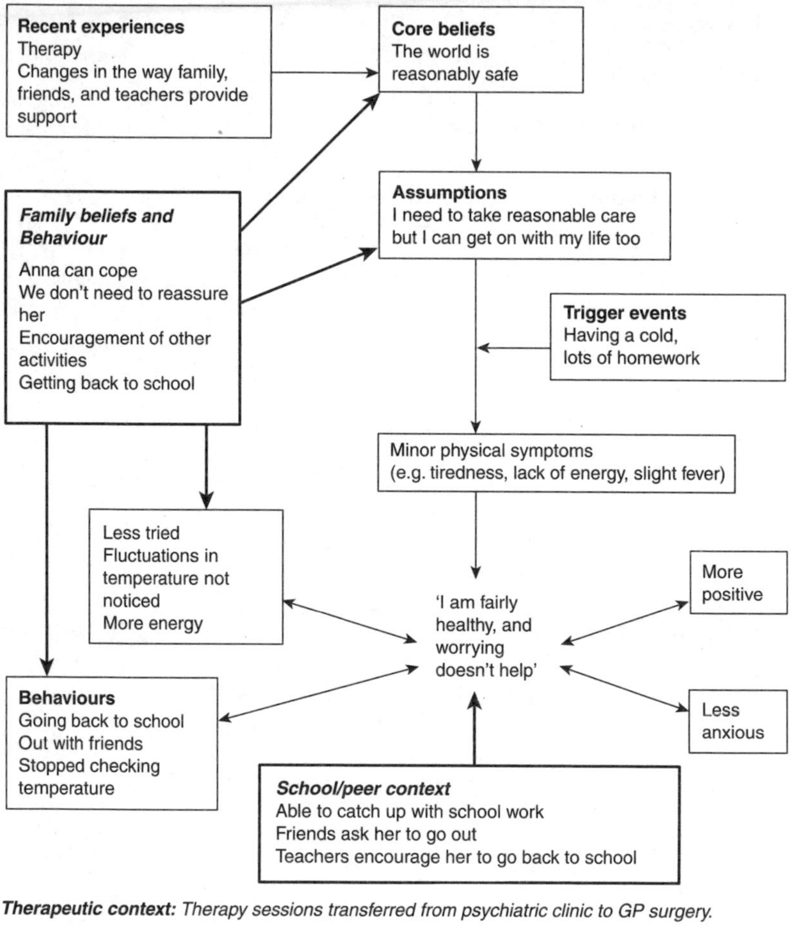

Fig. 9.6 Anna's re-formulation.

With children and adolescents, family meetings are generally routine alongside individual CBT. With an adult, it is also important to make this opportunity available, as there is now considerable evidence suggesting a psychoeducational approach with the family can be useful, for example, in psychosis (Burbach and Stanbridge, 1998). Increased understanding of the patient's problems can assist the family and others in the social network in being supportive and sensitive, promoting more helpful responses.

Anna: As the whole family was affected by Anna's difficulties there were meetings with the family early on in therapy to provide information on Anna's problems and the treatment recommended. This included a discussion of the nature of health anxiety and what keeps it going. This helped the family begin to appreciate their role and what they might do to help.

Family/partner-assisted CBT

More active involvement with the family may involve using the family or significant others to support the treatment, for example, assisting with behavioural experiments (Baucom et al., 1998). This is particularly helpful where there is a supportive parent or partner. Enlisting the help of other family members can make a difference to the outcome of the therapy (Scaturo, 1994).

Malcolm: Although Malcolm refused, initially, to have others directly involved in the therapy, he and his therapist discussed how other people could help him increase his activity levels. Following a discussion outside the session, Malcolm and his brother agreed to go swimming together. This became a regular occurrence and not only helped Malcolm but also gave his brother a better insight into Malcolm's difficulties.

Family/couple CBT

In situations where problems have been directly triggered or are being maintained by events/people within the family/wider system, incorporating the family or significant others directly in your therapy sessions can be productive. This may involve addressing beliefs and behaviours that originate within the system as well as within the individual. These beliefs may be preventing others in the social network from providing helpful support. You may find it helpful to invite significant others to explore the formulation together, to discuss the impact of other people's beliefs, and to agree specific strategies which enable change.

Anna agreed with her therapist that it may be helpful to have some sessions with her parents. The aim of these sessions was to present and expand the formulation and use this as a basis for agreeing useful interventions involving the family. Although Anna's parents had been initially asked to assist in getting Anna back to school they found this difficult because of their own anxieties. When they were invited to join a CBT session and to explore the formulation together with Anna, they were able to see that their own beliefs were impairing her ability to change. By understanding and readjusting their own beliefs they were able to alter their behaviour in a way which helped Anna to move forwards.

Malcolm: It became apparent that Malcolm had perceptions about his wife's beliefs that were affecting his view of himself. She was invited to join a couple of sessions and he reluctantly agreed to this. He discovered that his wife did not see his problems as insurmountable and she viewed their childlessness not as his fault but as something they needed to tackle together. Making explicit her beliefs helped him see himself differently and he became more positive about the future.

Working with parents of young children

Parents' beliefs about their children's behaviour can shape how they respond to them. Cognitive distortions, which may be partly based on a lack of knowledge of child development, can lead to unhelpful parental behaviour. Moreover, parental mental illness can influence the way parents view their children. For example, behaviour that may be viewed by someone else as highly spirited may be viewed as pathological by a mentally unwell parent, leading to a sense of self-blame and unhelpful responses (Nicholson et al., 1998). In working with parents, either within the adult mental health service or within child and adolescent services, it can be helpful to identify parental beliefs and challenge those which are unhelpful, as well as promote the development of more useful beliefs by providing appropriate information. This could include recommending self-help literature for parents (Cartwright-Hatton, 2007).

Working with other systems

It may become apparent in the assessment that other systems are involved in maintaining the problem or alternatively have the potential to assist the resolution of the problem. This may be school, work, the local community, prison, or hospital settings.

Anna: Two of Anna's schoolteachers believed that she would benefit from extended time off to recover from her anxieties and had suggested home tutoring for her. This view was not helpful for Anna so a meeting was held at school to encourage different perspectives and maximise appropriate support.
Malcolm: Malcolm instigated a meeting with his neighbours to discuss how their behaviour impacted on him. Once they gained more understanding about Malcolm's difficulties, they became more friendly, and started meeting up socially with Malcolm.

Individual CBT

If the family/wider systems do not appear to have a marked influence on the presenting problem, individually focused CBT without involvement of others may be indicated. It is however, still important for you to continue to take into account systemic influences, in order to promote a more helpful perspective and to increase the likelihood that progress is maintained. For some patients, systemic influences are crucial to working with the problems and significant others may need, ideally, to be directly involved. However, even if this is not possible, you can still incorporate a systemic perspective in your individual work.

Malcolm: In sessions Malcolm stated that "I feel rotten to the core". This was initially addressed individually because Malcolm was unwilling to invite others to the meetings. However, this belief was difficult to shift, and Malcolm kept highlighting the impact of his difficulties on his family and work colleagues. We agreed to spend two meetings focusing on systemic issues with him as an individual. A systemic formulation was developed with the help of a genogram, circular questions (see below), and a discussion of the different contexts that were relevant to him. Following this Malcolm was able to have discussions outside therapy with his siblings about their early childhood, and discovered that they had a different perspective, enabling him to develop an alternative view of himself. He also talked to his work colleagues and his boss about some of his concerns, which enabled them to understand and support him better; this positive response further helped to change Malcolm's belief about himself.

Parallel family therapy

Your initial assessment may reveal significant family relationship problems which could be addressed in systemic family therapy, thus necessitating a separate referral. Individual CBT may or may not be useful alongside this. Expectations from the referrer and the service can shape your decisions. If individual CBT continues alongside family therapy, you need to acknowledge the issues discussed in family therapy and incorporate them within the formulation.

Engaging the family/others and conducting meetings

The decision to involve the family or others in the wider system jointly with the identified patient needs to be made jointly. When working with more than one person in the room you may find it helpful, although not essential, to enlist the support of other professionals working with you. Within family therapy the use of reflecting teams (Anderson, 1995), that is, colleagues discussing the case when people are seen, either behind a screen or in the same room provides a way of enhancing the perspectives on the patient and their problems.

- *Socratic questioning* can be useful within wider family sessions. It can help you to identify family cognitions and clarify the impact of family behaviour on the patient's beliefs, emotional state, and behaviour.
- *Circular questioning.* Systemic family therapy describes the use of 'circular questions', which help people explore relationships including being aware of the impact of power, difference, and changes over time (Selvini *et al.*, 1980). This style of questioning has a similar function to Socratic questions in the way that it helps people think differently about the problems and the solution, but they are relationship focused. A circular questioning style applied to families or significant others can complement your individual use of Socratic questioning. For example, circular questions involving Malcolm and his wife might be 'When you stay late at work, how does your wife respond; when she responds in that way, how do you respond?', or 'If you were to stop thinking that you would be an awful dad, what opportunities would that create for your relationship with your wife?'
- *Externalizing the problem.* Another technique, originating in family therapy, which you may find useful in CBT is that of externalizing the problem (White, 1989). The patients and their family are encouraged to view their 'problem' as an entity or object outside of the person. This can enhance

confidence in tackling problems by helping them to gain a more objective or detached perspective.

Malcolm: We initially focused on Malcolm's beliefs about depression, particularly the family story that mental illness is inherited and unchangeable. In meeting with Malcolm and his wife together it was possible to explore those beliefs and help them view the depression as an unwelcome visitor rather than a personality trait. This enabled them to be more optimistic about change.

Confidentiality

An important issue to consider when working with the system is that of confidentiality. It is essential that you, the patient, and involved others, are aware of, and have agreed to, what information will be brought to the wider meeting and what might be discussed outside meetings and with whom. An exception to this is when there is risk of serious self-harm or harm to others, when you may need to break confidentiality.

Anna: In order to maximize the effectiveness of the family meetings, the aims needed to be agreed by all and the parents were encouraged to see that joint meetings were not about blame but about working together to resolve the problems. It was important that Anna felt confident that information she shared in the session would only be disclosed in other settings with her permission. This was made explicit and her parents agreed to respect confidentiality. In turn, this liberated Anna who could be much more open in the sessions.

Therapeutic context

In understanding and making sense of the different influences on the patient it is important to pay attention to the therapeutic context (*cf* Chapter 1).

Personal context

Each patient is shaped by various factors, such as class, age, gender, culture, skin color, disability, and emotional state. Similarly, you come with your own individual contexts. Understanding the interaction of these contexts may be crucial for engagement and successful therapy. For example, a female victim of a rape by a man, may find it upsetting receiving therapy from a male therapist. Being sensitive to this issue may result either in changing the therapist or in continuing the therapy while acknowledging the difficulty and working with it. Involving patients in conversations about the impact of different contexts on their presenting problem can be hugely beneficial in promoting engagement. When considering systemic aspects of CBT the influence of the personal context is much more complex as you need to be sensitive to several persons' preferences and needs. Making these issues explicit and discussing them within therapy can promote engagement.

Institutional context

The resources available for CBT within a department can influence the number of sessions as well as their frequency and length. These constraints have to be worked with and indeed can be useful in increasing motivation to work more efficiently. However, there are situations in which the limitations on numbers of sessions can be detrimental; in this case you may need to approach people in the wider system, such as managers of the service, to make a case for extending the therapy. There are also attitudes within institutions which might need to be recognized and addressed. These might be attitudes which undermine your patient ('... self- injury is attention seeking, that's all.') or attitudes which reinforce your patient's concerns ('... it is unwise to focus on traumatic memories, the patient might get suicidal.')

Context of expectations

The expectations of the patient, yourself as the therapist, the referrer, and wider team can impact on therapy. For example, the referrer may have 'prescribed' CBT in order to fix a problem located within an individual. This may cause the patient to feel that their experiences of negative life events have been ignored and that they are to blame for their difficulties. In order to help the patient make use of the CBT strategies and build their self-esteem your acknowledgement of the wider context of the patient may be crucial. Understanding the referrer's expectations will also benefit the professional relationships that provide the context for therapy. Not infrequently, a patient comes to therapy expecting to be 'fixed' and is disappointed that change requires hard work between sessions. This expectation will need to be resolved before therapy can proceed. Therapist demands can also impact on the treatment, for example, as a trainee therapist you might be expected to write up a number of case studies. This may shape the length and content of therapy and will need to be addressed so that patient care is not compromised.

Malcolm was surprised that the therapist suggested inviting others into sessions, as he expected to be seen individually, and believed that only he was to blame for his difficulties. Discussing wider systemic issues with him on his own, then with his wife and outside the session with his siblings, his work colleagues and boss, enabled him to develop an alternative understanding of his difficulties which enhanced his progress.

Environmental context

The place in which therapy occurs can impact on the patients' perception of therapy and the problem. For example, patients receiving CBT in a psychiatric hospital may come to therapy with a belief that their condition is serious, requiring long-term therapy, as opposed to someone attending anxiety management classes in a college classroom. It is therefore important that you ask your patient what their views are about the setting they are seen in.

Anna was initially seen in a Child & Adolescent Mental Health Service. However, she opted to continue sessions at her GP surgery because it was more accessible and less stigmatising for her. The therapist had the flexibility to do this; if this is not possible the effect of being seen in the clinic may need to be discussed.

Outcome of the cases

Malcolm enlisted the help of others. He wrote a complaint to one shop about their disabled toilets, and wrote to his MP regarding views about people with mental health problems. Including Malcolm's wife in sessions helped clarify the couple's beliefs about his difficulties and their relationship. Malcolm was surprised to discover that his wife did not see this problem as unfixable, and that she viewed their childlessness as a problem they needed to tackle together. Instead of siding with her family and community, she wished they would back off. Malcolm came to believe that he had the power to deal with his low mood. At his six month follow-up appointment Malcolm no longer saw himself as a "depressive" or a potentially awful father, which was timely as his wife was pregnant. By including systemic aspects in therapy he had recognized the influence that his family and society had had upon his beliefs and both he and his wife shared with the therapist how they had begun to create new family beliefs.
Anna: The involvement of Anna's family meant that her parents were able to see the impact their behaviour had on her and consider other ways of approaching her health concerns. They developed different beliefs about the nature of health anxiety and Anna's ability to cope with it. As a family they worked with the therapist to react differently, in particular not providing Anna with reassurance, and encouraging her to engage in other activities rather than focus on her physical symptoms. Although this initially caused stress, they kept going and Anna's anxieties began to diminish. Individual CBT continued and was also crucial in helping Anna to deal with her anxieties and modify her unhelpful behaviours. Linking in with her school facilitated a school return. Anna gradually became less anxious and started going out again.

Conclusion

CBT can be enhanced by taking into account the wider contexts of both you and your patients and drawing on systemic ideas at every stage of therapy. This can be done in various way including reflecting on systemic influences from the point of referral onwards, drawing up a systemic formulation with your patient, considering the impact of the wider context, or actively involving significant others in sessions. This in turn will enable your patients to acknowledge systemic factors impacting on their lives, and either draw on these as sources of support or develop a more helpful perspective on them.

Key points

1. Evidence suggests that involvement of families is important in the development and maintenance of many mental health problems and that it can also lead to improved outcome.
2. Partners and the wider systems can also have an impact on development and maintenance of the problem and the potential for recovery.
3. A careful assessment of the role of the family/systemic factors can be helpful in determining their impact and how this can be managed or maximized.
4. A systemic formulation done collaboratively with the patient can clarify the relevant issues and highlight the need for specific work which takes these factors into account.
5. There are a range of ways in which the family and wider system can be involved including psychoeducation with carers, family-assisted CBT, family/couple CBT, working systemically with the individual, and working with the wider system.
6. Identifying and modifying the cognitions and behaviour of relevant others involved in the patient's life, as well as changing structures in unhelpful environments/systems can facilitate progress.

Further reading

Carter, B. and McGoldrick, M. (2005). *The Expanded Family Life Cycle Individual, Family and Social Perspectives.* Third edition. Boston: Allyn and Bacon.

Cartwright-Hatton, S. (2007). *Coping With an Anxious or Depressed Child.* Oxford: Oneworld.

Dallos, R. and Draper, R. (2000). *An Introduction to Family Therapy*. Buckingham: Open University Press.

Dattilio, F.M. (2001). Cognitive behaviour family therapy: contemporary myths and misconceptions. *Contemporary Family Therapy*, **23**, 3–18.

Dummett, N. (2006). Processes for systemic cognitive-behavioural therapy with children, young people and families. *Behavioural and Cognitive Psychotherapy*, 34, 179–189.

Fact sheets for families and carers. Available at: http://www.mind.org.uk/information/factsheets/carers (accessed 1 September 2009), http://www.rethink.org/living_with_mental_illness/caring/index.html (accessed 1 September 2009).

NICE Guidelines. Available at: http://www.nice.org.uk (accessed 1 September 2009).

References

Anderson, T. (1995). Reflecting Processes; Acts of Informing and Forming, in Friedman, S. (ed.), *The Reflecting Team in Action*. New York, NY: Guildford Press, pp. 10–37.

Bandura, M. and Goldman, C. (1995). Expanding the contextual analysis of clinical problems. *Cognitive and Behavioural Practice*, **2**, 119–141.

Barrett, P.M., Duffy, A.L., Dadds, M.R. and Rapee, R. (2001). Cognitive-behavioural treatment of anxiety disorders in children. Long term (6-year) follow-up. Journal of *Consulting and Clinical Psychology*, **69**, 135–141.

Baucom, D., Shoham,V., Mueser, K., Daiuto, A. and Stickly, T. (1998). Empirically supported couple and family interventions for marital distress and adult mental health problems. *Journal of Consulting and Clinical Psychology*, **66**, 53–88.

Beck, A.T., Rush, A.J., Shaw, B.F. and Emery, G. (1979). *Cognitive Therapy of Depression.* New York, NY: Guilford Press.

Burbach, F. and Stanbridge, R. (1998). A family intervention in psychosis service integrating the systemic and family management approaches. *Journal of Family Therapy*, **20**, 311–325.

Carr, A. (2009). The effectiveness of family therapy and systemic interventions for child-focused problems. *Journal of Family Therapy*, **31**, 3–45.

Cartwright-Hatton, S. (2007). *Coping With an Anxious or Depressed Child.* Oxford: Oneworld.

Cartwright-Hatton, S., McNally, D. and White, C. (2005). A new cognitive-behavioural parenting intervention for families of young anxious children: a pilot study. *Behavioural and Cognitive Psychotherapy*, **33**, 243–247.

Chu, B.C., Choudhury, M.S., Pincus, D.B., Creed, T.A. and Kendall, P.C. (2004). Alliance, technology and outcome in the treatment of anxious youth. *Cognitive and Behavioural Practice*, **11**, 44–45.

Dattilio, F. (2005). The restructuring of family schemas: a cognitive-behavioural perspective. *Journal of Marital and Family Therapy*, **31**, 15-31.

Department of Health (1999). *National Service Framework for Mental Health: Modern Standards and Service Models.* Available at: http://www.dh.gov.uk/prod_consum_dh/groups/dh_digitalassets/@dh/@en/documents/digitalasset/dh_4077209.pdf (accessed 1 September 2009).

Department of Health; Department for Education and Skills *(2004). Framework for Children, Young People and Maternity Services: Core Standards.* Available at: http://www.dh.gov.uk/prod_consum_dh/groups/dh_digitalassets/@dh/@en/documents/digitalasset/dh_4090523.pdf (accessed 1 September 2009).

Emanuels-Zuurven, L. and Emmelkamp, P. (1996). Individual behavioural-cognitive therapy v. marital therapy for depression in martially distressed couples. *British Journal of Psychiatry*, **169**, 181–188.

Emmelkamp, P. and Foa, E. (1983). Failures are a challenge, in Foa, E. and Emmelkamp, P. (eds.), *Failures in Behaviour Therapy*. New York, NY: Wiley.

Kaufman, N.K., Rohde, P., Seeley, J.R., Clarke, G.N. and Stice, E. (2005). Potential mediators of cognitive-behavioural therapy for adolescents with comorbid major depression and conduct disorder. *Journal of Consulting and Clinical Psychology*, **73**, 38–46.

Kendall, P.C. (1994).Treating anxiety disorders in children: results of a randomized clinical trial. *Journal of Consulting and Clinical Psychology*, **62**, 100–110.

Kuipers, E. (2006). Family interventions in schizophrenia: evidence for efficacy and proposed mechanisms of change. *Journal of Family Therapy*, **28**, 73–80.

McGoldrick, M., Gerson, R. and Petry, S. (2008). *Genograms. Assessment and Intervention.* Third edition. London: Norton & Co.

NICE (2004a). *Eating Disorders: Core Interventions in the Treatment and Management of Anorexia Nervosa, Bulimia Nervosa and Related Eating Disorders.* Available at: http://www.nice.org.uk/nicemedia/pdf/CG9FullGuideline.pdf (accessed 1 September 2009).

NICE (2004b). *Depression: Management of Depression in Primary and Secondary Care.* Available at: http://www.nice.org.uk/nicemedia/pdf/CG23fullguideline.pdf (accessed 1 September 2009).

NICE (2005). *Post-traumatic Stress Disorder: The Management of PTSD in Adults and Children in Primary and Secondary Care.* Available at: http://www.nice.org.uk/nicemedia/pdf/CG026fullguideline.pdf (accessed 1 September 2009).

NICE (2006a). *Bipolar Disorder: The Management of Bipolar Disorder in Adults, Children and Adolescents, in Primary and Secondary Care.* Available at: http://www.nice.org.uk/nicemedia/pdf/CG38fullguideline.pdf (accessed 1 September 2009).

NICE (2006b). *Obsessive Compulsive Disorder: Core Interventions in the Treatment of Obsessive Compulsive Disorder and Body Dysmorphic Disorder.* Available at: http://www.nice.org.uk/nicemedia/pdf/cg031fullguideline.pdf (accessed 1 September 2009).

NICE (2009a). *Schizophrenia: Core Interventions in the Treatment and Management of Schizophrenia in Primary and Secondary Care (update).* Available at: http://www.nice.org.uk/nicemedia/pdf/CG82FullGuideline.pdf (accessed 1 September 2009).

NICE (2009b). *Attention Deficit Hyperactivity Disorder: Diagnosis and Management of ADHD in Children, Young People and Adults.* Available at: http://www.nice.org.uk/nicemedia/pdf/ADHDFullGuideline.pdf (accessed 1 September 2009).

NICE (2009c). *Borderline Personality Disorder (BPD): Treatment and Management.* Available at: http://www.nice.org.uk/nicemedia/pdf/CG78FullGuideline.pdf (accessed 1 September 2009).

NICE (2009d). *Antisocial Personality Disorder: Treatment, Management and Prevention.* Available at: http://www.nice.org.uk/nicemedia/pdf/CG077FullGuideline.pdf (accessed 1 September 2009).

Nicholson, J., Sweeney, E.M. and Geller, J.L. (1998). Focus on women: mothers with mental illness: 1. The competing demands of parenting and living with mental illness. *Psychiatric Services*, **49**, 635–642.

Norcross, J. (2005). A primer on psychotherapy integration, in Norcross, J. and Goldfried, M. (eds.), *Handbook of Psychotherapy Integration.* Second edition. Oxford: Oxford University Press.

Scaturo, D. (1994). Integrative psychotherapy for panic disorder and agoraphobia in clinical practice. *Journal of Psychotherapy Integration*, **4**, 253–272.

Selvini, M., Boscolo, L., Cecchin, M. and Prata, G. (1980). Hypothesizing-circularity-neutrality. *Family Process*, **19**, 3–12.

Uebelacker, L., Weishaar, M. and Miller, I. (2008). Family or relationship problems, in Whisman, M. (ed.), *Adapting Cognitive Therapy for Depression. Managing Complexity and Comorbidity*. London: Guilford Press.

Vetere, A. and Dallos, R. (2003). *Working Systemically with Families: Formulation, Intervention and Evaluation.* London: H. Karnac (Books) Ltd.

White, M. (1989). Pseudo-encopresis: from avalanche to victory, from vicious to virtuous cycles, in White, M. (ed.), *Selected Papers.* Adelaide, Australia: Dulwich Centre Publications, pp. 115–124.

Chapter 10

Doing CBT through others

Harriet Montgomery, Alison J. Croft, and Ann Hackmann

Introduction

Growing awareness of the evidence base for the effectiveness of cognitive behavioural therapy (CBT) inevitably leads to increased demand on CBT services, which can be difficult for therapists to meet. The publication of NICE (National Institute for Clinical Excellence) guidelines makes it increasingly important that health professionals other than CBT therapists are aware of CBT and its indications, so that they can identify suitable referrals or perhaps implement the initial stages of stepped care models. Scarcity of trained CBT therapists, long waiting times, and high 'did not attend' (DNA) rates mean that there are often significant difficulties with delivering therapy within a one-to-one framework even in cases where cognitive therapy ideas, formulations, and methods might be extremely useful.

Doing CBT through others also implies dissemination of skills so that patients with emotional difficulties can benefit without necessarily having to wait to see a highly qualified therapist. This can mean that patients are treated by workers they already know, in settings with which they are already familiar. The treatment they receive may be more specific to their needs, and they may therefore be able to benefit from a more intensive or highly targeted intervention than they would receive by attending a more general psychological therapies service. Doing cognitive therapy through others is central to the concept of widening access to CBT for groups of people who might benefit from, but would not usually be able to gain access to, such treatment.

There is therefore an increasing number of reasons why it might be a good idea to disseminate CBT skills to staff who are not qualified CBT therapists, who may then be able to deliver CBT interventions while working under careful supervision.

Aims and limitations

It is essential to be realistic about what can be achieved when working through others. In this chapter, we are not talking about providing comprehensive CBT training (see Chapter 17 on CBT training for guidance), but rather training others in specific, often very circumscribed sets of skills or therapeutic interventions to equip them to work with specific problems or groups of patients, for example, providing 'cognitive first aid' (Mannix *et al.*, 2006, see Section Using practitioners' existing skills and experience). The aim is often to broaden access to CBT, but the level of skill you aim to disseminate may sometimes be quite modest (e.g. in Example 10.2, one of the aims was to educate medical students about CBT so that they could formulate problems using CBT principles and have sufficient knowledge to make appropriate referrals to existing services).

Clarity about your aims is likely to result in greater success in working through others. You will then be able to communicate clearly both to the staff you are training and to those who may refer to the new CBT resource, what they are expected to do, and what the limits of their competence are. You will also be more able to select suitable patients for the CBT intervention, according to what staff are and are *not* trained to do.

What are the benefits?

1 Access to treatment may be improved and waiting times reduced. There may be keen but untrained staff or volunteers available who, with a minimum of CBT training, can reduce the numbers of patients needing to be referred on to an oversubscribed specialist psychological service.

2 The stigma of contact with a mental health service may be reduced or avoided altogether.

3 With careful screening, interventions can be targeted to patients with specific psychological problems and therapy can be delivered by people with limited training specific to those problems. Potential referrers to a specialist service may have their triaging skills much enhanced by having a small amount of CBT training.

4 Existing non-CBT specialist skills may be used to allow emotional problems to be addressed alongside physical or other problems.

5 There is the possibility of 'cognitive first aid' to prevent emotional difficulties from becoming exacerbated and interfering with someone's ability to cope with other ongoing difficulties, or to provide a first step for someone who may go on to use other services.

6 Working through others is often cost-effective.

7 People with large numbers of professionals already involved in their care may be spared the necessity of forming yet another new therapeutic relationship.

This chapter will highlight the key considerations in setting up CBT work through others, such as how to develop training packages, the role of continued supervision and risk management, and the importance of assessing current levels of competence, illustrated by examples from CBT therapists who have worked successfully in this way.

Who might benefit?

There are some groups of people who may be likely to access the benefits of CBT through non-specialist therapists and even be more amenable to this approach to service delivery. For example, Mannix *et al.* (2006) suggested that people with life-limiting illness, or with very complex needs, may have a great many professionals already involved in their care, and a limited capacity for new therapeutic relationships. There may therefore be very good reasons why CBT should be offered to such patients by someone they already know.

If patients are able to access CBT in a familiar setting from professionals used to working with their specific physical illness this may be advantageous. Staff such as general practitioners (GPs; Heatley *et al.*, 2005), volunteers, unqualified assistants, and nurses may be in a much better position to offer an appropriate level or type of CBT intervention more rapidly, alongside a more sophisticated understanding of specific health problems than generic CBT therapists would have.

Further examples of patient groups who might benefit could include people who do not need a highly specialist psychological therapies service, people who would rather not be associated with a psychiatric service at all, people who find it hard to access care through the usual channels, or people known to be vulnerable to mental health problems or the effects of stress but not often referred in their own right, such as carers.

It is clear that some patients respond to relatively circumscribed interventions. For these responders, treatment duration and intensity can be matched to need more efficiently when staff other than CBT therapists have skills to intervene. For example, patients who attend a GP surgery with panic-related chest pain are likely to do much better if they are given a cognitive formulation at primary care level rather than being given generic reassurance and then referred to a psychological therapies service. Generic reassurance, waiting while continuing to feel anxious and potentially practising a range of safety behaviours, as well as the suggestion that they are mentally ill, may all have seriously negative effects on the patients' emotional well-being, while an immediate understanding of the panic cycle may just be enough to enable them to break it.

Sometimes the benefits of working through others may actually be to deliver a more intensive treatment. In the example of home treatment for agoraphobia (Example 10.1) below, psychology graduate volunteers were used because they were less costly, while at the same time being able to offer a higher intensity of treatment in the form of home visits, longer treatment sessions, and being present during behavioural experiments.

Example 10.1 Training psychology graduate volunteers to treat clients with agoraphobia: using an untrained resource to provide a high-intensity treatment

Patients suffering from panic disorder with agoraphobia are often severely disadvantaged when it comes to accessing traditional clinic-based CBT services, as many are housebound and highly avoidant.

Graduate volunteers were selected from local research and clinical assistants, and from enquiries to the service of those seeking clinical experience. Training consisted of a two-day long workshop in CBT for panic disorder and agoraphobia. The emphasis was on the specific therapeutic skills required to treat this group of clients, including assessment, formulation, challenging misinterpretations of physical symptoms and behavioural experiments. The workshops included formal teaching, video demonstrations, role-plays, and experiential elements. The volunteers were also given instruction about ethical and governance issues relating to their new role as therapist.

Volunteers saw patients at home and carried out behavioural experiments in feared situations (e.g. in busy supermarkets, on public transport or journeys to collect children from school). This enabled patients to address directly the specific fears maintaining their problems via powerful experiential methods. Most of these patients would have been unlikely to have accessed effective CBT had they not been seen at home, and traditional services were not able to offer such a service. The volunteers were supported through fortnightly group supervision with the CBT therapist.

Patient satisfaction was high, and dropout rates low. Clinical outcomes have been as good as those obtained with similar patients seen by fully qualified therapists locally.

There are certain clear advantages to offering patients with agoraphobia this specific, targeted service: it improves their access to psychological treatments by offering home visits; it reduces waiting times for treatment by training highly motivated and available psychology graduates, who often go on to further training; and it makes use of a specific CBT model that is known to be clinically effective. It relies for good success rates on careful screening and triaging of potential patients, as volunteers are *only* trained to treat one disorder. Ongoing supervision of the volunteers is also essential and this is an important consideration in all this work (see Section 'Supervision' below). The model may be applicable with different client groups such as those with obsessive compulsive disorder (OCD) or social phobia, who would also benefit from *in vivo* behavioural experiments during the course of their CBT treatment.

Who might be available to deliver CBT in this way?

Emotional disorders are seen in many settings other than traditional mental health or psychological services. People working in such settings may be frustrated at their inability to deal with emotional reactions to stressful or traumatic events, and glad to learn some basic or specifically targeted CBT skills. Many unqualified people embarking on a variety of careers may be keen to learn some skills for dealing with emotional disorders, and may be an untapped resource.

Clinicians in training or those contemplating training often have relevant clinical skills and are keen to gather clinical experience. These individuals can often be trained in specific interventions and can work under your supervision to deliver care to clients, some of whom would have difficulty accessing CBT through other routes. They are also likely to have more time to spend with a patient than a fully qualified therapist, and may be able to provide encouragement for and modelling of behavioural experiments, that patients might otherwise struggle to do (see Examples 10.1 and 10.2).

GPs are often the first point of contact for clients seeking help and hold a key position in making referrals to overstretched services. The introduction of the stepped care model for depression within mental health (NICE, 2004) assumes that primary care clinicians will be responsible for delivering the initial steps of the model, yet most medical training programmes at best offer only minimal teaching about CBT.

Example 10.2 Teaching CBT skills to medical undergraduates: keen available therapists who will go on to be major referrers

A CBT therapist set up a programme for undergraduates in collaboration with a GP and teaching fellow and the medical school. The major benefits of teaching CBT skills to medical students were thought to be: awareness-raising regarding the potential value of CBT interventions, educating future referrers, and teaching basic CBT skills to future doctors. It was recognized that some 'hands-on' experience of CBT would enhance the learning experience of students, but also offer an additional, if limited, CBT resource for patients with mild-moderate problems. This was set up by the CBT therapist and her GP colleague as follows:

- *Two introductory CBT skills-based workshops.*
- *A small group of students were able to sign up for the CBT clinical experience.*
- *Patients were referred by GPs from one practice to facilitate ease of communication among students, CBT therapists, and GPs.*
- *The CBT therapist carried out an initial joint assessment with each patient and a student. Assessment included the patient's suitability for a brief CBT approach with a student, risk assessment, initial formulation, and the selection of appropriate self-help materials. It also allowed the CBT therapist to observe the student's competence in conducting a therapeutic interview.*
- *Students saw patients for up to 4 individual sessions of CBT-based guided self-help, using literature suggested by the CBT therapist.*
- *Students attended weekly group supervision sessions offered by the CBT therapist.*

In an evaluation of the programme (Kearley and Croft, in press), the students reported they had increased their knowledge of CBT, were more convinced of the credibility of the therapy, and had improved their general clinical skills.

Patients seen by students benefited from more rapid access to CBT materials and support in applying CBT strategies. All those surveyed believed that they had benefited from the interventions they received and this was confirmed by clinical outcome data.

The programme has also become an established, albeit small, clinical service within the GP practice, offering a different type of access to CBT for patients and with virtually no waiting time. This relieves pressure on the qualified CBT therapists offering longer-term therapy in the same practice.

This example highlights that educating other medical professionals about CBT can result in both short- and long-term benefits to patients. Working through trainee clinicians has the potential to add to the availability of CBT, and also equips them to function as better clinicians when qualified.

Another group who may be able to deliver CBT with training are people from voluntary organizations. There may be many opportunities to form partnerships with organizations such as MIND. While people working in voluntary organizations will often not have formal clinical training, they may have excellent insight into the needs of their service users, as well as providing a point of access that patients find less stigmatizing or intimidating than a statutory service. Some of the volunteers may themselves be patients who have recovered from, or learned to live with, their mental health difficulties, and can pass on their experience very constructively to others.

Example 10.3 Working in partnership with the voluntary sector: first-line interventions outside mental health services

As the result of a working party over 20 years ago, the first MIND day centre in Oxfordshire was set up, with an experienced CBT therapist involved in the planning. In 2009, there are MIND Day Centres in 14 towns in Oxfordshire, and there are frequent MIND CBT groups in Oxford City, and in towns in North and South Oxfordshire.

Topics include learning how to cope with depression and anxiety, building self-esteem, withdrawal from tranquillizers, and assertiveness techniques. Mindfulness-based cognitive therapy has also been offered. A 'piggy-back' model has been used. A CBT therapist has developed each group treatment program and has initially run the groups, with a MIND worker sitting in as an intern. When the group has run successfully several times the MIND worker takes a more active role, until they are running the group without professional input.

The group program has produced excellent results, monitored carefully with relevant questionnaires. Participants are screened beforehand, and group leaders are offered regular supervision. CBT has been seen as compatible with MIND values, as it is transparent and explicit, and empowering for participants, who take away skills from the group. It has been cost-effective for the National Health Service (NHS) as it involves only the development of the packages, initial training, and ongoing supervision.

What this and the previous example also highlight is the need to take note of certain key considerations in setting up CBT work through others. These include:

- Making work through others cost-effective.
- The level of skills other people already have, and what training they require.
- How to train them.

- How to ensure that those delivering CBT are offering safe and effective interventions.

The following sections will expand upon these areas.

Cost-effectiveness

It is important to achieve the right balance between the time spent training and supervising others, versus the time you spend doing therapeutic interventions that other therapists are unable to do. Working through others should not be *assumed* to be cost-effective. Some ways of ensuring cost-effectiveness may be:

- Offering training for a limited range of problems (e.g. agoraphobia, or the stress of caring for someone with dementia) or with a clearly defined skill level in mind (see Example 10.4).
- Having a 'critical mass' of trainees and only repeating training when there are enough participants.
- Developing good teaching materials, perhaps using material with proven effectiveness such as an adaptation of a research protocol, or piloting teaching material and adapting it following trainee feedback.
- Considering whether 'piggy-back' training (see Example 10.3), where the trainee first acts as an observer but gradually takes more responsibility for the treatment, is appropriate (this may be most suitable in a group format).
- Offering group supervision and considering how frequent this needs to be, based on the level of intervention being offered, the previous skill level of staff and the amount of CBT they are undertaking.

Even with the best plans, circumstances sometimes intervene to make a project less cost-effective than anticipated (e.g. staff moving on or not being able to commit in practice to something they were enthusiastic about in theory). Sometimes these factors cannot be anticipated, but it pays to take time to research thoroughly the practical implications of adding to the demands on staff time, securing management support for staff to take on new responsibilities, and getting a commitment to release staff and provide funding for ongoing supervision.

Training staff

In any project in which you are handing on skills, considerable thought and time needs to be devoted to the selection of suitable staff to train (e.g. through interviews, references, or recommendations from more senior staff) and what training is actually offered. Usually, the people you will be training will have some existing skills or experience that make them good candidates for this approach. It is important to be aware of what these skills are and the range of competence within groups of learners when planning training (see Chapter 17 on CBT training).

Manualized treatment packages may be very useful, but the degree of theoretical background to be given, and formulation skills to be taught, will need careful thought. It will be very important to be clear what you are aiming for in terms of skill level for your trainees. In practice, for trainees who are not professionally qualified, the training being offered may need to start with basic general skills such as group management, keeping to time boundaries, keeping other therapeutic boundaries that are appropriate to visiting people in their own home, and maintaining good rapport. Specific CBT skills such as agenda setting, monitoring of mood and behaviour, thought recording, thought challenging, and doing behavioural experiments, are likely to be central to much of the training for doing CBT through others, particularly when specific conditions are being targeted and a fairly uniform model of common emotional problems in the target group is to be used. The formulation skills needed will vary considerably, from the ability to draw out a simple vicious circle maintenance process to making the links between past experience, personality, and coping mechanisms and current strategies or difficulties. You need to tailor the level of training to your trainees' existing knowledge, and to the key skills required to carry out the intended CBT interventions. You can achieve this in several ways, such as setting criteria for the level of skills or knowledge required prior to training in CBT, getting candidates for training to fill in application forms before training, making sure that during training exercises less experienced trainees are partnered with more experienced ones, and at a more formal level, interviewing trainees before offering them the training.

It will be very important for those delivering the care to recognize the limits of their competence, and ongoing supervision will play a fundamental role in assuring this.

Using practitioners' existing skills and experience

When working through non-CBT therapists, one key principle is to use the skills people already have, their knowledge about particular illnesses or conditions, and their understanding of the difficulties and stresses of people in that situation. There are several advantages of doing so:

- It saves time in training.
- It builds confidence in learners. Learning new approaches can be de-skilling, and making use of their pre-existing skills helps to minimize this.

- Their existing skills put them in touch with patients who could benefit from CBT.
- Their existing skills and experience mean they have special insight and empathy with patients and will be better able to engage them in CBT.

It may be very much in their favour if their patients do not see them as mental health workers, therefore avoiding the stigma that is unfortunately still associated with mental illness. In some cases, such as physical illness, patients may be relatively robust emotionally but dealing with a stressful situation. They may not wish to be seen as emotionally disordered, or as having a mental illness, as might be implied by having to see a qualified mental health professional. Their ability to engage in challenging their perceptions and interpretations of events may be much greater if they believe their therapist understands and has experience of their situation, and sees their emotional difficulties as a normal reaction to the stress they are experiencing.

Mannix *et al.* (2006) trained nurses in a palliative care unit in CBT skills to help them deal with distress in the terminally ill. This allowed some of those working most closely with the clients to carry out what they called 'cognitive first aid'. These patients would be very unlikely to have the time to wait to see a qualified cognitive therapist, but immediate interventions by staff giving them their day-to-day care could enable them to optimize their adjustment to bad news, maximize coping skills, 'gain insight, change behaviour, and regain a sense of control', thus reducing distress for them, their families, and indeed the staff working with them.

Staff working with physical health problems that make people more prone to anxiety and depression might well be in an excellent position to use CBT skills with their clients to great effect. Their knowledge of the conditions they deal with every day may give them a better understanding of common psychological and emotional reactions to these conditions, compared to a therapist who rarely sees them. For example, physiotherapists may be in an excellent position to help people design behavioural experiments when anxiety impedes recovery during rehabilitation from accidents; and practice nurses may have greater access to patients with chronic physical health problems and be able to offer brief CBT input to help them manage their conditions better.

The skills such staff bring to CBT training can be utilized and built on by asking them to bring the cases they are most familiar with, or struggle with on a daily basis, into training role-plays. Staff groups who work with similar patient groups can share their experience and help each other find new ways of approaching them, based on the CBT principles they are learning.

Example 10.4 Practice and specialist nurses using CBT with patients in primary care: 'cognitive first aid' for people adjusting to chronic health problems.

Through informal discussion with members of the primary care team, a CBT therapist working in primary care became aware that the practice and specialist nurses (in diabetes and respiratory illness) were often working with patients with chronic physical illnesses who also had emotional difficulties, or who were struggling to make behavioural changes to adjust to their illnesses. These difficulties were not usually severe enough to warrant referral for psychological therapy, but the nurses felt they wanted to be able to offer something to these patients and were not skilled to do so. The CBT therapist suggested that she could offer some training in CBT skills for anxiety and low mood and this was received enthusiastically.

The therapist developed a brief training programme over two sessions, focusing on basic CBT skills for managing thoughts and behaviour change, including linking thoughts, emotions and behaviour, activity scheduling, goal-setting and graded approaches to behaviour change, behavioural experiments, and the basic concepts of challenging negative thinking. The nurses then began to identify suitable patients via their routine clinics. They carried out brief interventions with patients using the skills they had been taught and attended monthly peer supervision groups with the CBT therapist for support and ongoing skills development.

The nurses valued having specific CBT tools to manage common emotional and behavioural problems. In addition, their confidence in managing more difficult patients grew and they felt valued as a result of the investment in their training.

In this example, staff had existing specialist skills that were respected by their clients. Their experience allowed them to demonstrate an understanding of how difficult it is to adjust to living with particular health conditions, while being plausible in their expectations that adjustment is both possible and desirable. They also have generic clinical skills, such as the ability to assess and engage patients, which provide a good foundation for new CBT skills. A minimal cognitive intervention (cognitive first aid) may make a great deal of difference to the speed with which patients adjust to diagnoses that significantly affect their lives, and may even reduce the necessity for a future referral to a more specialist CBT service.

Another example where CBT has been shown to be effective is with carers of people with dementia (Marriott *et al.*, 2002). This is a group who live with high levels of stress and are known to have higher than average levels of depression (Donaldson *et al.*, 1997). Recent research (Zarit and Femia, 2008) suggests that although carers benefit from a wide variety of interventions, including education about the illness, stress management, etc., a psychological component to this is very important. CBT fits very well with an approach that combines psychoeducation, stress management, behavioural analysis and management, and emotional adjustment to loss. In Example 10.5, a manualized package of CBT for carers of people with dementia has proved very popular with team community nurses and occupational therapists.

Example 10.5 CBT with carers: development of a training package based on a research protocol

Carers of people with mental health problems are known to be vulnerable to anxiety and depression (Donaldson et al., 1997). They are prone to neglect their own health and to see their emotional problems as a normal part of the caring role. They are also acknowledged to be providing very valuable care and support to a needy population, and government guidelines have emphasized the importance of supporting their mental health to enable them to continue caring.

We set out to adapt the clinical trial protocol used by Marriott et al. (2002), which had originally been carried out by three researchers, to train staff working with carers of people with dementia. The result was a 3-day workshop and therapy manual. The training is divided into 3 sections:

- *How to offer psychoeducation (about dementia) in the way that most meets the needs of the carer.*
- *Stress management, including relaxation, thought recording, and challenging and behavioural management of stress using activities.*
- *Coping skills, including behavioural management of challenging behaviour, and further cognitive therapy skills for managing feelings of loss.*

Trainees were taught to start each section of treatment with assessment, to allow flexibility in tailoring the contents of the section to the carer's need. Community nurses and occupational therapists interested in working in this way with carers did the 3 days of training, including introductory CBT concepts and formulation skills, familiarity with the manual, and how to adapt the materials in a flexible way to the needs of each carer.

The trainees brought examples from their own clinical experience to use in role-play. They found that the CBT approach effectively formalized interventions that they were already attempting to use with the carers they were seeing, and added a CBT approach to the emotional difficulties arising from the situation the carers found themselves in.

Supervision was provided in group format, usually led by the team CBT therapist who also had done the training in order to be familiar with the manual. Supervision groups met every 4–6 weeks.

Feedback from training workshops suggests that this package is seen as highly relevant to staff, and that they value the chance to discuss how to apply the format to their clients. It has proved necessary to be flexible with how the package is used, as it is often unnecessary to use the whole protocol. It may be more appropriate to select the parts that address the carer's particular needs: for example, some carers are able to access a wide range of information resources about the nature of dementia, so the focus may be much more on coping with their emotional reactions, or managing their relative's difficult behaviour.

In this example, a research protocol was turned into a training package and therapy manual. It was tried out in early versions on groups of clinical psychologists working with older adults, and underwent a number of revisions before being finalized. It uses a model of training that includes role-play and familiarization with the materials in the manual by practising them on other attendees at the training workshop.

Carers are a group who are often very anxious to avoid being labeled as mentally ill; they see the problem as their relative's illness and the lack of resources available to support them in coping with it. This sort of approach allows for an acknowledgement of the stresses they are under from a staff group who are seen to have a wide experience of their difficulties. The intervention is therefore highly targeted, attempts to avoid stigmatizing carers, and makes good use of highly motivated staff who may otherwise feel frustrated at how to help carers cope with the emotionally very difficult situation they are in.

Ensuring interventions by others are safe

Assessment

You will need to consider how best to assess the patients coming for treatment with unqualified therapists, particularly in matters of safety. Some patients may need a full assessment from a qualified professional, including risk assessment, before being offered treatment under supervision by a less experienced worker. In other cases, assessment may be carried out by the non-CBT therapists themselves, provided there are good enough protocols and measures that indicate under what circumstances backup needs to be called in or a patient referred on. The ability to recognize changes in levels of risk will be important, particularly for unqualified and inexperienced staff. If the treatment is being carried out outside regular mental health services, you will need to consider what policies and procedures are in place for the management of risk, as well as what backup is available for less experienced workers from more experienced staff.

Screening as to suitability for the treatment being offered is extremely important, and you will need to offer guidance on this both during initial training and ongoing supervision. Draw up inclusion criteria for treatment, as well as criteria for referral on to more specialist services or those offering higher levels of skills for more complex problems. Formal assessment tools such as the Beck Depression Inventory (Beck *et al.*, 1961), Geriatric Depression Scale (Yesavage *et al.*, 1983), PHQ-9 (Kroenke *et al.*, 2001), or GAD-7 (Spitzer *et al.*, 2006) can help decide whether patients meet criteria either for the service being offered by the non-CBT therapists, or for referral onward. Such measures are relatively easy to administer, and can be interpreted with a minimum of training.

Supervision

Supervision helps therapists to adhere to the model they are using, which in turn may improve the outcome for the patient. It also means that those delivering the therapy are more likely to maintain their skills and stick to the protocols they have been taught, which in turn is likely to improve outcomes (Grey *et al.*, 2008). Supervision is particularly important when therapy is being provided by those without formal therapeutic qualifications. Mannix *et al.* (2006) showed that nurses trained to use CBT techniques in palliative care maintained their skills longer and applied them more effectively if they had regular supervision, compared to those without such supervision. Supervision can be provided very effectively in groups, allowing those receiving the supervision to learn from each others' experience as well as their own (see Examples 10.1 and 10.2). The supervisor can also decide whether it is appropriate to transfer care to a more experienced practitioner if the patient's problem lies outside the competencies of the therapist.

Monitoring outcomes

Auditing and monitoring are important in ensuring that the desired outcomes are being achieved. This is increasingly important as cost-effectiveness becomes more of a consideration in every area of healthcare. In statutory services, outcome measurement is required in order to justify the availability of the treatment. In other areas, such as the voluntary sector, such monitoring of outcomes may help ensure the funding needed to continue the work. GPs will only purchase extra services for their patients if there is evidence of cost-effectiveness and good outcomes, alongside good feedback from patients. You can do a small scale evaluation simply by gathering some clinical outcome measures and other feedback from patients, carers, or staff as part of everyday practice (see Chapter 18). Ongoing measurement also provides invaluable feedback about clinical progress for individual patients and those delivering CBT. Given these potential benefits, thought should be given at the outset to how interventions will be monitored.

Conclusion

The clinical examples in this chapter demonstrate that working through others can result in creative and innovative service models which are clinically effective and which widen access to CBT. Trainees give very positive feedback about their experience of widening their therapeutic skills, reporting improved confidence and enthusiasm. For the CBT therapist offering the training and/or supervision, the opportunity to share skills that are known to be effective and useful can be a very positive experience. Nevertheless, embarking upon work of this type requires careful thought and planning in order to safeguard all parties. When this is done, working through others can be a deeply rewarding experience both for the CBT therapist and those delivering the therapy.

Key points

- Doing CBT through others allows people to benefit from CBT who might not otherwise access it.
- CBT principles and techniques can be taught to non-CBT therapists.
- The level of skills to be taught will need to be carefully judged.
- Training may be manual based, use role-play, and include homework exercises.
- Screening of patients for treatment by less experienced practitioners should be carefully carried out by a more experienced professional.
- Modelling, with gradual assumption of therapeutic responsibility, is appropriate for groups.
- Ongoing supervision is very important to keep up skills.

Further reading

Kearley, K, and Croft, A. (in press). Cognitive-behavioural skills training for medical students: development and evaluation. The Psychiatrist.

Mannix, K.A., Blackburn, I.M, Garland, A., Gracie, J., Moorey, S., Reid, B., Standart, S. and Scott, J. (2006). Effectiveness of brief training in cognitive behaviour therapy techniques for palliative care practitioners. *Palliative Care Medicine*, **20**, 579–584.

Marriott, A., Donaldson, C., Tarriet, N. and Burns, A (2002). Effectiveness of cognitive behavioural family intervention in reducing the burden of care in carers of patients with Alzheimer's disease. *British Journal of Psychiatry*, **176**, 557–562.

References

Beck, A.T., Ward, C.H., Mendelson, M., Mock, J. and Erbaugh, J. (1961). An inventory for measuring depression. *Archives of General Psychiatry*, **4**, 53–63.

Donaldson, C., Tarrier, N. and Burns, A. (1997). The impact of the symptoms of dementia on caregivers. *British Journal of Psychiatry*, **170**, 62–68.

Grey, N., Salkovskis, P., Quigley, A., Clark, D.M. and Ehlers, A. (2008). Dissemination of cognitive therapy for panic disorder in primary care. *Behavioural and Cognitive Psychotherapy*, **36**, 509–521.

Heatley, C., Ricketts, T. and Forrest, J. (2005). Training general practitioners in cognitive behaviour therapy for panic disorder: randomised control trial. *Journal of Mental Health*, **14**, 73–82.

Kearley, K. and Croft, A. (in press). Cognitive-behavioural skills training for medical students: development and evaluation. *The Psychiatrist.*

Kroenke, K., Spitzer, R.L. and Williams, J.B.W. (2001). The PHQ-9: validity of a brief depression severity measure. *Journal of General Internal Medicine*, **16**, 606–613.

Mannix, K.A., Blackburn, I.M., Garland, A., Gracie, J., Moorey, S., Reid, B., Standart, S. and Scott, J. (2006). Effectiveness of brief training in cognitive behaviour therapy techniques for palliative care practitioners. *Palliative Care Medicine*, **20**, 579–584.

Marriott, A., Donaldson, C., Tarrier, N. and Burns, A. (2002). Effectiveness of cognitive-behavioural family intervention in reducing the burden of care in carers of patients with Alzheimer's disease. *British Journal of Psychiatry*, **176**, 557–562.

National Institute for Clinical Excellence Practice Guideline (2004). *Depression: Management of Depression in Primary and Secondary Care* (amended 2007). Available at: http://www.nice.org.uk/nicemedia/pdf/CG23fullguideline.pdf (accessed 10 September 2009).

Spitzer, R.L., Kroenke, K., Williams, J.B.W. and Loewe, B. (2006). A brief measure for assessing generalized anxiety disorder: the GAD-7. *Archives of Internal Medicine*, **166**, 1092–1097.

Yesavage, J.A., Brink, T.L., Rose, T.L., Lum, O., Huang, V., Adey, M. and Leirer, O. (1983). Development and validation of a geriatric depression scale: a preliminary report. *Journal of Psychiatric Research*, **17**, 37–49.

Zarit, S.H. and Femia, E.F. (2008). A future for family care and dementia intervention research? Challenges and strategies. *Aging and Mental Health*, **12**, 5–13.

Chapter 11

Working in multidisciplinary teams

Alison J. Croft and Helen Close

Introduction

Most cognitive behavioural therapy (CBT) therapists will work in a team at some point in their career. The Care Quality Commission NHS National Staff Survey (2008) found that more than 90% of staff described themselves as working in a team. Multidisciplinary teams (MDTs) are the most common form of team working in social and healthcare settings, serving diverse populations and having various functions. CBT practitioners may be part of primary (mental) healthcare teams, community mental health teams (CMHTs), early intervention teams, assertive outreach and crisis resolution teams, and psychological therapies teams made up of therapists from different therapeutic modalities. Additionally, there may be MDTs in inpatient mental health settings (see Chapter 12) or physical health settings (see Chapter 13).

Team working can provide many great opportunities, with the potential to enrich both your clinical work and that of your colleagues. Working alongside colleagues from other disciplines will allow you to learn about other therapeutic approaches and how they can benefit patients. Your colleagues' unique perspectives can help you to broaden and deepen your knowledge of the patient population you are working with. When an MDT is functioning well, patients receive more comprehensive and better quality care; this adds a rewarding dimension to your work as a CBT therapist that lone working never can. In addition, although you may be employed primarily as a therapist, your CBT skills can also be used to benefit the MDT more broadly, for example, through your contributions to MDT case discussions and indirect working. In this way, you may have a wider influence over patient care than you could through your own face-to-face clinical work alone.

However, there are also specific challenges and difficulties that can arise from working in MDTs. You may be faced with additional tasks, responsibilities, and dilemmas that arise from working closely with other professionals in a team, rather than as a more autonomous therapist. You may be fortunate enough to join a team as it is forming, meaning that you can be a part of the process of clarifying objectives, procedures, and roles. However, in most cases, clinicians join teams that have been in existence for some time, where a proportion of the team membership may be well established, and where the team 'culture' and working practices are fairly fixed. This can make it difficult for you to integrate successfully as a newcomer to the MDT, particularly if you suspect that others' expectations of you don't match with your own ideas!

Here are some of the most common dilemmas:

- Do I have a unique role in the team, and if so, what is it?
- How can I communicate/demonstrate this role to my colleagues effectively?
- To what extent should I integrate with the working practices of the rest of the team?
- How do I develop constructive working relationships with my MDT colleagues, particularly those from different professional or theoretical backgrounds?
- How can I best deal with conflicts of opinion and rivalry?
- How can I manage excess demand for CBT within my MDT?

This chapter will explore these issues and discuss possible ways of resolving them, using examples of how other CBT therapists have resolved these problems in their own clinical practice.

Establishing your role

Establishing your distinct role as a CBT therapist in an MDT is key. Onyett (2007) stresses that having clear and distinct roles within an MDT is essential if the team is to function effectively. When the roles of team members are clear, the team is able to benefit from the specialist knowledge and skills that each discipline brings, which in turn benefits the patient. Sometimes there are expectations that all team members should be involved in the same generic team tasks: for example, contributing to duty rotas or carrying out generic assessments. This runs the risk of team roles becoming blurred to the extent that the benefits of MDT working are lost. Nevertheless, there *is* value in contributing to the core functions of the team, not just for the rest of the team, but for the CBT therapist as well: for example, a sense of belonging; being regarded as a true member of the team by others; and a greater sense of the core work of the team and the pressures on colleagues. A balance needs to be struck between integrating with the team and practising your specialist skills. The following sections will consider how these issues may be addressed, and in doing so highlight the specific contribution you can bring to an MDT.

Be clear about what you can offer

If you are recently qualified, or have never worked in an MDT before, you may be a little unsure or tentative about your unique role within the MDT. This can make you reticent in asserting it, perhaps thinking that your skills are not unique at all or not developed well enough to want to shout about! However, this reticence is usually unfounded. To communicate your specialist skills to others, *you* must first be clear about what they are. Here are some suggestions of how you might become more clear and confident in this respect:

1. Establish a clear idea of what 'added value' you bring to the MDT as a CBT therapist. What is unique about your contribution to the MDT? For example:
   - Your knowledge of the evidence base regarding what CBT protocols and techniques have been shown to be effective. Keeping up-to-date with new developments in CBT will increase your confidence in using this knowledge when making decisions about treatment.
   - Your clinical skills in implementing these treatments with patients, either directly or by working through other staff members in offering supervision and consultation.
   - Your skills in structured and individualized assessment and formulation of problems.
   - Other CBT clinical skills that can be used more generally in the team such as working collaboratively, taking a Socratic approach, agenda setting, etc.
2. Consider what you can offer from your skills and experience as an individual as well as your training in CBT. For example:
   - What do you bring from your past clinical experience in other settings that will enrich your work with the team?
   - Do you have special interests in a particular area or way of working (e.g. CBT for psychosis, group work, etc.)?
   - Does your core professional training mean you have other generic skills to bring?
3. Discuss these ideas with your supervisor or a more experienced clinician who may have trodden the same path before you and have more confidence in their skills. He/she may also be able to help you to identify your individual strengths and how these could be used in your team.

Communicate with others about your role

One of the problems in working with colleagues from other disciplines is that they may have little understanding or experience of CBT. This can lead to misconceptions about CBT and your role as a CBT therapist. Although other clinicians may have a general knowledge of different psychological therapy models, this is often too cursory to allow for a good understanding of the relative strengths of different ways of working. In order to work constructively with colleagues who are approaching their work from other perspectives it is important to know what beliefs and assumptions underpin their work. For example, they may believe that CBT is 'superficial' (and prior experience of staff who lacked adequate training and offered CBT ineffectively may serve to reinforce this myth), or conversely that CBT can cure all ills (Veale, 2008). The development of 'third-wave CBT therapies' (e.g. acceptance and commitment therapy [ACT] or mindfulness-based cognitive therapy) means that CBT is now a diverse family of allied therapies rather than one coherent approach (Mansell, 2008). This diversity could add to the potential confusion of MDT colleagues as to what CBT is and what it can offer. Clarifying such questions can be achieved both directly and indirectly, as follows.

Case discussions/team meetings

The primary forum for MDT clinical decision-making is usually the team meeting (see section 'Time management and MDT meetings' for discussion of prioritizing attendance). It is often here that referrals are allocated and the assessment and treatment of patients discussed. This is a great opportunity for you to communicate through case discussion how you work and which referrals are appropriate. It helps to be well-prepared for these opportunities by being familiar with the latest guidance and evidence base (e.g. NICE guidelines, general literature). Knowing who is most likely to be helped by CBT (see Chapter 1), and being able to back this up with evidence, are extremely important in discussions where clinical decisions are being made (see Example 11.1).

Example 11.1 Working with psychological therapists from different theoretical models

In a newly formed team of psychological therapists, a series of seminars was set up where each team member was invited to describe some recent clinical work. The CBT therapist outlined a CBT case formulation and described the intervention strategies and their results. In addition, he was able to offer a CBT perspective during discussions of his colleagues' case presentations, highlighting similarities and differences in therapeutic models and techniques. The therapists also shared information about their training and specific interests. The seminars led to more effective team working and more informed discussions on resource allocation.

Shadowing

Allowing others to observe your clinical work can be an effective way of communicating CBT skills to members of the MDT. Although this kind of shadowing is commonly used for training purposes, colleagues from other disciplines, both junior and senior, may also benefit. Just as behavioural experiments add a different dimension to our patients' learning in therapy, so seeing for themselves how you work as a CBT therapist can be a great learning opportunity for your colleagues. It may also be a behavioural experiment for you as a therapist, if the prospect of being shadowed provokes negative predictions about your performance and how it will be judged! However, the benefits usually outweigh the costs.

The following guidelines will help both you and your colleagues get the most from shadowing:

- Make sure your patient is fully informed and gives his consent to observation.
- Live observation is preferable, as this allows the observer to pick up on the subtleties present in the interpersonal process in the session and is likely to be more engaging. Where live observation is not possible, recorded sessions (either audio or video) can be used.
- Plan the observation. Be aware in advance of your observer's knowledge and experience of CBT, and any beliefs and assumptions he/she may have. Take time before and after the session to discuss what you were doing and how this fits with the case formulation and treatment plan for the patient. A debrief can provide an opportunity to clarify and if necessary challenge assumptions further.
- It would be ideal to plan a range of cases for observation, spanning different levels of complexity and diagnosis. Observation over the course of a whole clinic may make this possible. If it is not, discussion of the range of cases on your caseload may serve the same function.

Joint working

Opportunities for joint working with your colleagues often present themselves naturally as part of the team's everyday practice. By 'joint' working we mean actually seeing the patient together with your colleague rather than merely that more than one MDT member is working with a patient. Where true joint working is not possible, you should seek opportunities for more detailed discussion of the work you and others are doing with the patient in team meetings, CPA reviews, or on an *ad hoc* basis. These are opportunities to demystify how you work, to clarify your role, and to add a psychological perspective to the overall care of the team's caseload (see Example 11.2).

Example 11.2 Demonstrating the value of CBT via joint working

A CBT therapist joined a recently formed team working in a psychiatric day hospital. There was no precedent for having a CBT therapist on the team, so it was necessary for her to establish a role. The rest of the team was keen for the CBT therapist to set up groups for patients. She could not run these alone, as the group numbers were too large and were made up of patients with complex problems who often needed substantial support. No one else had CBT training or skills. The therapist developed materials for two groups and began running these jointly with a couple of staff members who were willing to contribute (mainly through offering support to group members). The same staff members then took a more active role in the next cycle of groups, gradually taking on a more shared role with each new cycle as they felt more confident.

Working in this way allowed other team members to develop a better understanding of how CBT could be applied to specific problems in a group setting. They were able to develop some specific CBT skills through the mentoring offered by the CBT therapist and were subsequently better equipped to offer ongoing support to patients who had attended the groups.

Modelling core CBT skills

Many MDTs will have regular meetings where more difficult cases are discussed at greater length. If your team does not, you may be able to introduce this idea. Most team members will value the opportunity to discuss cases that they find challenging—not least you yourself! As well as providing further opportunities for presenting examples of CBT work, meetings like this can also be an opportunity to demonstrate clinical skills that you may take for granted, but that some other disciplines may not use either so explicitly, or at all. Examples might be:

- Agenda setting
- Case formulation
- Socratic questioning
- Collaborative problem-solving

One example of such a process is described by Lake (2008). His 'team formulation approach' was used in MDT settings and aimed to foster an atmosphere of open discussion and discovery. He describes using an eclectic model of formulation, but it would be possible for you to use a CBT model to facilitate team formulation of complex cases. A more specifically CBT approach is described in Example 11.3.

Such 'in-depth' case discussions can also provide a useful means of resolving differences of opinion regarding interventions as well as offering support to clinicians who are feeling the strain (see Section Conflict within MDT's below).

Example 11.3 A CBT case formulation discussion

One CBT therapist introduced the idea of a regular time slot in the MDT meeting to facilitate discussion of complex cases. An agenda was set at the beginning which would include identifying key questions or dilemmas about the patient's care. Through Socratic questioning, a CBT case formulation was developed and drawn out on a whiteboard. This process stimulated discussion and helped to identify areas for further assessment, treatment targets, and possible interventions. This approach helped the MDT to develop a greater awareness of the value of CBT case formulation as an alternative perspective to medical diagnosis. Having a shared understanding of a patient's difficulties often enhanced the team's understanding of and empathy with the patient, leading to better and more consistent treatment.

Skills training and supervision of MDT members

Training and supervising others in the MDT can help both in communicating the value of CBT, and in managing excess demand for CBT (see Section Improving access to CBT in MDT settings, also refer to Chapter 17 on Training, Chapter 16 on Supervising, and Chapter 10 on Working through others).

Some MDT members may have CBT skills already and be keen to apply those skills within the team. The evidence points to supervision as being crucial in helping staff to consolidate CBT skills and successfully use treatment protocols in the workplace (e.g. Mannix *et al.*, 2006; Grey *et al.*, 2008). You may not yet be experienced in providing supervision and training but you will probably have some skills to offer your colleagues in this area.

There are different models for offering training and supervision in MDTs:

- Using peer group sessions or the occasional MDT meeting for specific CBT skill training.
- More formal CBT training sessions for the whole MDT.
- More experienced CBT therapists supervising less experienced CBT colleagues, or those undertaking CBT training.

- Generic supervision or case consultation with colleagues' cases, perhaps using CBT skills as part of this process, even when a non-CBT approach is being used (e.g. Socratic questions, case formulation, behavioural experiments).
- CBT supervision groups for staff who have attended the same training programmes.
- *Ad hoc* supervision of colleagues, or one-off consultations regarding particular clients.
- Consultation or supervision 'clinics' (see Example 11.4).

Offering supervision, at whatever level, is a very valuable contribution to the work of the team and can indirectly benefit clients. When your colleagues accept you in this role it may also indicate that you have been successful in establishing a valued role within the team.

Example 11.4 Offering consultation to MDT members

An experienced CBT therapist worked in a CMHT alongside a psychotherapist colleague. They were each being approached regularly by team members wanting to discuss cases and potential referrals. They agreed to set up a weekly drop-in consultation session at a regular time that was known to all team members. Clinicians attended on an ad hoc basis whenever they had a case to discuss. These might be potential referrals or clinical problems within their ongoing work with a patient. Both therapists would engage in a discussion with their colleagues and would make suggestions about how to formulate and resolve the presenting problems. This was a more efficient use of their time. It also provided an opportunity for case discussion from more than one theoretical perspective, deepening the understanding of team members and the therapists themselves as to what the two models had to offer.

Conflict within MDTs

Conflict is a natural and inevitable part of the life of any group (Tuckman, 1965). If handled well, it can be a great opportunity for MDT members to develop a better understanding of each others' perspectives and to work together more effectively. Common ways to manage conflict apply to MDT work as much as any other, and may include the following:

- Take time to understand both perspectives.
- Try to adopt a collaborative problem-solving approach.
- When conflicts arise concerning differences of opinion about clinical approaches, you need to able to argue your case knowledgeably, clearly, and with conviction—so again, be clear about the evidence base for CBT.

- When conflicts concern more organizational issues, seek support and advice from your supervisor or your line manager.

There are some conflict 'hot spots' for CBT therapists working in MDTs. These include:

- Role conflict and others' expectations of what you will do in the MDT.
- Differences between those using different therapeutic models.
- Conflict resulting from having limited CBT resources.

These will be discussed below with some of our solutions.

Role conflict

This describes the kind of dilemma that can arise from having more than one role to fulfil (e.g. generic team member and specialist therapist). You may be employed within an MDT primarily as a nurse, social worker, OT, or doctor, with a therapist role that is explicitly part of your contract, or it may be less clearly defined. Conflicts may therefore arise between carrying out your core professional functions and the expectations of others (or yourself) that you should also use your CBT skills. No one model will apply to every context, but some of the following strategies may be helpful:

- Understand the expectations other team members have of your role.
- Clarify via your contract, job description, and your manager specifically what is expected of your role within the team (e.g. CBT therapist and care coordinator).
- Be clear about the time allocated for your CBT therapist role.
- Clarify the level of demand for CBT relative to the time available.
- Establish what other CBT resources are available both within the team and in other local services.

Following a thorough assessment of the situation, the nature of the dilemmas regarding how your time should be spent should be clearer. You should now be in a better position to problem-solve and negotiate how the conflict can be resolved. Try doing some initial problem-solving with CBT colleagues from other teams who may have encountered similar difficulties, or with your clinical supervisor. It may then be useful to approach your team manager and, if possible, to discuss possible solutions or compromises with the team as a whole (e.g. how you prioritize your roles or the balance between CBT-specific and generic time). Other team members may not be aware of the constraints on your time, so communicating this clearly may help them to adjust their expectations. Collaboratively sharing responsibility for such decisions fosters open communication, builds trust, and understanding and can circumvent potential conflicts. Build in a review of any new model of working to assess its utility (See Example 11.5). This creates a new forum for tackling any remaining difficulties. Your line manager and/or CBT supervisor may be able to support you if disagreements cannot be resolved at team level. Supervision and peer support from CBT colleagues *outside* the team may be invaluable in retaining role clarity in the longer term (see Onyett, 2007).

Example 11.5 Participation in a team duty rota

A CMHT introduced a duty rota to manage telephone calls from patients in crisis. The CBT therapist discussed with the team whether it would be helpful for her to be involved in this rota. Although she could see that participation might foster greater integration with her team, her role was different from the care coordinators', in that she was the only team member employed specifically to deliver CBT. There was also a waiting list for this service. However, it was agreed that it would be helpful to try participating in the duty rota as an 'information gathering' behavioural experiment, over a period of 6 months.

It soon became clear that the CBT therapist was only able to fulfil this duty if she was not seeing patients and had the majority of the day set aside for office-based tasks. Finding a whole day each week to participate in the rota was difficult to manage. The team recognized that this was not the best use of her skills and of the limited CBT resource. A decision was made to withdraw from the rota, with an agreement that this decision could be reviewed at a later date.

Differences in therapeutic approach

Conflicts often exist where one model, for example the medical model, prevails. Onyett (2007) argues that there is a need for explicit theoretical discussions to occur within teams, so that decision-making is reasoned and theoretically grounded. He suggests that those working psychologically in teams often have a role in upholding a non-medical perspective in these discussions, which is valuable in helping the MDT to think more broadly (see Example 11.6).

Example 11.6 Helping the MDT to resolve conflict over the clinical management of a patient

A CMHT was struggling to work with a very challenging patient with psychosis. The patient had persistent delusional beliefs which made it very difficult to engage him in any form of support, and he was reluctant to take medication. The care coordinator had a good relationship with the patient, but was feeling unsupported and undermined because when she tried to adopt a more psychological approach to the patient's problems—for example, talking to the patient about his delusional beliefs and trying to understand the basis for them—these interventions were questioned by more senior team members who had a fairly rigid medical model of the patient's problems and thought that the patient just needed to be taking more medication.

The CBT therapist was able to facilitate a longer discussion in the team meeting when all the clinicians involved in the case were encouraged (via Socratic questioning) to articulate their implicit formulations of the patient's presenting problems and how these related to the types of intervention they believed should be carried out. He helped the care coordinator to formalize her implicitly psychological formulation, and enabled her to develop this into a more coherent individualized CBT formulation, backing this up with some theoretical evidence supporting the effectiveness of this approach. This provided a more robust challenge to the medical model. The discussion resulted in better understanding on both sides, recognition of some common ground, and more explicit and collaborative problem-solving about how to proceed. In addition, the care coordinator felt better understood and supported by her colleagues.

Limited resources and conflict

The problem of excess demand can lead to difficulties around your integration with the MDT and your relationships with your colleagues. As a CBT therapist you may need to adopt different working practices to the rest of the MDT: for example, being clinic-based and offering time-limited interventions. You may find that the bulk of your caseload differs significantly from that of your colleagues, and that you have to prioritize the patients you see according to who you think will benefit most from your skills. This can result in interprofessional rivalry and conflict.

Typical examples of the questions this raises include:

- What is the best use of your time?
- Which of the MDT's patients should be selected for CBT?
- Should there be a waiting list for CBT when there are more referrals than you can deal with?
- Which patients should be prioritized for treatment?

These are discussed below, with some possible solutions.

Time management and MDT meetings

When CBT resources are limited, there is a dilemma concerning how far to prioritize attendance at MDT meetings over other demands such as patient clinics. As the sections above suggest, attending meetings has so many benefits that doing so on a regular basis is usually a good investment of time; but it may be necessary to ration the time spent on this, particularly if team meetings proliferate! Again, allocating time is best done collaboratively with the MDT. This need not be a problem so long as you are clear about when you will be available to meet and you keep to those commitments, so that colleagues can plan when to discuss issues with you. Potential benefits of prioritizing meeting attendance include:

- A greater sense of integration with the team.
- Opportunities to communicate your role.
- Enhancing your clinical work through discussing and debating issues with your colleagues.
- Enhancing the work of others through the unique perspective you can bring to clinical discussions.

Which patients are offered CBT?

You may find that the MDT's referral criteria do not always fit well with offering an effective and evidence-based CBT service. MDTs often ration access to services by adopting more stringent referral criteria, which may mean that those people who are most likely to benefit from CBT are least likely to receive treatment (this will be less of an issue when alternative services are available and patients can be signposted there instead, e.g. in stepped care systems: see Chapters 6 and 7).

Even within the MDT's referral criteria it is likely that demand for CBT will exceed the resource available, so it is likely you will still need to make difficult choices about who to treat when. This may mean not seeing patients who could benefit from your input, or at least being very selective. For example, when there are potentially many patients who may benefit from CBT, you might be stricter in assessing a patient's motivation to engage in CBT. This may then be perceived as 'cherry picking' by colleagues who have less freedom to choose whom they see.

Some suggestions for managing these difficulties include:

- Being clear about the evidence for CBT for specific problems, and what the recommended treatment protocols are. This may not reduce the number of referrals but it may curtail cherry picking accusations! It may also help you to consider length of treatment and the preferred mode of delivery—factors which may also impact on decisions about what to offer to whom. You will also be better placed to communicate with confidence to your team about waiting times.

- Adopting CBT-specific referral criteria based on the evidence may lead to more appropriate referrals, although it may also increase the number of referrals.
- Being up-to-date regarding alternative CBT resources such as online resources, self-help literature, and other appropriate clinical services so that patients can be signposted elsewhere.
- Communicating clearly to your colleagues that if there is no alternative resource, people will have to wait for treatment.
- Being aware of the skills of your colleagues, who may be able to offer alternative and effective approaches.
- Using innovative strategies to improve access to CBT in MDT settings (see section 'Improving access to CBT in MDT settings').

Waiting lists

The level of CBT resources in an MDT will influence whether or not you need to have a waiting list. The alternative of accepting referrals only when a treatment space is available does not provide an equitable system to all, which many therapists find ethically unacceptable, and amounts to a waiting list anyway, since patients who are in need will usually be re-referred. Not having a waiting list for treatment may also mask excess demand for a service, thus reducing the likelihood of resources being increased to match the actual demand. Therefore, for many CBT therapists in MDTs, as in other services, waiting lists are the lesser of two evils.

Offering assessment to patients soon after referral is usually good practice in order to clarify that they are suitable for CBT and to identify which modality of treatment may be most appropriate. This triaging process can help to identify suitable patients for junior colleagues, trainees, and for groups.

Government and local service targets to reduce waiting times have encouraged CBT therapists to consider new and different ways of working (see Section Improving access to CBT in MDT's). Having *some* waiting time for CBT may actually have some advantages:

- Where patients have had some form of early assessment involving sharing a preliminary formulation of their problems, or being given self-help materials, they may have the opportunity to think these through or begin to make changes on their own, thus increasing their readiness for therapy when it is offered.

- An awareness that the demand for CBT is high may enhance patient engagement in CBT and also encourage therapists to adhere to CBT protocols (Waller, 2009).

Nevertheless difficulties clearly arise when waits for treatment are excessive and patients do not receive appropriate treatment in a timely fashion. This can lead to pressures from colleagues to prioritize some patients.

Pressure from colleagues to see patients

You may be under pressure from other MDT members to see a specific patient more quickly than others who are further up the waiting list. This presents an ethical dilemma as prioritizing one patient means another has to wait even longer (see Chapter 4). Although the general rule should be to see people in order of referral, there may be a number of good reasons to prioritize some patients over others. Reasons to prioritize may include:

- Risk of suicide or harm to others
- Risk of significant deterioration of psychological state
- Risk of adverse changes to life circumstances (e.g. loss of job or educational opportunities, or breakdown of family or other relationships)

Such decisions will depend on other resources available in the team, and should be made with the MDT as a whole, taking into account the other patients on the wait list, what their needs and current supports are, and what other resources are available in the team. This encourages collaborative working within the MDT and means that the responsibility is shared, so that you are better supported.

Where there are less clear reasons to see people sooner, despite the fact that they may be helped by the CBT, you could consider other options to improve access to CBT in MDT settings.

Improving access to CBT in MDT settings

Other chapters in this book describe how to use innovative methods of delivering CBT in order to improve access for patients (see Chapters 6, 8, and 10). Many of these principles can be adopted by CBT therapists in MDT settings and some examples are outlined below.

Guided self-help

CBT therapists are often in the position of providing self-help materials for MDT colleagues to use with their patients. If they are going to be able to use these materials successfully, you need to take time to explain how to use self-help and, ideally, to supervise or support your MDT colleagues in working with patients in this way. This could be done via team-wide education slots or on an individual basis, as described in Example 11.7.

Example 11.7 Assisting a colleague to deliver CBT guided self-help

John, a community psychiatric nurse (CPN), was seeing a patient who had been recently discharged from an acute inpatient ward. The patient still had moderate levels of depression and was relatively inactive. The first stage of psychological treatment for this patient was for the CBT therapist to provide the CPN with an appropriate CBT self-help guide on managing depression and advise the CPN on working through the booklet with his patient. The CBT therapist guided the CPN to review each section of the self-help with his patient and to actively practise the exercises outlined. With support from the CPN, the patient was able to read the booklet and succeeded in becoming more active, resulting in an improvement in his mood.

Example 11.7 shows how you can work through others to provide guided self-help with the added bonus of improving awareness of CBT techniques.

CBT groups (See also chapter 8 CBT groups)

A specific advantage of running groups in an MDT is the opportunity to involve other MDT staff in their planning and delivery, which can offer opportunities for joint working and skills training. Working with other MDT staff enhances the quality and diversity of skills on offer to patients, particularly those with more complex and severe problems. It can also be great fun and can help to forge strong working relationships with your colleagues. In order for groups to be cost-effective you will need to identify a 'critical mass' of patients who would be suitable and will attend, and ideally for groups to be repeated so that preparation and planning time is recouped (see Example 11.8).

Example 11.8 A CBT group for people with bipolar disorder

In one service the wait for treatment had become lengthy. When the CBT therapist reviewed the waiting list, he identified 8 people needing treatment to help manage mood swings. These people were invited to attend a group. The group was also opened up to other patients in the MDT. Ultimately, 15 people were invited to attend, 10 attended and 8 completed group treatment. This group used 2 hours of a CBT practitioner's time for 8 weeks, treating 8 patients. An additional half hour was spent before and after the group to plan the session and debrief. Although more time was invested initially in planning the group programme, the materials were then available as a resource to provide a 'rolling programme' to this team and other teams in the region. Further advantages included two MDT colleagues gaining some training in CBT techniques for people with mood swings.

For the MDT, therefore, the group represented both the provision of a cost-effective clinical resource for patients with mood swings and an opportunity for skills development for staff.

Drop in or rapid access clinics

This approach requires skill and resilience from the CBT therapist. It was important to allocate adequate time after the clinic to complete notes, reflect, note possible plans for the next session, and generally have a breather! The benefits of such an approach when resources are scarce include the following (see Example 11.9):

Example 11.9 CBT drop-in clinic

Patients were offered rapid access through attendance at a drop-in clinic run by a CBT therapist. The group ran for one morning a week and offered half-hour appointments. Following an appointment, patients could book their next appointment with the therapist or ring the MDT secretary who had a list of available slots in the clinic. Appointments were on a first come first served basis. Patients were not able to book more than one appointment at a time. The frequency of drop-in appointments was determined by the number of patients using the clinic (i.e. more patients led to less availability of appointments). Where appropriate, patients were also given CBT self-help materials which they were encouraged to use in conjunction with the clinic. CBT interventions in the clinic focused mainly on conceptualizing difficulties, offering guided self-help, problem-solving, or behavioural activation strategies.

- Waiting times for at least some CBT input are reduced.
- The therapist can carry out the triaging tasks identified above more efficiently (e.g. assessing motivation, and identifying those who may benefit more from another therapy, those who need more intensive CBT interventions, or those who may require support from other MDT members).
- It also creates opportunities for more informed case discussion and care planning with MDT colleagues.

You will have to make careful judgements about whether investing the time to establish and run novel models of service delivery is justified, taking account of the somewhat reduced availability of individual therapy that may result from you using your time in this way, and the clinical outcomes attained. Evaluation of service innovations is vital, as is negotiation with the MDT, so that the implications of changes to service delivery are clear and can be supported (see Chapter 18).

Key points

- MDT working can be enormously rewarding. It provides you with opportunities to work much more broadly and to have a greater impact than would be possible working alone. It can enable you to use and develop your knowledge and skills as a CBT therapist and become more effective.
- The main challenges for the CBT therapist working in the MDT are role clarity, resolving conflicts, and how to manage limited resources. Solutions may include:

  Role clarity:

  - Clarify your role and communicate this to your colleagues through attending team meetings, joint work, consultation and training, and supervising others.

  Role conflict:

  - Be alert to possible role conflicts around being both a generic team member and a CBT therapist.
  - Clarify what is expected around both aspects of your role and communicate this to the MDT.

  Conflicting theoretical models:

  - Your non-medical approach adds value to team clinical discussions.
  - CBT skills (e.g. formulation) can be used to help teams resolve conflicts about clinical issues.

  Limited resources in MDTs

  - Waiting lists allow for greater equity of access but need to be minimized.
  - Patients must be prioritized according to clear rationales and in collaboration with the MDT.
  - Improving access to CBT in an MDT setting may require adapting new ways of working. Any such innovations should be carefully evaluated.
  - Access can be improved further through disseminating CBT skills via training and supervision.

Further reading

Lake, N. (2008). Developing skills in consultation 2: a team formulation approach. *Clinical Psychology Forum*, **186**, 18–24.

Onyett, S. (2007). *New Ways of Working for Applied Psychologists in Health and Social Care: Working Psychologically in Teams.* British Psychological Society. Available at: http://www.bps.org.uk/document-download-area/document-download$.cfm?file_uuid=12B7C9B9-1143-DFD0-7E1C-75AEDF90F941&ext=pdf (accessed 3 September 2009).

Veale, D. (2008). Psychotherapy in dissent. *Therapy Today*, February Issue, 4–7.

References

Grey, N., Salkovskis, P., Quigley, A., Clark, D. and Ehlers, A. (2008). Dissemination of cognitive therapy for panic disorder in primary care. *Behavioural and Cognitive Psychotherapy*, **36**, 509–520.

Care Quality Commission (2008). *NHS National Staff Survey.* Available at: http://www.cqc.org.uk/_db/_documents/NHSStaffSurvey_Nat_briefing_final_200904233323.pdf (accessed 5 September 2009).

Lake, N. (2008). Developing skills in consultation 2: a team formulation approach. *Clinical Psychology Forum*, **186**, 18–24.

Mannix, K., Blackburn, I.M., Garland, A., Gracie, J., Moorey, S., Reid, B., Standart, S. and Scott, J. (2006). Effectiveness of brief training in cognitive behaviour therapy techniques for palliative care practitioners. *Palliative Medicine*, **20**, 579–584.

Mansell, W. (2008). The seven C's of CBT: a consideration of the future challenges for cognitive behaviour therapy. *Behavioural and Cognitive Psychotherapy*, **36**, 641–649.

Onyett, S. (2007). *New Ways of Working for Applied Psychologists in Health and Social Care: Working Psychologically in Teams.* British Psychological Society. Available at: http://www.bps.org.uk/document-download-area/document-download$.cfm?file_uuid=12B7C9B9-1143-DFD0-7E1C-75AEDF90F941&ext=pdf (accessed 3 September 2009).

Tuckman, B.W. (1965). Developmental sequence in small groups. *Psychological Bulletin*, **63**(6), 384–399.

Veale, D. (2008). Psychotherapy in dissent. *Therapy Today*, February Issue, 4–7.

Waller, G. (2009). Evidence-based treatment and therapist drift. *Behaviour Research and Therapy*, **47**, 119–127.

Chapter 12

CBT with inpatients in mental health settings

Patsy Holly, Nicky Boughton, and Jill Roberts

You have recently qualified as a CBT therapist and are keen and enthusiastic to start your new job working in an inpatient unit. When you arrive you discover you have no idea what you are expected to do—the ward has never had a CBT therapist before and you need to decide what is the best use of your time on the ward. Should you run some groups for all patients to attend? Or offer individual CBT to a select few? If so, how do you decide which patients are most likely to benefit from your intervention? Or should you be working with the other staff to increase their skills or provide support in their work? Or should you be making a contribution to the overall organization and activity programme of the ward?

Although the evidence base for cognitive behavioural therapy (CBT) in inpatient settings is at a very early stage, National Institute for Clinical Excellence (NICE) guidelines recommend CBT as a treatment of choice for many of the diagnoses that cause people to be admitted as inpatients (e.g. eating disorders, depression). As many CBT therapists are employed in inpatient settings, opportunities arise for group and individual work as well as for teaching CBT skills to the wider team. This chapter outlines the main challenges in using CBT in inpatient settings and makes suggestions for how CBT protocols can be adapted for use in such settings. Clinical examples are used to illustrate key points with the aim of showing how CBT can make an invaluable addition to standard nursing and medical care.

Background: inpatient settings

Inpatient mental health services accommodate the full age range and specialist (tertiary) services are available to treat conditions such as eating disorders, personality disorders, and forensic problems. Inpatient admissions are often preceded by negative life events and/or crises and the admission may be against the patient's will. The main challenges associated with using CBT in inpatient settings are outlined below.

Patients who are admitted for inpatient care tend to have more chronic, severe, and complex problems, and frequently have co-morbid diagnoses or physical health or social issues too. Often safety is a more immediately pressing issue for inpatients because symptoms commonly include severe depression, psychosis, serious self-neglect and self-harm. Because of their severity, these problems can carry an attendant risk of suicide, and in some cases, risk of harm to others. Inpatients may be in poor physical health, sometimes as a consequence of their disorder: self-neglect associated with depression or psychosis, starvation associated with anorexia nervosa, self-harm in the context of heightened distress or the effects of substance misuse. The greater severity of symptoms and the inpatient setting pose particular challenges for the CBT therapist. Some difficulties relate to the types of patient that are typically seen in inpatient settings—the difficulties inherent in working with more severe problems/fragile patients who may not have given the same degree of consent to treatment as those who receive CBT on an outpatient basis (e.g. those admitted involuntarily or who are [at best] ambivalent about the need to be an inpatient). Some arise from the setting itself—those relating to integrating CBT within the overall treatment approach and team, to issues of privacy/boundaries, and the 'artificiality' of the environment. These challenges are outlined and addressed below.

The case for inpatient CBT

Although the evidence base for CBT in inpatient settings is at an early stage, initial studies report promising results for inpatient CBT for psychosis (Drury *et al.*, 1996; Lewis *et al.*, 2002; Startup *et al.*, 2004; Tarrier *et al.*, 2004) and for the cognitive behavioural treatment of low self-esteem in patients with psychosis (Hall and Tarrier, 2003) and for acceptance and commitment therapy in an inpatient setting (Gaudiano and Herbert, 2006). Stuart and Bowers' review of inpatient CBT (1995) concludes that CBT has benefits both as a primary treatment and as an adjunct to antidepressant medication. In addition, NICE guidelines strengthen the case for inpatient CBT by recommending it for people with depression (2004a), eating disorders (2004b), self-harm (2004c), post-traumatic stress disorder (PTSD; 2005a), bipolar disorder (2006), and schizophrenia (2009): all problems with which inpatients are frequently admitted. NICE also recommends the use of CBT for obsessive compulsive disorder (OCD; 2005b) and anxiety (2007), which are common additional problems for inpatients (http://www.nice.org).

All the reasons why we use CBT in outpatient work apply to inpatient settings too, but particular benefits to using CBT in inpatient settings include the following:

- The theoretical basis of CBT and its formulation-driven nature mean that it is well-placed to help inpatient teams adopt a coherent approach by providing a coherent rationale for treatment decisions and developing a team formulation.
- CBT therapists can make full use of all their skills and knowledge when working with patients and staff teams in inpatient settings: providing individual and group therapy, teaching ward staff about CBT and supervising them putting it into practice; as well as using CBT techniques to support staff in their work.
- CBT interventions can complement other forms of inpatient work, such as occupational therapy or psychoeducation, which promote attainment of the patient's goals, making the ward a more therapeutic environment and helping the patient on the road to recovery. The ongoing challenge for you may be how to integrate the various facets of treatment, such as group work, and psychiatric monitoring, with individual CBT.
- CBT skills, and the focus on collaboration, may be particularly effective in motivating and engaging patients who are ambivalent about their admission to hospital: it enables you to come alongside and work with them, giving patients a sense of having some say in their treatment, rather than feeling they have no control over it.

General principles

Severity of symptoms

Inpatients are typically more mentally and physically fragile, with lower distress tolerance than community patients. Being mindful of this heightened susceptibility to distress and perhaps acting upon it when necessary is amongst the most important principles for carrying out CBT in inpatient settings. Close liaison with the wider team, who might be dealing with the 'fallout' of your individual or group therapy session, is crucial. Important information needs to be communicated to the team, to enable increased support to be provided after a difficult therapy session, where there might be an increased risk of self-harm; or the background provided to some otherwise unaccountable behaviour. For example, if a normally passive patient runs off the ward and comes back drunk, the staff may be left mystified. If, however, the individual therapist shares with the ward staff the fact that an incident of abuse has been discussed for the first time in the individual session, then the mystery is solved and ward staff are able to offer the appropriate support and understanding.

The presence of severe symptoms, problems with concentration, or cognitive impairments might necessitate modification to standard CBT protocols, at least at the start of treatment, when the patient is severely ill. These modifications could include working at a more behavioural level to begin with; for example, the use of activity scheduling with lethargic patients, or an increased focus on coping skills training for patients with severe and distressing symptoms. In longer-stay units, where patients may have secondary social impairments, an increased focus on social awareness and developing social skills may be helpful, with the aim of giving the patient the best chance of being rehabilitated into the community.

The inpatient setting

CBT with inpatients may be distinguished from the average outpatient treatment, by the very fact that patients receive multidisciplinary input into their care and as a result the work is more intensive. For the patient, CBT sits within a mixture of treatment influences, any of which can reinforce a sense of hope that change is possible, and that problems can be resolved. This may mean that therapists find it difficult to isolate the effects of CBT from those of other treatment influences: thus making it more difficult to evaluate and plan what to do next in a session.

So, to summarize, there are three main additional treatment influences to think about when using CBT in an inpatient environment: the provision of 24-hour care within a structured environment; the combination of treatments available; and greater attention to social and occupational functioning.

The provision of 24-hour care within a structured environment

The patient is supported in the process of recovery, and nursing staff in particular can support patients through any untowards effects of CBT; for example, distressing flashbacks and urges to self-harm following a disclosure of sexual abuse. This allows for therapy to continue with safety mechanisms in place. This higher level of structure provided may be of particular benefit to the more severely ill patients and those with disorganized or chaotic thinking.

The combination of treatments available

An example of the combination of treatments typically available is the provision of regular meals and physical health checks, the closer monitoring of pharmacological interventions, and supportive counselling provided by ward staff as well as input from other professions such as occupational therapy, physiotherapy, or even chiropody. These interventions can effect a change in the patient's state and symptoms, allowing the patient to make better use of specific CBT techniques, such as thought challenging. Improved physical health is helpful, and often especially relevant to those patients who are admitted to hospital. Being in hospital means that physical neglect can be directly addressed, which is not so easily achieved in an outpatient setting. A strength of CBT in this setting is that it directly addresses the interaction of physiology, thoughts, emotions, and behaviour: we know that changes in one domain will impact on the others. From the start of treatment, the need for overall self-care can be reinforced. This can bring up powerful self-beliefs, such as 'I am not worth looking after' or 'I don't deserve to be well', which can be addressed with CBT techniques and with team input. The increased focus on physical well-being is also helpful for inpatients who find it difficult to articulate their thoughts and feelings. Inpatient staff can observe the patient 24 hours a day, and are able to gather information on bodily symptoms. Bodily symptoms can be a powerful prompt to attend to emotions before they escalate. Anxiety, depression, or anger can be picked up through an awareness of somatic symptoms, and this awareness can increase the patient's understanding of their emotional state. A simple question such as 'where do you feel it in your body?' can be useful. Working at a physical level, perhaps through mindfulness approaches or relaxation techniques, can decrease arousal, agitation, and fatigue; it can, therefore, make flexible thinking more of a possibility, as indicated in Examples 12.1 and 12.2.

Example 12.1 Being in the here and now

A regular slot is set aside for some gentle stretches on an inpatient unit. It has been valuable not only in reducing levels of arousal and anxiety, but in allowing people to give themselves the opportunity to stop—a space to 'be' rather than 'do'. There is a powerful message here about the importance of focusing on the here and now, and it being okay to give some time to one's own well-being. Thoughts relating to 'I don't deserve this' or 'I have to keep striving all the time' can be addressed, and a different perspective sought.

Example 12.2 Benefiting from structured activity

A group of young men on an inpatient unit were all experiencing motivational problems as a consequence of psychotic illness and the impact of sedating anti-psychotic medication. They were encouraged to join a gym group and shown how to fill in ratings of their mood, pleasure, and satisfaction levels, both before and after the gym session; they were asked to focus on how they felt 'in their body'. Over time, this enabled the men to think more carefully about how they felt before and after exercising, about their goals for exercise, and how the use of exercise might help them to feel better physically and mentally in the longer term. Another benefit was that after having this positive experience they became more amenable to joining in other therapeutic activities on the ward.

Inpatient units pay greater attention to social and occupational functioning

Examples include help dealing with financial matters and housing issues, and identifying occupational goals. These are often key issues when working with complex cases. There are also inherent challenges for patients being admitted to inpatient units, such as having to share living space, having to deal with other distressed patients, fluctuating staff levels, and not having the control over their own environment that most people have outside of this setting (e.g. choosing what time to get up and go to sleep, what and when to eat, and how to spend your time). CBT may be used to help the patient deal with these challenges effectively by developing skills in problem-solving and tolerating situations that one cannot change.

Inpatient CBT therefore offers opportunities to work with the system at various levels, going beyond the normative community model, which has emphasized individual once-a-week-for-an-hour CBT. You can work with staff teams, in groups, and with individual CBT. In any event, it is worth thinking about your level of intervention in advance, consulting colleagues and patients, and setting a review period, in order to evaluate the benefits of the model adopted, or to amend the approach taken where necessary.

Indirect ways of working

It can be helpful for the wider inpatient staff team to learn more about CBT for four main reasons: to support staff in delivering CBT interventions and to embed CBT within the ward milieu; to provide a safe setting for behavioural experiments; to develop a coherent approach to the patient's treatment by utilizing CBT formulations, and as a tool for staff reflection.

Supporting staff delivering CBT

The structure offered by inpatient units lends itself to using staff members to reinforce CBT principles and techniques and staff members can find this beneficial in their work. CBT principles and methods can be readily assimilated into inpatient units' standard working practices; for example, you can train and supervise staff in the delivery of specific techniques such as diary keeping, activity scheduling, and positive data logs. These can be introduced into patients' care-plans, and regularly reviewed. In this way, team members can reinforce CBT principles and techniques, making the intervention more powerful. Example 12.3 illustrates the benefits of integrating CBT in the inpatient environment.

Example 12.3 Benefits of integrating CBT in the inpatient environment

Fiona was struggling during her second admission for depression. She had powerful, self-critical thoughts related to her admission; for example, 'I am failing, I am not good enough, I am not trying hard enough, it is all going wrong again'. Starting a positive data log was extremely valuable, particularly as all members of the multidisciplinary team could be involved. The CBT therapist worked with her to develop a record sheet for recording relevant information, and her named nurse and other staff helped her to identify relevant information—any evidence that things were going well, that she was putting effort into her recovery, or that she was engaged with those who were trying to help her. Having input from the nursing team and from the occupational therapist to help her record when things were going well made the written work she was doing much more meaningful. These weekly sheets were also very useful to look back on, in order to challenge more catastrophic thoughts such as 'I have achieved nothing while I have been here'.

A safe setting for behavioural experiments

Inpatient settings provide an excellent opportunity to assess the validity of fresh perspectives through experience in a safe, controlled, and supportive environment. Behavioural experiments are a particularly powerful method for bringing about enduring change in unhelpful thinking and related unhelpful behaviours because they include an active as well as a reflective component (for more information on designing effective behavioural experiments, see Bennett-Levy *et al.*, 2004). Behavioural experiments can be used to optimize learning from the work with the wider inpatient team in the absence of formal CBT by encouraging patients to actively test the impact of changes in routine, medication, self-care, social support, or activity levels. They are, of course, also an integral part of individual or group-based CBT.

The inpatient setting uniquely provides the supportive environment necessary for behavioural experiments which may be too difficult or unsafe in other, less supported environments. It can be especially helpful to use behavioural experimentation to test:

- Facilitative beliefs that fuel self-injurious behaviour and avoidance of affect.
- The utility of adaptive coping strategies.
- Interpersonal beliefs and coping styles, including unhelpful beliefs about withdrawal and social isolation.

This obviously requires good communication between team members in order to ensure consistency of approach, and handover of important information. As we have already noted, effective team communication is an important goal for the inpatient CBT therapist. Example 12.4 shows a behavioural experiment to test interpersonal safety.

Example 12.4 Behavioural experiment to test interpersonal safety

Jane's mood had dropped profoundly after a violent incident at her place of work triggered severe and disabling flashbacks to abusive experiences in childhood. The primary goal for her admission to an acute ward was to keep her safe while she learned adaptive coping strategies to manage her unwanted memories.

Original cognition: If I allow a male nurse to sit with me when I am distressed, he will take advantage of my vulnerability, or I'll end up falling apart.

Alternative: I'm much more able to manage the flashbacks now so I won't fall apart and not all men are abusers.

Experiment: Jane allowed a male nurse to sit next to her and offer support following her individual CBT session.

Results: Jane was able to apply her discrimination skills well. She found the male nurse's supportive use of humour really helpful, in recovering from an intensive CBT session. This experience allowed Jane to carry out further experiments to address her fears about the company of men in the safe and controlled environment of the ward.

CBT case formulation

You can use your CBT knowledge and skills to develop cognitive behavioural case formulations with inpatient teams; this can make a uniquely valuable contribution in the ward environment. Kennedy (2009) argues that case formulation provides a more compassionate narrative than the traditional medical model in inpatient settings, thereby benefiting both patients and those in helping roles. Berry *et al.* (2009) also report that CBT case formulations have a positive influence on staff perceptions of inpatients with psychosis. As well as progressing beyond diagnostic conceptualizations, CBT case formulations are important in developing hypotheses about an inpatient's problems. These hypotheses can be tested and refined over time, and you can support the team in this process. Furthermore, because inpatients are observed on a 24-hour basis, there is richness and detail to the case formulation that may not be achievable in outpatient settings. The usefulness of a formulation in developing the team's understanding is illustrated by Example 12.5.

Example 12.5 Case formulation in developing the team's understanding

Since her admission Valerie had remained isolated on the ward and she did not respond to offers of 'one-to-one' time with the nursing team. During group supervision sessions with the wider team, the CBT therapist was able to share Valerie's developing formulation of her difficulties. Valerie's early experiences of abuse led her to have very fixed assumptions about both asking for and receiving help. She believed 'if I ask for help I will be ridiculed', as sadly this had happened in her childhood. She also had deep-seated beliefs about her own lack of worth, and so she felt she did not deserve help, even if it was offered. By linking her present behaviour to past events, and deep-seated beliefs, the CBT therapist was able to help the team to make sense of her perceived unresponsiveness and rejecting stance, and devise ways of encouraging her to accept the help that was offered and thus be able to meet her goals of being more open and able to accept help.

For more information on developing and using CBT formulations, see Kuyken *et al.* (2009).

CBT as a tool for staff reflection

The team can also be encouraged to think about their own reactions to a patient, which could hinder the patient's progress. Inpatient staff can be asked to reflect on 'what we observe in a patient'; then, 'what the patient pulls from us'; then, to complete the process, 'how we unhook from this'. This is an excellent example of a technique that has been developed from CBT, which allows all members of the team to work together in order to increase their understanding of individual patients (Safran, 1996).

Direct work with inpatients

CBT inpatient settings can involve direct work with inpatients, as in CBT group therapy and one-to-one work, which we shall discuss in turn.

Group work

Issues relating to group CBT are discussed in more detail in Chapter 8. CBT therapy groups can run alongside individual CBT or independently of it. CBT groups can increase access to CBT for a wider body of inpatients, who might not otherwise have access to it. For example, it might just be possible to envisage trying a CBT group for patients suffering from psychosis when they are inpatients, when scheduling and attendance and safety issues might render this difficult in an outpatient setting. The type of group offered will depend largely on the nature of the unit, and the average length of inpatient stay. For example, a brief 'open' group with a very specific stand-alone agenda for each session might be suitable on an acute admission unit, where the length of stay is relatively short. By contrast, long-stay units, such as forensic units, offer opportunities to develop 'closed' groups with long-term agendas, addressing specific problem areas, such as cognitive distortions in relation to offending behaviour. Group programmes on inpatient units can create a greater visibility for CBT than individual therapy alone, thereby contributing to the increased recognition of the scope and potential of CBT approaches (Hill *et al.*, 2009). Groups have the additional benefits of peer support and learning from each other (see Chapter 8), as illustrated by Example 12.6.

Example 12.6 Benefits of peer support and learning from each other

In the final session of a 10-week self-esteem group, patients circulated sheets of paper (one for each group member) and wrote down one positive comment about that group member. Then each person read out the list of positive comments that had been compiled for them. This challenged many deep-rooted beliefs about having no good qualities at all, and also the fear that developing a more robust view of the self would result in becoming 'big headed and arrogant'. Generating alternative viewpoints from fellow patients, rather than staff members, had great value, as staff comments are sometimes discounted—'you have to say that; it's your job to be nice to me'—although these thoughts too can be considered and discussed. In addition, the fact that these patients spent considerable amounts of time in each other's company allowed for the comments to be more evidence based, and examples of the positive qualities could be elaborated upon.

Individual therapy

The unpredictability of the length of inpatient stays presents a challenge for individual CBT—you may need to set your therapy goals with the length of stay in mind. However, many inpatient units now have some facility for continuing CBT as an outpatient and some brief, focused CBT interventions can be achieved even in short inpatient admissions. For example, you might work on developing a formulation to understand the events that precipitated the admission, or carry out a specific behavioural experiment, such as examining the effects of sleep on elevated mood or irritability. Opportunities to build the therapy relationship may be limited where the length of stay is relatively brief, but the relationship has a chance to develop with longer-stay patients (e.g. in specialist units treating eating disorders, OCD, or forensic problems). There are several additional factors to think about before commencing one-to-one work on inpatient units, which are broadly applicable to other aspects of CBT inpatient work.

Getting started

Given the constraints of the inpatient setting, assessing suitability for individual CBT is of paramount importance. Factors likely to influence the viability of individual CBT include both the likely length of stay and the patient's current state. Both of these will impact on the setting of appropriate goals for therapy, which may not be to achieve complete remission from severe depression in a 3-week admission, but to develop a CBT formulation and/or learn some specific CBT techniques for managing low mood.

To begin, it can be hard to find a suitable room for the therapy, as any therapist working in the NHS (National Health Service) will know. In addition, privacy may be compromised on an inpatient unit, owing to lack of space, and requirements for increased observation. A calm environment and dedicated therapeutic space is desirable, if not always available. As a last resort, it might be possible to see a patient in his or her own bedroom, but you need to gauge the suitability of doing this. If the therapy involves uncovering difficult memories, it may be better not to associate this with the patient's private space and to keep this as a place of sanctuary. It is worth giving special thought to the factors that can inhibit disclosure, while trying to create a trusting therapeutic relationship. Inpatients have little autonomy, and they understandably fear that disclosing symptoms may be met with overreaction from professionals, with further consequences for their liberty, such as loss of leave into the community. Given that a patient's cooperation is crucial if progress is to be made, it is useful to discuss this in an upfront manner. It is always best to be clear about the limits of confidentiality. Where information does need to be handed over, the patient's understanding and involvement should be sought, even if agreement is not always possible. It goes without saying that it remains crucial to follow the policies and procedures of the particular inpatient environment, for safety reasons.

As we have already noted, inpatients are typically distinguished from community patients by the severity of their symptoms. Thus, it may be better to wait until the patient's mental health is at a receptive level before embarking on a course of CBT. This can be discussed with the inpatient treatment team, who are well-placed to contribute to an informed decision about starting individual CBT, because they see patients intensively on a day-to-day basis. It is naturally important where severe symptoms are involved not to focus too soon on upsetting thoughts. Shorter sessions are advisable for patients who struggle to concentrate, and written summaries may help patients to retain the content of the session. The 'pacing' of the session needs to be closely monitored, while engaging the patient in assessing what is suitable. Simple enquiries are important as is delivering the message that shows you are interested in the patient's experience of therapy. At the same time, it is useful to pay attention to non-verbal communications that may contradict ostensible agreement, such as distraction or agitation. Clearly, the matters discussed in this section relate equally to outpatient work, but they take on increased significance in an inpatient context, because inpatients are more likely to be distressed, agitated, or physically unwell, not least as a result of living in an artificial environment with lack of access to the everyday interactions of normal life.

Both voluntary and involuntary admissions can evoke a mixture of feelings, which can affect motivation to engage with treatment on any level. An outpatient might choose, of course, not to turn up to a session, but the inpatient therapist can seek out a patient who does not arrive at an allotted time. It is especially helpful to give careful thought to the matters of consent and maintaining the essential collaborative stance of CBT. A good way to set about ameliorating problems is to discuss with the patients their feelings about their admission, and about seeing you. It is also helpful to explore their previous experiences of treatment, including what has worked before, their strengths and assets, and to watch out for any patterns of relating that could affect engagement; for example, the tendency to withdraw when upset, or the tendency to agree to treatment without necessarily knowing the full implications.

Remain goal focused

As always, the goals of CBT need to be agreed with the patient; even more so where a patient has been detained in hospital against his/her will. CBT therapy goals should be consistent with the broader package of inpatient interventions, in order that the full program of treatment and care operates in unison. Goals need to be realistic and achievable. Long-term goals may seem distant, but these can be broken down into a set of more readily achievable short-term goals. Remaining goal-focused with inpatients can be difficult; digressions frequently occur and there may be times when the patient's goals are superseded by more urgent and immediate concerns surrounding the patient's safety. This contradiction exists in outpatient work but is more pronounced with inpatients because of the greater fragility in the patient's mental state. Agreement on the goals of therapy may also prove difficult if the patient and therapist do not share a conceptualization of the problem (or even that a problem exists!): this is particularly relevant where a patient has been involuntarily admitted. One way of overcoming this disparity is to ensure that the team gives clear and consistent information to the patient about what needs to be done to achieve the patient's goals. It is always helpful to allow the patient time to think about what goals he or she would like to achieve, and whether a trial of CBT might help in attaining those goals.

Other obstacles to change include the inpatient's (and possibly your) fluctuating motivation, the slow pace of change, and the increased potential for ruptures to the therapy relationship where an inpatient has an increased sense of vulnerability in interpersonal relationships. When working with inpatients, change occurs slowly, crises are common, fluctuations tend to be more marked, and progress can be affected by events on the ward, or the adverse effect of being surrounded by other distressed patients. We frequently see people who have had more than one admission (the so-called 'revolving door' patients): individual CBT can be a real opportunity to explore specific beliefs and thoughts about repeated treatment. Beliefs about staff attitudes—'they have given up on me' or 'they are fed up with me'—can be explored and discussed to prevent them from getting in the way of the patient making the most of the admission. It is important to instil a sense of hope that change can occur, but without making false promises. Seemingly modest gains are an important and significant step forward for many inpatients. For therapists working in this setting, it is important not to get caught up in feeling defeated or self-critical thinking. Therapists can be helped by attending to their own self-care, utilizing supervision and support, and applying basic CBT to their own practice; for example, examining beliefs around perfection (see Chapter 20).

When problems arise in individual CBT in an inpatient setting, it may be more than usually difficult to know when and how to challenge a patient's belief or behaviour (e.g. about not completing homework), owing to the greater fragility of his/her mental state. Once the relationship has been established, and the patient understands that you have his or her best interests at heart, you ought not to be afraid to challenge the patient constructively, as illustrated by Example 12.7.

Example 12.7 Challenging constructively

Karen was receiving treatment on an acute admission ward, following an episode of psychosis that had been triggered by separation from her boyfriend, money worries, and stopping prescribed medication. She was well-known to the therapist who had worked with her in the community. Karen's mood fluctuated during sessions, alternating between sadness and angry outbursts. Entries in her clinical notes made reference to episodes of shouting, and ward staff described her behaviour as intimidating. Invariably, this resulted in a negative cycle of loss of leave into the community, increasing her frustration levels, which triggered further outbursts. Empathizing with Karen's distress and frustration was an important first step in getting her to think about how to move forward. Although ward staff were intimidated by her behaviour and thus avoided challenging her angry outbursts, the CBT therapist was able to draw out a maintenance cycle of frustration leading to shouting, which in turn produced negative reactions from others and consequently greater frustration. Karen was able to reflect that this was unhelpful, and left her feeling 'out of control'. Karen agreed to try some more adaptive ways of managing feelings of frustration; these included using thought records and problem-solving techniques to manage feelings of frustration, seeking support, and joining relaxation sessions. Her shouting diminished, and with it, she and the team were able to build more positive relationships with the consequence that staff gained confidence in her ability to stay safe and calm inside and outside of the ward, and thus she had more control over the situations that triggered her frustration.

Work with the complex network of relationships

CBT with inpatients is distinguished by the greater need to attend closely to a whole network of relationships: therapist and patient, patient and team, and therapist and team, so personal self-awareness is required in terms of relating to the team and to the patient. Challenges to any one relationship can affect another: for example, lack of agreement between you and the team can be an obstacle to progress for the patient, owing to inconsistent care (see also Chapter 11). Disagreement among team members tends to be more pronounced when working with patients with complex needs, and where care is given by several professionals simultaneously (as happens on inpatient units). Disagreements and contradictions are therefore inevitable on inpatient units. Ultimately, agreement needs to be reached, so taking time to understand each other's position is desirable. Generally, the best way of achieving this is to stand outside of difficult dynamics, attempt to understand why people think as they do, peruse any evidence supporting alternative points of view, and review as objectively as possible one's own viewpoint. Use of the CBT case formulation is advisable, as illustrated by Example 12.8.

There are some important qualities that therapists can bring to their work

Example 12.8 Use of the CBT case formulation

Lesley was approaching the end of a period of intensive in- and day-patient treatment. Her commitment to the treatment programme had been erratic, and she had been strongly advised to commit fully to the final 3 weeks of the intensive programme. However, in her individual CBT session, Lesley argued that her daily time on the ward should be reduced, so that she could have meals at home with her children. She had resisted spending time with her children, so as to avoid the activation of her underlying belief that she was not a good mother. By now choosing to address this belief—by spending more time with her family—she was working towards one of her overall goals in a definite way. Her therapist was able to discuss this hypothesis with the wider team, and present Lesley's wishes as a way of working towards important therapy goals, thereby minimizing the risk of polarized responses within the team. The team agreed that this strategy was a good behavioural experiment: it enabled Lesley to work on her beliefs, with ongoing support from staff on the ward.

with inpatients. Literature about the use of CBT with people with personality disorder makes a number of useful suggestions that are relevant to working with the kinds of patients that end up as inpatients. For example, Beck *et al.* (2004) suggest a range of desirable therapist characteristics, which include: a non-judgemental stance; the ability to set boundaries and to remain problem-focused; the ability to guide the patient towards realistic goals; sensitivity to the role of the patient's culture; a clear sense of personal limits and good personal awareness; the ability to model prosocial behaviour, and good use of self-care and coping strategies, including stress management strategies. These characteristics are equally useful when using CBT with inpatients, especially the qualities of personal self-awareness and the ability to set boundaries: because inpatients are very ill, their ability to set interpersonal boundaries may be compromised. You may also find that patients get to know more about you, perhaps through comparing experiences with other patients you see, and there is plenty of time for fellow patients on the ward to discuss their experiences in therapy, which can also have a negative effect. You may have shared more personal information with members of the ward team, which filters down to patients through the ward 'grape vine'. Practically speaking, if you see your patient around the ward, outside of a therapy session, other issues are going to arise. It may be useful to consider how you will respond to one patient's query about how another patient is being treated. The important thing is to be clear about boundaries; for example, you might say to a patient: 'I can't discuss Mary's situation with you; we need to focus on your situation'.

Inpatient units where long-term CBT is a feature bring greater familiarity with a patient, thereby running the risk of gradual erosion of boundaries, or of neutrality. Worrying signals include: special treatment being given to the patient, increased therapist self-disclosure, and failure to follow the rules or obligations of the unit. It is important that you make time to reflect on your work with distressed or severely ill patients, with a view to avoiding the problems detailed above. Broadly speaking, reflective practice involves reflecting on workplace practice and behaviours, with the aim of increasing confidence in dealing with the kind of ambiguous situations that often occur on inpatient units. Increasingly, reflective practice is seen as relevant for staff working on inpatient settings (Cowdrill and Dannahy, 2009). Ongoing and regular supervision, as always in CBT, is vital.

Attend to evaluation and termination issues

Terminating therapy with inpatients raises specific issues. In outpatient settings the boundaries tend to be clear; most services have a set number of sessions, which are offered and then come to an end, but in inpatient settings this is less clear, owing to the greater need to pace the therapy and the protracted engagement period. In addition, the decision as to when therapy should come to an end is more than usually difficult when patients have complex and multiple needs. Reviews with the patient and the team can be a key influence on the decision about when to terminate CBT. As always with CBT, it is important to collaborate with the patient and the team, and to have a clear rationale for stopping CBT, particularly if the decision is an unwelcome one for the patient, as illustrated by Example 12.9.

Example 12.9 Attending to termination issues

Jean was being seen for weekly CBT for her eating disorder, but therapy seemed to have reached an impasse: she could not complete homework tasks, keep a diary, or change her meal plan, and so she started to lose weight. She did, however, regularly attend, and she wanted to continue to do so, although she really was not making any progress. Eventually, her weight dropped to a dangerous level and her mental state deteriorated, so she was admitted for a short period of stabilization. She had been admitted to the same service many times in the past, and her treatment had included numerous sessions of cognitive therapy with experienced therapists: she thus expected to continue CBT as an inpatient. Reflecting on what had happened in the past, it was evident to the team that she had not been able to benefit from cognitive therapy. So, when she requested further individual CBT, the multidisciplinary team supported a decision not to offer it. Jean was hurt and angry and her reaction left her previous therapist feeling guilty. However, the whole team worked together to resist her demands and instead were able to consider how best to offer her support, primarily from the nursing team and occupational therapist, and help her gain the most from her time in hospital and prepare her for a different approach on discharge. This was carefully explained to Jean as a failure of matching appropriate treatment to her situation, rather than a failure on her behalf.

Towards the end of any admission, the CBT therapist can help the patient to plan behavioural experiments related to increased time at home, and use remaining therapy sessions to consolidate skills and generalize strategies to handle situations outside hospital. Common challenges following discharge include re-establishing relationships and explaining absences from work, or for young people, school. With inpatients it is especially important to effect the transfer of skills from the ward to the community, owing to the artificiality of the inpatient environment. Inpatients can find it difficult to reintegrate into society after separation from it, especially if the separation is prolonged, and they can feel stigmatized about having gone through the experience of hospitalization, and anxious about others' reactions on their return. The final therapy blueprint is particularly valuable, as discharge involves going home to a completely different setting and maybe a completely different therapist as well. Some useful questions for the blueprint include: 'What have you learned in hospital?' 'How can you apply this learning outside of the hospital?' 'What kinds of situations or events are likely to trigger a setback?' 'How can you best cope with these situations?' It is important to remind inpatients to revisit the blueprint after discharge from hospital. Relapse prevention work can also involve rehearsal of specific plans for dealing with setbacks.

Evaluating progress

Progress in CBT in inpatient settings can be evaluated using all the standard methods, such as: whether the goals of therapy have been achieved, measures of symptom change, specialized psychometric assessments, the use of therapist and patient opinions, and patient/team satisfaction ratings. Increased confidence in being able to cope with mental health difficulties, or perceived improvement in quality of life, may also be important measures for inpatients. Evaluation of CBT with inpatients can be difficult owing to its sitting within a mixture of therapeutic influences. It can also be difficult to evaluate progress where this is slow, or where fluctuations occur (as often happens on inpatient units). You may struggle to tease out the effects of specific factors (such as specialized techniques), from non-specific factors (such as being responded to with care and compassion), which may be equally important to inpatients.

Key points

1. While doing CBT with inpatients can be challenging, it is also especially rewarding to work with those with more severe and complex difficulties.
2. There is a case for CBT with inpatients, not least because NICE guidelines recommend it as the treatment of choice for the difficulties commonly found on inpatient wards. More research in the area is needed.
3. Careful thought has to be given as to how CBT is applied in inpatient settings. The interaction among individual CBT, group work, and other medical and psychiatric interventions needs to be considered.
4. Issues such as engagement and motivation, pace of therapy, and agreement on goals are more complicated in an inpatient setting, and so deserve special consideration.
5. CBT case formulation can be helpful in enabling team members to understand disagreements about care that can arise when working with inpatients, and has a special value on inpatient units.

Further reading

Clarke, I. and Wilson, H. (2009). *Cognitive Behaviour Therapy for Acute Inpatient Mental Health Units.* East Sussex: Routledge.

References

Beck, A., Freeman, A. and Davis, D. (2004). *Cognitive Therapy of Personality Disorders.* Second edition. New York: Guilford Press.

Bennett-Levy, J., Butler, G., Fennell, M., Hackmann, A., Mueller, M., Westbrook, D. and Rouf, K. (2004). *Oxford Guide to Behavioural Experiments in Cognitive Therapy.* Oxford: Oxford University Press.

Berry, K., Barrowclough, C. and Wearden, A. (2009). A pilot study investigating the use of psychological formulations to modify psychiatric staff perceptions of service users with psychosis. *Behavioural and Cognitive Psychotherapy*, **37**, 39–48.

Cowdrill, V. and Dannahy, L. (2009). Running reflective practice groups on an inpatient unit, in Clarke, I. and Wilson, H. (eds.), *Cognitive Behaviour Therapy for Acute Inpatient Mental Health Units.* East Sussex: Routledge.

Drury, V., Birchwood, M., Cochrane, R. and Macmillan, F. (1996). Cognitive therapy and recovery from acute psychosis: a controlled trial II. Impact on recovery time. *British Journal of Psychiatry*, **169**, 602–607.

Gaudiano, B.A. and Herbert, J.D. (2006). Acute treatment of inpatients with psychotic symptoms using acceptance and commitment therapy: pilot results. *Behaviour, Research and Therapy*, **44**, 415–437.

Hall, P.L. and Tarrier, N. (2003). The cognitive-behavioural treatment of low self-esteem in psychotic patients: a pilot study. *Behaviour, Research and Therapy*, **41**, 317–332.

Hill, G., Clarke, I. and Wilson, H. (2009). The 'Making Friends with Yourself' and the 'What is Real and What is Not' groups, in Clarke, I. and Wilson, H. (eds.), *Cognitive Behaviour Therapy for Acute Inpatient Mental Health Units.* East Sussex: Routledge.

Kennedy, F. (2009). The use of formulation in inpatient settings, in Clarke, I. and Wilson, H. (eds.), *Cognitive Behaviour Therapy for Acute Inpatient Mental Health Units.* East Sussex: Routledge.

Kuyken, W., Padesky, C. and Dudley, R. (2009). *Collaborative Case Conceptualisation.* New York: Guilford Press.

Lewis, S., Tarrier, N., Haddock, G., Bentall, R., Kinderman, P., Kingdon, D., Siddle, R., Drake, R., Everitt, J., Leadley, K., Benn, A., Grazebrook, K., Haley, C., Akhtar, S., Davies, L., Palmer, S., Faragher, B. and Dunn, G. (2002). Randomised controlled trial of cognitive-behaviour therapy in schizophrenia: acute phase outcomes. *British Journal of Psychiatry*, **181**, 91–97.

NICE (2004a). *Depression: Management of Depression in Primary and Secondary Care—NICE Guidance.* Available at: http://guidance.nice.org.uk/CG23/NiceGuidance/pdf/English (accessed 30 August 2009).

NICE (2004b). *Eating Disorders: Core Intervention in the Treatment and Management of Anorexia Nervosa, Bulimia Nervosa and Related Eating Disorders.* Available at: http://guidance.nice.org.uk/CG9/Guidance/pdf/English (accessed 4th March 2010).

NICE (2004c). *Self-harm: The Short-term Physical and Psychological Management and Secondary Prevention of Self-harm in Primary and Secondary Care.* Available at: http://www.nice.org.uk/nicemedia/pdf/CG016NICEguideline.pdf (accessed 30 August 2009).

NICE (2005a). *Post-traumatic Stress Disorder (PTSD): The Management of PTSD in Adults and Children in Primary and Secondary Care.* Available at: http://guidance.nice.org.uk/CG26/NiceGuidance/pdf/English (accessed 30 August 2009).

NICE (2005b). *Obsessive Compulsive Disorder: Core Interventions in the Treatment of Obsessive-Compulsive Disorder and Body Dysmorphic Disorder.* Available at: http://www.nice.org.uk/nicemedia/pdf/cg031niceguidelines.pdf (accessed 30 August 2009).

NICE (2006). *The Management of Bipolar Disorder in Adults, Children and Adolescents, in Primary and Secondary Care.* Available at: http://www.nice.org.uk/nicemedia/pdf/CG38niceguideline.pdf (accessed 30 August 2009).

NICE (2007). *Anxiety (amended): Management of Anxiety (panic disorder, with or without agoraphobia, and generalised anxiety disorder) in Adults in Primary, Secondary and Community Care.* Available at: http://www.nice.org.uk/nicemedia/pdf/CG022NICEguidelineamended.pdf (accessed 30 August 2009).

NICE (2009). *Core Interventions in the Treatment and Management of Schizophrenia in Primary and Secondary Care (update).* Available at: http://guidance.nice.org.uk/CG82/Guidance/pdf/English (accessed 4th March 2010).

Safran, J. (1996). *Interpersonal Process in Cognitive Therapy.* Washington, DC: Jason Aronson.

Startup, M., Jackson, M.C. and Bendix, S. (2004). North Wales randomized controlled trial of cognitive behaviour therapy for acute schizophrenia spectrum disorders: outcomes at 6 and 12 months. *Psychological Medicine*, **34**, 413–422.

Stuart, S. and Bowers, W.A. (1995). Cognitive therapy with inpatients: review and meta-analysis. *Journal of Cognitive Psychotherapy*, **9**, 85–92.

Tarrier, N., Lewis, S and Haddock, G. (2004). Cognitive Behaviour Therapy in first episode and early schizophrenia: 18 month follow up of a randomised controlled trial. *The British Journal of Psychiatry*. **184**, 231–239.

Chapter 13

Physical health settings

Diana Sanders, Christina Surawy,
Daniel Zahl, and Heather Salt

You may have started working as a CBT therapist in psychological medicine, or be attached to a specific medical department and want to learn how to adapt CBT to the needs of your patients. How does the medical condition impact on therapy? Are the psychological problems, depression or panic, the same as those without coexisting physical problems? Can CBT be adapted for people with chronic pain? Your local hospice may have contacted you to ask for supervision for palliative care staff, and you need to know how to adapt CBT to the needs of people at the end of their lives. You are working in primary care, and are referred a teenager who is not complying with insulin medication. Working with medical patients present us with a range of issues which differ from those of patients we see in mental health settings—issues of engagement, physical health problems impacting on both psychological state and treatment, finding realistic goals, working with realistic cognitions, and working with multidisciplinary medical teams who are not necessarily psychologically minded. In this chapter we look at how to adapt CBT to meet the needs of the patient groups in medical settings, and give examples of how things can go wrong as well as those which go well.

Introduction

People with health problems face a number of difficulties, such as depression from loss of health, anxiety about the future, trauma of sudden illness or medical interventions, and difficulties adjusting to a new diagnosis or chronic ill health. CBT can be tailored to the needs of those with physical health problems, and we have a number of informative models and effective approaches for problems such as chronic pain, chronic fatigue, medically unexplained symptoms (MUS), and health anxiety (BACP, 2005; Sage *et al.*, 2008; Taylor and Asmundson, 2004; White, 2001). CBT and other psychological therapies are becoming increasingly available in many medical specialities, and are offered by a range of healthcare professionals. CBT can help people manage long-term and chronic conditions such as diabetes, renal failure, disfigurement, multiple sclerosis, amputation, head injuries, cancer and heart disease, and with depression and other psychological problems arising from chronic ill-health (BACP, 2005; NICE, 2009).

People with physical health problems have a range of issues and difficulties which differ from patients in mental health services. Some of our patients find it difficult to understand the relevance of psychological therapy, and we need to take into account the impact of their physical problems on both psychological well-being and CBT. The format of CBT varies and you need to work creatively according to the medical setting. For example, you may offer fairly standard CBT for a specific psychological difficulty, such as depression arising from a chronic illness, or panic following a heart attack: in these cases the medical problem is a trigger for the problems but not the main focus of therapy. At the other extreme, you may be offering a specialized form of CBT for chronic fatigue syndrome (CFS; Burgess and Chalder, 2005) or chronic pain (Ogden, 2007; Cole *et al.*, 2005), or training palliative care staff to offer CBT 'first-aid' to patients in hospice settings (Mannix *et al.*, 2006).

Our aims in CBT with medical patients vary depending on the individual, medical problem and setting. For some conditions such as CFS, chronic unexplained pain and other MUS, psychological approaches such as CBT offer the best form of evidence-based treatment currently available. Some people have complex interactions between their primary physical problem, such as diabetes or cancer, and their psychological difficulties (Kennedy and Llewellyn, 2006). For other patients, CBT may be short-term and focused, such as helping people adjust to changes as a condition deteriorates, or reduce anxiety and panic following a heart attack. The aims of CBT in physical health settings are:

- To reduce and treat mental health problems, such as anxiety, depression, and post-traumatic stress disorder (PTSD).

- To reduce treatment costs and hospital admissions, by enabling patients to better manage their condition and associated psychological distress.
- To help people with pre-existing mental health problems cope with medical problems.
- To improve adherence to treatment and management of the physical illness, and compliance with medical treatment.
- To help people reduce behaviours which are impacting on their health.

In this chapter we look at how to adapt CBT to the needs of medical patients, using examples from our work with people with CFS, unexplained medical problems, cystic fibrosis, and diabetes, and those seen in cardiac rehabilitation and palliative care. We have organized the chapter to reflect the journey our patients take through our services, from referral, assessment, and engagement in therapy, to treatment issues, endings, and relapse prevention. The overall message is that the work is varied and interesting. The psychological difficulties our patients face—depression, anxiety, panic, PTSD, and even extreme health anxiety—are no different from those you see in primary care and mental health patients, and can be independent of their health problems. You need to adapt your approach to take into account the medical diagnoses, focus especially on engagement and formulation, and then use a wide range of methods and approaches from general CBT.

Referral

Managing the referral process

The patient pathway to seeing CBT therapists will of course vary depending on your work setting. If you work in condition-specific medical or health services you will no doubt have a defined referral pathway and selection criteria—for example, patients with CFS might be referred by the consultants in the CFS medical services, whereas those with cardiac problems might be referred by the nurses who run the cardiac rehabilitation service. In these cases, the referring physicians and nurses have a good idea about which of their patients may do well with CBT, have clear referral guidelines, and refer appropriately (see Fig. 13.1). Other services may refer people with difficulties not suitable for CBT, or who do not want psychological support or therapy.

In medical and physical health services, it is not unusual for people to find their need for psychological help unacceptable or shameful in some way, and patients' views about being referred to you depend on the way in which the referrer discusses the option for psychological treatment. When medical staff give patients the clear message that CBT is part of the integrated medical care,

Phase 1 Intervention: Cardiac nurse assessment and advice based on CBT (supervised by CBT therapist) for patients with:

- Hospital Anxiety and Depression (HAD) score of 10 or above for either anxiety or depression.
- Past or current mental health problems.
- Ongoing family or social problems.
- Difficulties coping, now or in the past.
- Anyone who has had an ACS episode out of area.
- Any patient who expresses distress which is considered more or less than expected during cardiac rehabilitation.
- Any patient who causes concern to staff.

Phase 2 Intervention: Referral to CBT therapist for patients with continuing problems:

- Very high or persistently high levels of anxiety or depression.
- Persistent dysfunctional beliefs, attitudes or behaviours.
- Continuing problems identified by the HAD score.
- Functional impairment out of proportion to the extent of the coronary heart disease.

Fig. 13.1 Referral criteria for cardiac service.

patients are generally pleased to be offered treatment. In other cases, you might come across patients who have been told, 'I can't find anything physical, therefore it must be psychological', and are understandably upset and puzzled about their problems and referral.

In order to facilitate appropriate referrals, it is extremely helpful to work with medical and nursing staff to increase their understanding of CBT, by giving talks, inviting staff to sit in with you when you see patients, or offering supervision sessions using elements of CBT. Try to provide clear referral guidelines, with examples of when and when not to refer, and enable staff to decide which patients are appropriate for CBT (see Example 13.1).

Example 13.1 Using appropriate referrals in CBT

In our work with cardiac services, the nurses and physiotherapists offer patients who have had a heart attack, surgery, or other cardiac interventions, a course of 10 rehabilitation sessions at the local gym. During this time, they keep a careful eye on physical and psychological progress, and can identify those who are finding it difficult to cope or continuing to feel anxious or low. We meet the nurses every 2 months for CBT training and supervision. During the training sessions, we cover basic CBT formulation and methods, normal adjustment reactions, and how to identify anxiety, panic, and clinical depression, which gives the nurses some 'first aid' methods to help patients. During supervision, we discuss how best to manage the difficulties patients are encountering, and whether or when to refer to us for formal CBT. When the nurses encounter extreme distress in patients shortly after a heart attack, we encourage them not to refer straightaway, but instead we advise on how they can best help the patients themselves, by validating and normalizing the distress and encouraging the patients to talk to family and friends about how they are feeling. Similarly, greater understanding of normal grief reactions means that patients' distress isn't 'pathologized' in the early stages of bereavement. Regular teaching, supervision, and support enable medical staff to feel more confident in their ability to manage psychological issues and to make more appropriate referrals.

Assessment, engagement, and formulation

Core therapeutic skills

For medical patients (particularly those who are shocked by a diagnosis or unexpected decline in health), having the chance to talk things over, experience what is going on and tell their story to a non-judgemental outsider is enormously helpful. Although CBT focuses on unhelpful or distorted ways of thinking, for some patients thoughts such as 'I might die; I may have to face great pain; this is terrible; my family are going to suffer' are realistic. Our job, therefore, is not to help patients find more positive ways of thinking, but instead to focus on what is helpful during such difficult times. The core skills to remember are empathic and non-judgemental listening to enable patients to tell their stories and come to their own solutions (Moorey and Greer, 2002), being more Rogerian than perhaps is usual in CBT. We are on the lookout for places where patients are 'stuck' in affect or behaviour. For example, someone doing much less than is realistically possible, constant rumination or worry, unhelpful health beliefs, or where depression or anxiety are getting in the way of coping with difficulties.

Assessment—building the relationship

Although in many respects CBT assessments with medical patients are similar to general mental health CBT assessments (White, 2001), this patient group differs in terms of their expectations, and impact of the physical problems. The initial one or two meetings that you have with your patients are in many ways the most important in both engaging the patient and beginning the process of therapy. As we have discussed, the way the patient has been referred can set up expectations about treatment. Patients may feel sceptical, worried, or sometimes angry about coming to see us. One of our first tasks, therefore, is to help patients feel that it is normal and acceptable to see a therapist, and that you may have something useful and effective to offer and therefore it is important to start the first meeting with a question about how the patient feels about being referred to your service.

John, aged 25, had cystic fibrosis, and as his condition deteriorated, he became very anxious about how his father would cope when he became much more unwell or died. John wanted to talk to him about practical arrangements, such as care of his dog while he was in hospital, and wanted his dad to know how bad his health really was. However, John's mother had died of cancer when he was a young boy, and his dad, though visibly distressed, had never talked about it. John grew up thinking it was best to keep difficulties to himself in order to protect his dad. John was initially reluctant to talk to a therapist, believing it was a sign of weakness. The first session was focused on how he felt about coming for CBT, and gave him the opportunity to begin to tell his story. His feedback at the end of the session was that it had been helpful, to his surprise, and he was happy to come again to look at ways of coping with his anxiety about his future.

Assessment aims to help the patient understand how behavioural, emotional, and cognitive as well as physical factors are involved in triggering and maintaining their problems, and see a clear path out of their problems. Assessment also enables us to assess whether CBT is right for this patient, or whether another approach might be helpful. For example, if the patient has been referred for specific reasons, such as stopping smoking following a heart attack, it is not unusual for the referrer to be more keen on treatment than the patient, who comes along to the session because the referrer had insisted. In such a case, motivational interviewing methods can enable the person to consider changing their mind as a prelude to changing behaviour (Fig. 13.2).

Motivational interviewing has parallels with CBT, involving similar strategies to help people develop a new view of their situation and behaviour and to increase motivation to change, using carefully chosen Socratic questions such as:

- "What do you think are the advantages of you smoking?"
- "What do you think the disadvantages are?"
- "What are the obstacles for you to stop smoking?"
- "How might you be able to overcome these?"
- "Who would be the best person to support you?"
- "What might happen if you don't stop smoking?"

Fig. 13.2 Motivational interviewing.

The individual is helped to consider a specific behaviour, such as 'smoking' in relation to other aspects of life such as family, social, psychological, medical, and cultural factors. Weighing up the pros and cons and targeting how obstacles can be overcome may help the individual to see a way forward and be more empowered to try to change. The therapist can collaboratively develop a plan that will help the individual develop and attain their important goals. For further information, see Rollnick *et al.* (2008).

It is usually helpful to have a long assessment session, say 90 minutes in order to give patients time to tell their stories, and begin to construct a formulation and plan for treatment. Start with the physical problems, with full description of the main symptoms and then begin to broaden the agenda to cover emotional, cognitive, and behavioural factors. An initial focus on physical symptoms is particularly important for patients whose symptoms are 'medically unexplained' or for people with complex conditions such as CFS or irritable bowel syndrome who may be particularly sensitive to the idea that the symptoms are 'all in the mind' or primarily psychological and therefore not worthy of discussion. Only when you have fully assessed the physical symptoms, broaden the agenda to consider cognitive, behavioural, and emotional factors. For example, with patients with CFS, we focus on the various symptoms of the illness, such as fatigue, pain, muscle weakness, headaches, and any idiosyncratic symptoms, as well as the individual's explanation of the illness, such as viral causes or food allergies, before beginning to focus on what else is going on in life, mood, and behaviours related to the illness (Surawy *et al.*, 1995). Useful questions to ask yourself include:

- Does the patient know why they have come to see me?
- Do they understand what CBT is and how it can help them?
- What is their attitude to seeing me?
- Can I be sensitive to their understanding of their condition and incorporate it into a workable model?
- Do I know enough about their medical condition?
- Do I know enough about their family and social circumstances?

Formulation

The process of formulation begins at the first session. Aim to map the problems, even if in rudimentary form, so that both you and the patient have an idea of what might be keeping the problems going and what might be a possible way forward (Kuyken *et al.*, 2009; Grant *et al.*, 2008). In physical health settings, you can use many different kinds of formulation including Padesky's 'hot cross bun' (Padesky and Mooney, 1990) and longitudinal models taking account of how early and predisposing experiences have shaped beliefs and assumptions. For clear difficulties such as depression, anxiety, panic, or PTSD, you can use well-developed models of these difficulties (Grant *et al.*, 2008; Sanders and Wills, 2006; Westbrook *et al.*, 2007). For a number of medical problems, there are published models which can guide our individual formulation (Kennedy and Llewellyn, 2006; Ogden, 2007; Sage *et al.*, 2008). For example, the 'butterfly' model of CFS looks at how people develop a 'boom and bust' model of living, where they rest excessively following the illness, causing physical, emotional, and social deterioration. At the point where they start to feel better, their high expectations of themselves lead to increased activity, the 'boom', followed by a crash, and so on in a vicious cycle (Fig. 13.3).

For others, you need to develop an idiosyncratic formulation, which can include physiological and social elements, the healthcare system and the family. These formulations are as varied as the people you see, informed by our general knowledge of formulation, our understanding of the patient's illness, and information from the patient.

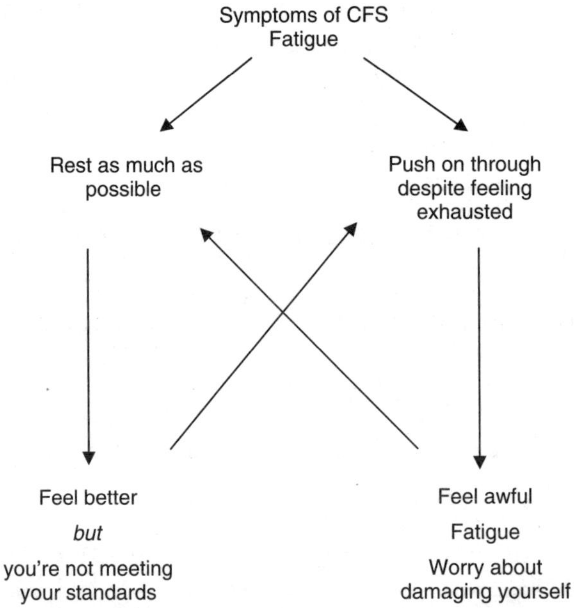

Fig. 13.3 Butterfly model of CFS.

Source: Surawy, C., Hackmann, A., Hawton, K. and Sharpe, M. (1995). Chronic fatigue syndrome: a cognitive approach. *Behaviour Research and Therapy*, **33**, 535–544.

Padmal, who has cystic fibrosis, was very anxious about his health and he and his mother were constantly telephoning the unit for advice and reassurance. Putting his difficulties in the context of how his family and the team might be contributing to his worries and constant phone calls enabled us to think of ways of involving his mother in therapy. In particular, we focused on how continually seeking reassurance was making both Padmal and his mother more anxious (Fig. 13.4). We suggested that his mother could encourage Padmal to go into consultations by himself and take responsibility for his own treatment. Unfortunately this was very difficult for his mother to do, but the formulation was at least helpful to the staff in that they could draw up guidelines for Padmal as to when it was really important to contact the team. It also helped staff understand what was going on and feel a little less frustrated by the constant demands of the family on their time.

A good formulation which fits well for the patients, and takes into account the wider system, including family and medical staff (see Systemic CBT, Chapter 9) is for many patients almost enough to begin the process of change. Some patients readily take to the model and can see where to make changes. For others, you need to introduce more methods and approaches from CBT.

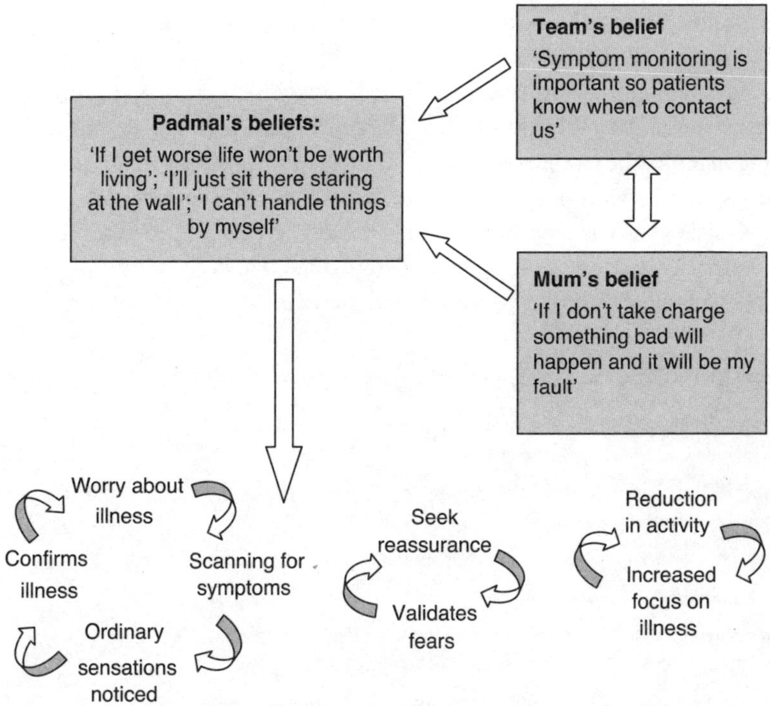

Fig. 13.4 Padmal's maintenance formulation.

CBT methods and therapy issues

Many methods and approaches from CBT are extremely valuable in physical health settings, although individuals' physical problems can mean that you have to be creative in your ways of working and adjust the methods, and setting, to the needs of the individuals. In this section, we look at ways in which you need to adapt CBT to the needs of medical patients, and some common problems (Sage *et al.*, 2008; White, 2001) and recent developments in mindfulness and acceptance in physical health problems.

The impact of the physical health problems on therapy

When working in physical health settings, you need to know enough about the patient's medical condition and prognosis in order to have a clear picture of current and future problems. You do not necessarily have to be expert in all medical problems; however, it is very helpful to know where to find out more, and which sources of information are reliable, particularly Internet sites. Table 13.1 summarizes some of the sites we have found useful. It is also helpful to have a good relationship with medical colleagues for when we need specific advice.

Our patients are themselves a good source of information, although you need to be cautious. Some people are expert in their conditions, and will know enough to be able to advise us on when particular courses of action are contraindicated. This is particularly true for those with chronic conditions which they have had for a long time or from birth. People with diabetes, cystic fibrosis, congenital heart disease, or post-transplant, for example, are trained to manage their own conditions and therefore knowledge is a necessary aspect of survival. People who have been through the 'expert patient' programme (www.expertpatients.co.uk) tend to be well-informed. However, others may have gained information from sources other than reputable, thanks to the creativity

Table 13.1 Useful websites for evidence-based medicine.

NHS Direct for patient information on common conditions and their management	www.nhsdirect.co.uk
National Institute of Clinical Effectiveness for evidence-based practice	www.nice.org.uk
British National Formulary for all medications	www.bnf.org
Cochrane library of evidence-based medicine	www.thecochranelibrary.org
Bandolier: compiles details of best evidence-based treatment for common medical problems	www.medicine.ox.ac.uk/bandolier/
Website from Oxford University research with people's stories of illness	http://www.healthtalkonline.org/

of the Internet, and we may need to tactfully check where the information originated.

You need to be aware of the potential conflict between the types of changes you suggest, such as graded activity or activity scheduling, and the individual's medical condition. For example, if you are helping someone with a chronic condition that involves ongoing treatment such as diabetes, you need to know about medication regimes, side effects, complications, and the interaction between variables such as food, stress, exercise, and blood glucose. It is also helpful to know relevant NICE or national guidance so that you can refer patients to these if necessary (http://www.nice.org.uk/). When using activity scheduling and behavioural experiments involving activity with cardiac patients, you are guided by advice from cardiac staff, and your patient's understanding of what is safe. Certain behavioural experiments such as the hyperventilation provocation test in panic are contraindicated in lung disease, breathing problems, heart disease, high blood pressure, asthma, and pregnancy. It is no longer recommended that patients breathe into a paper bag when hyperventilating, because it can cause serious cardiac problems in people with heart disease. Other sources of behavioural experiments with medical patients are given in Silver *et al.* (2004a; 2004b).

Unusual or worrying symptoms

Sometimes we come across symptoms that you may not have come across before, which cause alarm in both therapist and patient and you are not sure whether to take seriously or suggest that the patient sees a doctor. People with MUS can describe a range of bizarre symptoms, such as aching armpits or numbness in one leg. It is always important that underlying organic disease has been ruled out before starting psychological treatment. So long as the symptoms have been medically checked, try to avoid showing deep concern, so as not to worry the patient more. Bizarre or unusual symptoms can be understood as idiosyncratic physical responses to stress, anxiety, tension, or inactivity. However, if problems continue, and you have doubts that something might have been missed or a new problem developed, discuss with a medical expert or your supervisor before deciding on what to do.

Applications of CBT when health is very poor

In inpatient settings and palliative care, you may be working with people who are very unwell, and have limited concentration and energy. It is essential to work collaboratively with the patient, family, and medical staff, so ideally you are all working in the same direction. You need to adapt the methods to individual need. Examples include: very brief, 5- to 10-minute sessions, several times a week; enabling patients to find pleasure and purpose by making small changes such as getting dressed for visiting time rather than always being in bed; planning a 'memory box' for family left behind; or organizing photographs. We need to be creative about possible solutions or behavioural tasks to try. Knowing when not to use CBT and simply listen and be supportive is equally important for patients who are very unwell. For other suggestions, we recommend Moorey and Greer (2002) and Sage *et al.* (2008).

Dealing with uncertainty

Illness can be a time of great uncertainty for the future, compounded by the medical system, which often involves a long time of waiting for information, test results, or appointments. People can be preoccupied with thoughts such as 'am I going to die?', 'how long have I got?', 'what is going to happen to me?' causing unbearable anxiety, distress, and hopelessness. Some may begin to lead their life as though the worst has already happened.

For patients struggling to cope with uncertainty, encourage them to look at their fears and work out their specific fears. Sometimes, the anxiety itself is worse than the possible illness, and the problems can be understood as a form of health anxiety, amenable to CBT treatment (Wells, 1997). Identify the individual's specific fears, and look for behaviours which are not helping, such as continually seeking reassurance, checking symptoms, avoiding thinking about health, or constant worrying.

For others, it is very helpful to spend time discussing and planning how they would cope if the worse was to happen:

- What exactly are you frightened of? What do you imagine is the very worst that might happen? What is bad about it, for you?
- Is this the most likely or realistic possibility, or is some other scenario more likely?
- If the worst did happen, what would you do? How would you cope? Who can help you? What do you need to do now in order to plan?

It is also helpful to focus on areas of life where the individual can make a difference, such as taking medication regularly, doing exercise, and increasing time spent on valued activities, time with family, and so on. Doing a time-line can help, asking the following sequence of questions:

- If you had only 5 days to live, and you were definitely going to die then, what would you do now? How would you spend your time from now to then?
- If you had 5 weeks to live, what now?

- If it was 5 months?
- Or 5 years?

The questions enable patients to think about what is important and valued, such as time with family, focussing more on getting the best quality of life, however long it is. *Acceptance* of uncertainty as part of life is enormously helpful, drawing attention to the fact that none of us can be certain about the future, and the importance of the here-and-now.

Common therapy problems

What to do when patients are unable to get to appointments

There are a number of reasons why people may not be able to get to appointment. In some cases, patients may be too unwell or have limited mobility, or are unable to organize help with transport. Our patients are eligible for hospital transport, organized via the general practitioner (GP) or hospital. You can also offer CBT via the telephone or email, or use self-help materials backed up with regular phone calls. When doing work over the phone, it is essential to have at least one face-to-face session in order to get to know each other and not speak to a 'disembodied voice'. Alternatively, home visits might be an option.

Sometimes a patient experiences a relapse in symptoms, which makes it difficult to get to sessions. A relapse is often an ideal time to help your patient—assisting them with applying behavioural or cognitive strategies that they have used or practiced previously, and identifying and working with behaviours that may in fact maintain or worsen problems, such as resting too much or doing too much, or avoiding all social contact. Maintaining contact is therefore a priority, and calling patients as soon as there is a cancellation or DNA (did not attend) rather than writing a letter can help people stay engaged. In cases where relapses are frequent it can be useful to do some setback planning and behavioural experiments to try out different skills (Silver *et al.*, 2004a; 2004b).

Patients believe that you can't understand or help

On occasions, patients with physical health problems attend therapy not because they think it could be helpful, but because someone has put pressure on them to try, or because they feel there is really no where else to go. Occasionaly, the patient may choose to see you to show others that CBT is not going to help. As a result, you might feel put on the spot and frustrated or defensive, but it is essential to understand the patients' point of view—having lived with health problems for many years and made life choices based on their view of their capabilities, it can be hard to trust anyone else to be able to help. It is important therefore, to be very respectful of their feelings, by acknowledging how things have been difficult. You may want to gently enquire about why exactly they feel CBT will not help them. Sometimes it may be necessary to 'hold the hope' for patients. For example, you might say (see Example 13.2):

Example 13.2 Facilitating engagement

'I'm sorry to hear that you are feeling so pessimistic about the prospect of things improving for you. It sounds as though you have tried very hard to try to improve things for yourself and feel frustrated that nothing so far has worked for you. There may be things that you've not tried yet which may actually help. Could we work together for a few weeks to see if we can find ways to help you manage better, and if there is anything you don't want to do, that is fine too. Is it worth at least a trial?'

Showing empathy can be key to gaining the trust of patients—and may be the key thing that has been missing from other medical consultations they have had. Being enthusiastic about working with the patient, and gently positive about their prospects will help model an alternative attitude to their problems that in time they may be able to adopt themselves.

It is also very important not to expect too much, or discount small gains. Look for small activities which can make a big difference, and carefully monitor signs of change. For example, someone who is coping with a terminal diagnosis may be staying in bed all day because 'there is no point', but discounts the action of getting up as something 'anyone can do' and not a sign of progress. Simply getting up and getting dressed is a major achievement for someone who is very unwell, and paying attention to achievements helps to improve mood.

Emotional and cognitive avoidance

Being faced with physical illness and life-threatening problems is understandably a painful and distressing time for people. Many people may feel that the best way to cope is to deny the reality of a problem. They may be reluctant to ask for help, admit to limitations, or even adhere to medical treatment if it confronts their fears or compromises their relationships with others.

The way emotions are handled in medical settings and in society can encourage avoidance. In hospitals, medical staff tends to respond to tears or upset by hasty reassurance, advice, or medication, or referral to a psychiatrist, giving the message that strong emotions are not acceptable. Friends and relatives may also find it difficult to accept the expression of emotions and often report 'I don't know what to say'. It is very common for our patients to say that they do not feel they can talk to anyone about how they are feeling, and therefore do not have the chance to express, validate, or understand their feelings or thoughts.

Rob was referred by the cardiac rehabilitation team for depression after surviving a partial rupture of the wall of his aorta. The damage extended up his carotid arteries, which meant that he had very reduced blood flow to his brain, and therefore was unable to think or feel anything at the time. The event occurred when he was abroad and unable to speak the language, which further compounded his inability to talk about what was going on. It was a miracle that he had survived. He had told the story many times, to many friends and medics, and had to him always been just a story. By pointing out my reaction, of shock and sadness, Rob began to realize he had not really begun to believe what had happened to him. He felt as though all the emotion was trapped inside himself, stagnating, leading him to feel so heavy and low. He also feared verbalizing his feelings in case he was overwhelmed and unable to cope.

You can use a variety of methods to help people to label and express emotion appropriately. Your role is often to listen, empathize, and allow time for the patient to talk and reflect (Moorey and Greer, 2002). It may be tempting to rush in with thought challenging, advice, or tissues, but you may well reinforce the message that the emotion needs to be sorted out and got rid of. You also need to identify any beliefs patients have about expressing their emotions, such as 'it is weak to cry', 'people will think I'm stupid', 'I ought to be better by now', 'I survived, what have I got to feel upset about', and discuss these. For example, asking what the patients think about others who feel upset, or what they would do if a friend started crying, may reveal double standards. Rob believed that his family would not be able to deal with his emotions, thinking he was 'over it'. In fact, he did a behavioural experiment, talking to his wife one evening about how he felt, which ended with them both in tears about how he had nearly died. He noticed that he then started to feel much more emotional about all sorts of things, and began, for the first time, to tell his children how much he loved them.

Expressive writing has been shown as a highly effective means of working with emotion (Pennebaker, 2004). Rob found that writing for at least 15 minutes a day enabled him to process the trauma, as well as express the emotions connected with the aortic rupture, and improved after a few weeks. Mindfulness methods can also be helpful, giving the individual the opportunity to examine and reflect on emotions in a clear and non-judgemental way.

The other side of emotional expression is when the patient seems to be stuck in the emotion, inappropriately and unhelpfully, especially when angry. Suppressing anger may lead to later problems, but it can be very difficult to find an appropriate means of expression. Assertiveness methods may help, for example, in asserting a need for more help around the house. Some emotional expression methods may be useful in carefully time-limited means, such as writing an angry letter then tearing it up or punching cushions. The physical 'fight' response can be channelled into a brisk walk or other physical outlet, again in a time-limited way. Sometimes expression of anger leads to the hidden emotion: rage leading to grief about the loss of function, for example. Other 'stuck' emotions include hopelessness, helplessness, or fear. In these cases, we need to assess the extent to which they arise from clinical depression or general anxiety, which needs appropriate treatment targeted at the problem. Helplessness can arise from a changed role within the family, such as when the partner takes over the patient's work within the family, insisting the patient rests all the time. We need to look at this within the wider context of the family, and inviting the spouse or partner along to one or two sessions can be helpful.

Mindfulness-based cognitive therapy (MBCT) and physical health

Mindfulness has been successfully used for over 20 years for helping medical patients deal with chronic pain, life change, and disability (Kabat-Zinn, 2004). MBCT groups have been run for patients with CFS, with good results (Surawy *et al.*, 2005). Mindfulness offers a way of relating to our physical and emotional experiences, as well as thoughts and behaviours, which is non-judgemental and compassionate, and learning to break the cycles and patterns which maintain problems. For example, chronic pain is maintained not by immediate sensations of pain, but by long-standing patterns of negative thoughts, e.g. 'this is terrible, I can't cope'; behaviours such as extreme avoidance of activity, rest, or doing too much; social situations, e.g. being unable to work, or treated as an invalid in the family, as well as depression or anxiety. With mindfulness, these maintaining factors can be more clearly seen, giving the individual the possibility of choosing more helpful responses (McCracken and Keog, 2009). MBCT is likely to become a more widespread and useful addition to the repertoire of psychological interventions you can offer people with physical health problems, and for further information, we recommend Kabat-Zinn's work and Burch (2008).

The value of illness

The experience of life-threatening illness may not be all negative. Many people cope extremely well, and indeed feel that the experience has been valuable to them in many ways. We hear and read many stories about people with even severely limiting illnesses finding meaning and value in life. The ability to live in the present, and appreciate what one has, rather than does not have, are central themes to those who do well. A focus on what has been gained through illness can be extremely helpful. The areas where people have found value in illness include (Hefferon *et al.*, 2009):

- Reappraisal of life and priorities—realizing the value of family and relationships; re-evaluation of life goals and activities; focus on what is important.

- Improved relationships.
- Focus on healing previously difficult relationships while there is still time.
- Surprise at the devotion and help from other people, particularly strangers and healthcare staff.
- New relationships amongst other patients.
- New appreciation of life, finding it a 'gift'.
- Being thankful for the chance to realize what is important in life.
- Appreciation of the 'here and now'.
- Improved 'self', discovering a stronger self or a fighter, or more empathic self.
- New awareness of and respect for the body, realizing the importance of self-care.
- Impact on others, promoting more awareness of illness and need for screening and self-care in relatives and friends.

Although not all of our patients will find any benefit in their illness, it is very useful to ask an open question, such as 'Are there any benefits to what you have been through?' 'What have you learned from your experience?' A focus on the wider picture can enable patients to find meaning in what was previously construed as only painful or difficult.

Endings in CBT

With patients suffering from physical health problems, the ending of therapy may not be clear. You are likely to make a relationship with the patient, family, health professionals, and carers which lasts over the patient's lifetime. For example, in our work in cystic fibrosis, contact starts when the person is having difficulties negotiating the transition from adolescence to adulthood, and carries on throughout his/her subsequent treatment, ending when the individual has a successful lung transplant and can live independently. In palliative care, you may meet the patient at a late stage in his/her illness, and carry on seeing the bereaved family for several months after the person's death. At the other extreme, CBT in cardiac rehabilitation may be extremely short—one or two sessions to focus on the panic and anxiety experienced as a result of a myocardial infarction. If your contract is for very short-term CBT, you may need to refer the patient on to another service, such as one for patients with complex needs, or longer-term CBT.

Some patients work best with an open access system, or blocks of therapy followed by gaps, and the ability to work flexibly within your service is essential. Such a way of working can suit people who are likely to face changes due to their health condition (see Example 13.3).

Example 13.3 Working flexibly

A young diabetic woman was very ambivalent about seeing us, but would regularly become very ill due to non-compliance with medication. We left it open for her or her doctors to contact the service for regular top-up sessions, until she began to resolve some of the issues leading to harming herself.

Whatever the time course of therapy, constructive endings are an extremely important part of successful therapy. What we remember of events is often colored by the ending; a messy and unresolved ending is likely to hang around for some time in our, as well as our patients' or their family's mind. Ideally, a course of therapy of any length comes to an orderly and predictable ending, with a review of successes and learning, and a blueprint as a reminder of progress. In reality, endings can be more complex and evoke many emotions and difficulties. For patients facing many losses due to health problems—loss of function, loss of independence—ending the relationship with the therapist can be another loss. It is useful to bring up the ending at an early stage of therapy, to formulate any beliefs or thoughts that might arise and work out ways of dealing with them. For those for whom ending CBT is going to be particularly difficult, it is important to find out exactly what the difficulties are and try to problem-solve these. For example, the patient may have been feeling extremely lonely and cut-off from others because of the health problem, so preparing for ending therapy involves finding sources of external support such as a local patients group.

Sudden endings

We have all had the experience of patients who suddenly terminate therapy, leaving a sense of incompletion for us and uncertainty about 'where you went wrong'. Patients ending abruptly and not responding to letters or phone calls, can haunt us for some time: What has happened? Is he or she alright? Did I do something wrong? Could I have done better?

Sometimes we have indeed made mistakes which we have to learn from, painful though that may be. Sometimes, therapy has simply gone too fast for the patient to cope with. In our short-term CBT offered to cardiac rehabilitation patients, occasional patients drop out after discussing previously hidden trauma. It is not uncommon for near-miss health scares, such as heart attacks or emergency surgery, to remind us of our mortality and take stock, which can awaken unresolved memories and issues.

Keith came to see me after the cardiac rehabilitation nurses were concerned about his low motivation to engage in exercise following his MI. After a few questions from me, Keith started talking and was in full-flow most of the session.

He told me, in the nature of a confession, that he was sexually abused as a child, and had never spoken about it before. At the end of the session he reported being "drained, but relieved". He missed our two subsequent sessions, always telephoning afterwards to apologize because he "forgot". Although he returned a set of much improved questionnaires. I was left wondering if the one session had indeed been useful to him, or whether the shame of the confession meant that he could never return. We learned the importance of treading carefully when people start to fully open up in the first session.

We therapists are human, and make mistakes in our work. Such issues are best taken to supervision, and in our experience, are potentially a source of valuable clinical learning.

Another difficult ending is when patients die suddenly. You then have your own issues of grief and loss to work with, through supervision or support of colleagues. You may have questions about whether it is appropriate to attend the funeral or write to the family, again to be discussed with colleagues.

Key points

- People with physical health problems have the same psychological issues as those seen in other settings and you use many of the same methods—don't be frightened of the diagnosis.
- Spend time working on the formulation, understanding the role of the health problem and treatment in the overall picture without giving it more prominence than necessary. For example, not everyone with heart disease or cancer is depressed or anxious: what are the issues for this individual?
- Once you have the formulation, you can creatively use all the standard CBT methods.
- Get at least a basic understanding of the relevant medical problems and treatment. If in doubt, ask the patient, and cultivate good working relationships with medical staff.
- Be flexible and adaptable, prepared to work with different patients and clinicians in a variety of ways.

Further reading

Journal of Health Psychology, Psychosomatic Medicine, Journal of Psychosomatic Research.

Moorey, S. and Greer, S. (2002). *Cognitive Behaviour Therapy for People with Cancer*. Oxford: Oxford University Press.

Sage, N., Sowden, M., Chorlton, E. and Edeleanu, A. (2008). *CBT for Chronic Illness and Palliative Care: A Workbook and Toolkit.* Oxford: Wiley-Blackwell.

The Faculty for Healthcare Counsellors and Psychotherapists, and their journal, 'Journal of Healthcare Counselling and Psychotherapy' produce information relevant to working in physical health care. Available at: http://www.fhcp.org.uk/journal.html (last accessed 24 February 2010).

White, C. (2001). *CBT for Chronic Illness.* Oxford: Wiley-Blackwell.

References

BACP (2005). *Shaping Effective Counselling Services in Health care: Case Studies of Service Delivery and Outcomes.* Available at: http://www.fhcp.org.uk/pdf/shaping_effective.pdf (accessed 9 September 2009).

Burch, V. (2008). *Living Well With Pain and Illness.* The mindful way to free yourself from suffering. London: Piatkus.

Burgess, M. and Chalder, T. (2005). *Overcoming Chronic Fatigue Syndrome.* London: Constable-Robinson.

Cole, F., Macdonald, H., Carus, C. and Howden-Leach, H. (2005). *Overcoming Chronic Pain: A Self-help Guide Using Cognitive Behavioural Techniques.* London: Constable-Robinson.

Grant, A., Townend, M. and Mill, J. (2008). *Assessment and Case Formulation in Cognitive Behavioural Therapy.* London: Sage.

Hefferon, K., Grealy, M. and Mutrie, N. (2009). Post-traumatic growth and life-threatening physical illness: a systematic review of the qualitative literature. *British Journal of Health Psychology*, **14**, 343–378.

Kabat-Zinn, J. (2004). *Full Catastrophe Living.* London: Piatkus.

Kennedy, P. and Llewellyn, S. (eds.) (2006). *The Essentials of Clinical Health Psychology.* Oxford: Wiley-Blackwell.

Kuyken, W., Padesky, C. and Dudley, R. (2009). *Collaborative Case Conceptualization.* New York, NY: Guildford Press.

Mannix, K., Blackburn, I.M., Garland, A., Gracie, J., Moorey, S., Reid, B., Standart, S. and Scott, J. (2006). Effectiveness of brief training in CBT techniques for palliative care practitioners. *Palliative Medicine*, **20**, 579–584.

McCracken, L.M. and Keogh, E. (2009). Acceptance, mindfulness, and values-based action may counteract fear and avoidance of emotions in chronic pain: an analysis of anxiety sensitivity. *The Journal of Pain*, **10**(4), 408–415.

Moorey, S. and Greer, S. (2002). *Cognitive Behaviour Therapy for People With Cancer.* Oxford: Oxford University Press.

NICE (2009). *Depression with a Chronic Physical Health Problem.* Available at: http://www.nice.org.uk/Guidance/CG/WaveR/23 (accessed 9 September 2009).

Ogden, J. (2007). *Health Psychology: A Textbook.* Fourth edition. Milton Keynes: Open University Press.

Padesky, C.A. and Mooney, K.A. (1990). Clinical tip: presenting the cognitive model to clients. *International Cognitive Therapy Newsletter*, **6**, 13–14.

Pennebaker, J.W. (2004). *Writing to Heal: A Guided Journal for Recovering from Trauma and Emotional Upheaval.* Oakland, CA: New Harbinger Press.

Rollnick, S., Miller, W.R. and Butler, C.C. (2008). *Motivational Interviewing in Health Care: Helping Patients Change Behavior (Applications of Motivational Interviewing).* New York, NY: Guildford Press.

Sage, N., Sowden, M., Chorlton, E. and Edeleanu, A. (2008). *CBT for Chronic Illness and Palliative Care: A Workbook and Toolkit.* Oxford: Wiley-Blackwell.

Sanders, D. and Wills, F. (2006). *Cognitive Therapy: An Introduction.* London: Sage.

Silver, A., Sanders, D., Morrison, N. and Cowey, C. (2004a). Health anxiety, in Bennett-Levy, J., Butler, G., Fennell, M., Hackmann, A., Mueller, M. and Westbrook, D. (eds.), *The Oxford Guide to Behavioural Experiments in Cognitive Therapy.* Oxford: Oxford University Press, pp. 81–110.

Silver, A., Surawy, C. and Sanders, D. (2004b). Physical health problems and disability, in Bennett-Levy, J., Butler, G., Fennell, M., Hackmann, A., Mueller, M. and Westbrook, D. (eds.), *The Oxford Guide to Behavioural Experiments in Cognitive Therapy.* Oxford: Oxford University Press, pp. 309–330.

Surawy, C., Hackmann, A., Hawton, K. and Sharpe, M. (1995). Chronic fatigue syndrome: a cognitive approach. *Behaviour Research and Therapy*, **33**, 535–544.

Surawy, C., Roberts, J. and Silver, A. (2005). The effect of mindfulness training on mood and measures of fatigue, activity and quality of life in patients with chronic fatigue syndrome on a hospital waiting list: a series of exploratory studies. *Behavioural and Cognitive Psychotherapy*, **33**, 103–110.

Taylor, S. and Asmundson, G.J.G. (2004). *Treating Health Anxiety: A Cognitive Behavioural Approach.* New York, NY: Guildford Press.

Wells, A. (1997). *Cognitive Therapy of Anxiety Disorders.* New York, NY: Wiley.

Westbrook, D., Kennerley, H. and Kirk, J. (2007). *An Introduction to Cognitive Behaviour Therapy: Skills and Applications.* London: Sage.

White, C. (2001). *Cognitive Behaviour Therapy for Chronic Medical Problems.* Chichester: Wiley-Blackwell.

Chapter 14

Going it alone: working in private practice

Joan Kirk

Chapter overview

For some, private practice conjures up images of independence from management, freedom in setting working hours, a potentially higher salary; for me, the major attractions are being able to choose what sorts of patients I will see, to determine how I will spend my time, and to avoid bureaucracy after a long career of meetings and papers. If you were to consider a move of this magnitude, the reasons would be idiosyncratic. It is worth carefully considering them, as they will to some degree shape what you offer.

Many of the challenges of working in private practice are simplified if you work in an organization, where issues about whether there is a demand, what administrative systems to put in place, what and how to bill patients, etc. are taken care of. While this takes a burden off your shoulders, it is at the cost of your freedom to decide your clinical priorities, how much time to allocate to patients, and so on, thus it is worth reviewing if this is what you want.

This chapter focuses on working as an independent practitioner, possibly alongside one or two colleagues, but not supported by an external structure. The emphasis is on your deciding if and how to go it alone rather than on clinical matters as many of the clinical considerations of working in private practice parallel those in non-private practice. However, the clinical issues of continuing professional development (CPD), supervision, boundaries, and safety will be addressed towards the end of the chapter as these can be uniquely challenging for the independent practitioner.

Getting started

You will need to consider some basic questions:

- Would working independently suit me?
- Is independent practice feasible for me?
- How much income do I need to be financially viable?
- How will I let people know about me?
- What business/professional administration will be required?

Would working independently suit me?

Look at your reasons for considering this, and then check Table 14.1 to see whether there are other reasons that seem relevant. For each of the points in favour of working independently, it is worth considering what the drawbacks or difficulties might be, and working out what could be done to mitigate these. For example, working at home would reduce travel time and costs, and allow more flexibility in managing domestic affairs; on the other hand, space would be taken up, an additional level of tidiness would be demanded, and the boundary between work and home might be difficult to manage.

Put this into context by also considering what working in an established post offers that you value, as it would be helpful to build some of this into a future private practice. Again, try and set out your own ideas, then check these against those in Table 14.2.

At this point it is wise to consider if you will be able to deal with *significant* difficulties such as having no managerial support (particularly if you were facing a crisis such as a legal claim being made against you or a patient suicide) or working in isolation if you know that you have valued team work in the past. Such difficulties are not insurmountable—you could, for example, plan

Table 14.1 Some reasons for working in private practice.

Desire for:
Independence in setting priorities and deciding ways of working
Increased income
Flexibility in working hours
Improved accommodation
New challenge
Mixed range of referrals, from simple to complex
Long-term plan for career development
Work from home
Dislike of:
No established jobs available
Insufficient established sessions available
Immediate management
Internal politics
Stigma attached to mental heath services
Difficult relationships with colleagues in current post

Table 14.2 What work in an established post offers.

◆ Support from manager
◆ Supervision
◆ Accommodation
◆ Employer's contribution to superannuation
◆ Peer support
◆ Multidisciplinary working
◆ Social contact
◆ Career planning and advance
◆ Variety of work
◆ Team work

to build in sufficient time for networking with other professionals—but they merit your consideration.

Finally, reflect on your values in respect of working with patients as this will help you avoid stumbling later on in your private venture. For example, if you believe that it is important that help is available at the point of need, independently of ability to pay, you will need to think through how this would play out in your practice. If you assumed that you could offer 'a few' patients a reduced fee in order to allow treatment to proceed, you could find that your reputation as a 'fair-minded' therapist spread rapidly. You may instead, for example, have to decide on a fixed quota for how many reduced fee/free patients you would have at any one time.

It is worth doing a written pros and cons comparison for whether or not to go into private practice. This process is described well in the book *Manage Your Mind* (Butler and Hope, 2007). Do not qualify the pros and cons on the first draft, but drawing on the reflection you have already done, go through the list a second time, and add in possible solutions for the cons, and possible drawbacks for the pros. As Butler and Hope point out, once you have weighted the pros and cons in order of importance, the chances are that you will then need to make a decision based on how you feel about the issue, because the weightings will leave you undecided. However, the process of weighing things up will have informed your feelings, and will help you to decide.

Is independent practice feasible for me?

If you are ambivalent about the shift to private practice, there are a variety of ways that you could test out how it feels to work in this way. You could work privately during some evenings or at weekends; you could negotiate a reduction in your sessions with your employer, and use the freed time to work privately (in which case you should check with your Human Resources Department whether part-time work carries different terms and conditions of employment); you could work privately in your free time if you are already part-time; if you are not in a job, you could attempt to get sessional or part-time work to leave yourself space to build up some private work; and so on. If you work, for example in the National Health Service (NHS), it may be possible to negotiate to use a room for your private work, either in a hospital or community setting; or you could experiment with using a room at home—bear in mind that this will in neither case be cost free: the NHS would charge a fee, and the cost of using space at home is that it has to be made suitable for clinical use, which may be a significant cost in freedom and time for yourself and the family.

An advantage of a gradual approach of this kind is that you are reducing the risks that giving up a job otherwise carries, allowing you to work out what aspects of private working you enjoy or find satisfying, without, for example, committing yourself to a contract on accommodation. Furthermore, it takes time to build up referrals and a caseload when establishing a private practice, and a gradual change may reduce the requirement for a capital outlay while you have a reduced (or no) income.

If any of the aspects that you value seems so important that you would not want to work without them, despite the qualities that independent working would otherwise bring, then it may be worthwhile dipping your toe into the water of private practice, and doing it as a behavioural experiment. For example, if you were fearful that you would not cope with social isolation, you could operationalize what not coping would feel like (being anxious about seeing patients with no immediate opportunity to discuss them with a colleague, feeling miserable in free periods, spending time on the phone to people during work hours), and you could then keep ratings for a few weeks of the predicted moods, or a log of how often relevant events occurred.

If you decide that you are going to switch completely to independent working, you should first consider whether you are eligible for appropriate accreditation as a cognitive behaviour therapy (CBT) practitioner, for example by the British Association of Behavioural and Cognitive Psychotherapy (BABCP, www.babcp.com). This validation is necessary to protect the patients who seek out your services, and is one way of protecting yourself in the event of litigation concerning your competency to provide the services that you are offering. If you are qualified in one of the core health or social professions, it would also be sensible to retain or establish membership of your professional body as this will increase further your credibility for patients; will be a source of information for a whole range of issues—for example, whether you should accompany in her car a patient with a driving phobia; and provide you with CPD opportunities, both for clinical and professional development. Most importantly, it will provide you with a code of ethics, which will be invaluable when you are working without the close support of others.

It is then important to plan your venture thoroughly in advance, so that you maximize the possibility of finding work and support. You will need to consider:

- What you intend to provide.
- What your resources are.
- Whether there is a demand for the services that you are planning.

This may sound suspiciously like a business plan, but it can be as informal as you like, unless you are going to approach someone to ask them to lend you money for set-up costs. In that case you will need to draw up a more formal business plan, which is beyond the scope of this chapter, but is dealt with in Chapter 19.

What do you intend to provide?

What you plan to provide depends on your areas of expertise, and it is important to spell this out for potential referrers and patients. This is not only for the obvious reason that they need to know what areas you work in, but also because people may be keen to persuade you to take referrals that you do not feel competent to deal with. For example, there may be few local practitioners with experience of working with people with bipolar disorder, and a referrer may try to persuade you to take one of their patients, even though you explain that you do not have sufficient supervised experience with the problems presented by such patients. You can choose to decline the referral, or you have the freedom to choose whether you want to increase your skill base, by further reading, additional supervision, attendance at training events, and this can be planned within your own CPD programme, as discussed below.

An information sheet can be helpful, explicitly describing what you are offering, in addition to information about yourself, your approach, conditions of work, etc. Table 14.3 gives an example of part of such an information sheet.

Initially, you might want to concentrate on building up your client base, and getting yourself known as an independent clinician. However, you may have scope to develop and expand your service, and if you value variety in your work, you may plan to include supervision of other clinicians, or to consider teaching and training opportunities; legal work may also extend your potential referrals. You could consider gradually taking on associates, for whom you

Table 14.3 Information for users and referrers.

In general I offer treatment to individuals, broadly between the ages of 16 and 70 years. For over 35 years, my approach has been cognitive behavioural, applied to a wide range of problems such as those described below.
What is CBT?
CBT helps people understand the links between thoughts, feelings, and behaviour. The therapist and patient work together to identify the thoughts, attitudes, and beliefs that are associated with particular problems, and to discover if there are more realistic and helpful ways of seeing things. With the support of the therapist, patients are then encouraged to try out new ways of dealing with problems and to evaluate what works best for them.
The CBT approach is easily learned, and patients are encouraged to use it in their own way. CBT works best when the patient is actively involved in treatment, with a good working partnership with the therapist. There are usually assignments for the patient between treatment sessions, and these help to move treatment forward. It is helpful to bring a therapy notebook to sessions, both to note down any assignments or useful material from the sessions, but also to make notes of any relevant material between sessions.
Who does it help?
The effectiveness of short-term CBT is well-established for anxiety disorders, depression, obsessional problems, reactions to trauma, and eating disorders. The results of treatments for more complex problems requiring longer-term treatment are also showing very promising results.
What is the length of treatment?
The average length of a course of treatment is 6–15 sessions of 1 hour, but this is only a guide. Sessions are normally weekly to begin with, and gradually reduce in frequency.

could manage referrals; or you could plan to work in parallel with other practitioners who complemented your skills—for example, someone who worked with a younger age group, or who offered couple work while you did not.

Having considered what services you would offer, it would then be helpful to consider what resources you have available, many of which will reside in you.

What are your resources?

Skill and experience in CBT

These are your main resources. Drawing up a brief curriculum vitae is a good way of clarifying what you think you can offer to potential clients, whether patients or referrers. Useful information would include your qualifications and accreditations or registrations, and a brief summary of your experience and posts held. Reference to teaching and training, writing and research would be relevant for increasing your credibility.

Edie's patient information sheet contained the following information:

As a chartered clinical psychologist with 15 years of experience as a cognitive therapist, I am an experienced clinician. I trained in London and Oxford, worked within the NHS for 12 years and have been accredited with the BABCP for 10 years. I have experience with a wide range of clinical problems such as depression, anxiety disorders and, in particular, eating disorders. I am also trained in families and couples therapy. I maintain an active interest in developments in CBT and regularly attend conferences and specialist training events. I have been involved in research, have presented academic papers and now also supervise other CBT practitioners.

However, for independent working you will need additional personal qualities. It would be useful to spell out those that you consider relevant, before looking at Table 14.4 where there may be some additional ones for you to consider.

Flexibility in the way you work

You can be highly flexible and this can be very attractive to clients who find 'office hours' appointments difficult to attend. You can work early mornings, evenings, and weekends, but boundary and safety issues (which are addressed later in this chapter) need to be taken into account. Clearly you also have the advantage of being able to keep sections of the day and school holidays free.

Your physical environment

This is another very important resource. Your main choice is whether to work at or away from home. While some problems are minimized if you work away from home, this has to be set against the greater cost of renting or taking out a mortgage. Wright and Davis (1994) surveyed what patients valued in therapy, and of the 10 features that emerged, the first requirement concerned the physical space, specifically that the 'place we meet must be physically safe, private, confidential, free from distraction, and comfortable'. The room needed to reflect friendliness and authority, not to be carelessly untidy, with other people's files left openly around. The consulting room does not need to be as neutral as that

Table 14.4 Personal qualities useful in working privately.

◆ Organizational skill
◆ Self-reliance
◆ Optimism/realism
◆ Planning and attention to detail
◆ Drive
◆ Internal locus of control
◆ Physical health
◆ Flexibility in working hours
◆ Assertiveness

demanded by other therapeutic schools, but you should nevertheless bear in mind what impression the patient will get from features in your room. This is particularly relevant if you are working at home, and noises and smells should be included in this. This can be *particularly* difficult if children will be around for parts of the year, as it is clearly important that the patient is confident that your attention is undivided.

There needs to be a designated waiting area, similarly free of personal accoutrements. Although ideally patients will not be waiting, relatives/friends may accompany the patient, particularly if they are children or vulnerable adults.

The immediate neighborhood is also worth paying attention to, as patients will certainly do so—they are unlikely to attend if the area is threatening or neglected.

Your physical resources

These include handouts, books and booklets, monitoring forms, and questionnaires to supplement your clinical work, and you will need to build up a range of them, and keep them up-to-date. You should take care not to photocopy questionnaires or other forms that are copyrighted; they will need to be purchased. The loan of books carries a substantial financial risk, and unless you are prepared to carry that, it is wiser to recommend that your patient buys rather than borrows a book, or borrows it from a library.

Even though you have much to offer, there is not much point setting up your business unless there is someone out there willing to pay for your services, so it is essential to get a rough estimate of demand.

Is there a demand for your services?

There appears to be no hard data on how many people use private CBT services, and so you will have to rely on common sense, estimating how many people in your area are likely to be in a position to pay for treatment—your area in this context referring not to the local Primary Care Trust, but the distance that can be easily traveled, probably by car—and how many therapists are currently providing services.

The first step is to determine from census data how many people live in your catchment area, and assuming that approximately 20% are from social classes 1 and 2, (and hence possibly able and willing to pay for treatment), and further assuming that about 65% are the adults of working age range of say (16–70) if you are going to work with adults, this means that approx 13% of the total population would be in a position to pay.

The next step is to establish how many private CBT therapists are already working in your area, at what levels of experience, and with which populations.

The BABCP therapist list is a good place to start; the local psychological therapy services may have a list of private therapists; and your local health centre may also have such a list. Colleagues from the area will also have information. The Yellow Pages may list therapists, though probably not differentiated by approach.

The potential paying population in your area should then be divided by the known number of therapists in your area. A rule of thumb would be that a prospective population would support approximately one private therapist per 30,000. For a validation of this estimate, you could find out whether there are waiting lists for NHS and private CBT—bearing in mind that these may be affected locally by the presence of some effective therapists in your area, and may develop rapidly, for example, when the media publicize the efficacy of CBT. Consider that people will travel long distances to see a therapist with a good reputation, particularly if your hours are flexible.

You have so far considered whether you want to proceed with private practice, have clarified what you can offer, and where, and whether anyone is likely to want your services. You now need to establish how much you need to earn, and hence, how much you need to charge/how many patients you need to see.

Business affairs

How much income do I need to be financially viable?

In broad terms, you need to ensure that your income exceeds your expenses, including your salary. This part of your planning will include elements that you may have paid scant attention to while in an employed position, but will demand detailed attention once you become self-employed. For example, you may have found it irritating that you were expected to share a room in your existing job. Once you begin to include the cost of accommodation in your expenses, and hence in your income target, it will become apparent that the number of empty minutes for an office is highly relevant.

It is useful to consider the set-up costs of your new venture separately from subsequent running costs.

The set-up costs may include:

- The equipment to support the administration of your business, such as telephones (with answer phone), IT, secure facility for your current and past records
- Furnishing
- Initial advertising
- Deposit on rented accommodation

In other words, you may need capital that will not immediately be replaced. In addition to this, the running costs of the business will include:

- Your salary—you need to decide what you would find acceptable
- National insurance and pension contributions
- Payments to others (accountant, supervisor, administrator, secretary)
- Subscriptions to professional bodies
- Rent or mortgage
- Services (telephone, gas, electricity, water, council tax)
- Insurance (professional, property, sickness)
- CPD (workshops, books and journals, etc.)
- Stationery, postage, office equipment
- Advertising
- Tax, including VAT if your income is sufficiently high
- Repayment of capital costs (above)

The total estimated sum of all these components gives you the figure for the total income that you require. All of this has to be covered by work taking place over possibly 45 weeks of the year (this takes into account 4 weeks holidays and 2 weeks statutory holidays, and allows for 1 week's illness, when your earnings are zero).

If you are totally reliant on your private income, it is clear that for the first year or two, money may be very tight, and that you will need a good system to manage your finances. It is essential that you carefully monitor what income you receive, and what you spend, and that you keep these accounts separate from your everyday personal accounts, even though the salary that you take from the private practice then becomes your personal account.

It is probably worth seeking the advice of an accountant on what information you should collect, and what expenses are tax allowable. McMahon *et al.* (2005) give detailed guidance on how to set up systems to monitor cash flow, and hence how to avoid financial failure. It is important to remember that you will need to pay your tax bills, in advance, on two occasions a year, and hence it is reassuring if you put away each month a proportion of the tax you are likely to have to pay annually.

What fees to charge

Once you know what you need to earn, you can calculate how much you would need to charge for each treatment session. To do this, you must decide how many 'chargeable hours' you want to work each week, bearing in mind that other activities supporting the clinical work (e.g. letters and phone calls, reading, your own supervision, planning treatment sessions, dealing with crises, missed treatment sessions, etc.) will add substantially to these hours, probably by as much as 50%. It is unlikely that you will have administrative support early in your private working, and so you will need to create time for this aspect of your work.

Edie realized that she would need to earn £77,760 per year and she knew that she wanted to work a 36 hour week. She estimated the breakdown of her time as follows:

Time seeing patients	*24 chargeable hours*
Supporting activity (50% of 24 hours)	*12 hours*
Target for total activity	*36 hours*

She multiplied this by 45 weeks, which gave her the total number (24 x 45) of chargeable hours in the year: 1080 hours.

Thus she needed to generate £77,760 within 1080 chargeable hours (£77,760/1080) and calculated her hourly fee as £72.

It is helpful if you have friends or colleagues working in area, so that you can establish what fees are being charged by other CBT therapists, to check whether what you have calculated is in the right range.

The means of collecting fees is an issue for some therapists, although the lack of embarrassment shown by most patients means that you might quickly habituate to the situation. Invoicing monthly may be preferred by some patients, but immediate payment at the end of each session, either with cash or cheque, minimizes the number of sessions that are not paid for, and reduces your administrative tasks. Cash flow problems are also greater with invoiced payments, and so this is probably the least preferred option for most therapists. Although information about payment will probably be on the written information you provide for new patients, it is helpful to spell it out for them. You could say,

As far as payment is concerned, the most straightforward method is to simply pay me at the end of each session, either with cash or a cheque(/credit card). Some people prefer it if I send them an invoice on a monthly basis, but generally people pay as we go along.

The issue of a sliding scale was raised earlier. As you will not be governed by anyone else's priorities, you can charge each patient a different amount if you so wish. It is more likely that you may opt to have reduced rates for particular sub-groups, in the interests of equality of access. You can, for example, charge people less if they are self-financing, as opposed to being funded by an insurance company; or have a small quota of lower income patients, or students. It is wise to monitor how many patients fall into what fee category, so that you do not unexpectedly find your income dropping significantly.

Patients who do not turn up or do not pay

A patient not turning up for appointments is a fact of life. Build this into your calculations about your required income and develop a policy about how to respond. In your information leaflet, you could spell out, for example, that you will charge if an appointment is cancelled fewer than 24 hours in advance—and then you must decide how rigidly you will stick to that rule. If there appears to be a genuinely unexpected reason for absence, like an illness or a car accident, then you could waive the fee. If there seems to be a more casual approach to attending sessions, then you may charge half initially, but if it happens repeatedly, then charge the full amount. If for any reason a therapist misses an appointment, for example because of a clinical crisis, then it is worth charging a half fee or nothing for the next session, even though you feel the responsibility was not yours. Be sure you explain this clearly; a patient of mine was incensed when she thought I was charging her half the fee for a session I missed due to a lengthy hospital appointment, and did not understand that I was talking about the fee for a subsequent session.

A different issue is raised by people who default on payments. The first step is to repeat the request, but if this produces no response, it is worth threatening recourse to a debt collection agency (names of which can be found on the Internet). Although the author has been in this position three times in 8 years, the threat has always been sufficient; it has never been necessary to contact an agency. An alternative is to issue a small claim in a county court. This can be an inexpensive way of tackling the problem, as a major intention of this procedure is to simplify it as far as possible, without requiring assistance of solicitors. Nevertheless, this should only be a step of last resort when all other attempts at dispute resolution have been exhausted.

Insurance and pension

You will need to insure yourself, to protect your patients (in the case of negligence), or your own reputation if you feel that a complaint is unreasonable. Your professional organization will provide information about insurers experienced in this area of work.

You may also need buildings or office contents insurance. Even if you are renting a room, it is unlikely that the contents of your office would be insured by the landlord, and if you are using a room at home, it would be worth checking with your insurance company whether the terms of any insurance policy are altered by your home-working.

Finally, it is worth considering insuring against prolonged illness or other loss of earnings. Although it is improbable that you would be off work for more than 6 weeks, and you could put money aside to cover you for that, a longer illness can be devastating for an uninsured independent practitioner.

The amount you will need to put aside for your pension depends to some degree on how much you have already accumulated if you have been employed already and were in an occupational pension scheme. Whether or not this is the case, you will need at this point to begin or continue to build up a pension fund, or other potential income to cover your retirement, but it is beyond the scope of this chapter to discuss the relative virtues of different kinds of personal investment. The main point is that, because of the effect of compounding interest, it is important that you do not put off pension payments until later. You cannot easily catch up the interest of the missed years. You should seek independent financial advice, beginning perhaps with *the Which Guide to planning your retirement* (www.which.co.uk).

You have now considered what you will provide, and how much you will charge for it, and so it is time to consider how people will know that you are available.

How will I let people know about me?

Even if you have been working for some time in an area, you may be surprised by how little people are aware of you, or how quickly they forget. You will therefore need to take active steps to advertise that you are available for private work, that you have relevant skills and experience, and can be trusted. This will be even more important if you are new to the area. Your professional organization may have guidelines about how you can advertise yourself, and this is likely to warn you against making exaggerated claims about yourself, and unfavourably comparing alternative organizations or individuals with yourself. Among the ways of advertising yourself are the following:

- **Networking**: if you are moving from an established service, let your colleagues know, including those from professions other than your own. This should include relevant secretarial and administrative staff. You could send out a business card, or a short email message or a letter with information about what you are offering and how to contact you. Inform psychological therapy services (private and statutory) as well as individual psychiatrists, psychologists, nurse specialists, and counsellors within the local mental health services.
- **Local general practitioners (GPs)**: send a brief mail shot to all GPs in your immediate area, which is likely to total a few hundred. Sending information to each practice is less likely to be useful as the information may not be circulated.

- **Register as a private therapist with the BABCP and your professional body:** many patients will seek information about therapists from professional and accrediting bodies. The BACP Directory could be considered, although this is more general than the BABCP listing. The Yellow Pages should also be considered. If you treat a patient who is totally self-referred, it is useful to send his/her GP (with the patient's permission) information about yourself and CBT.
- **Voluntary organizations**: the staff of organizations such as MIND can be a helpful source of referrals.
- **Local media:** you could publicize yourself by, for example, offering to write an article for the local newspaper, or contacting the local TV or radio station to offer to comment on a current topic from the news.

Monitoring where your referrals come from is useful. You will then know where to put your marketing efforts. Bear in mind that some publicity (e.g. the BABCP Directory) will bear fruit in the short term, whereas other referral sources (e.g. two or three GPs or psychiatrists) will only gradually build up- and may then become of major importance.

How you respond to individual requests is important, and you should ensure that this is timely, informative, and pleasant, whether to a patient or to a referrer. If you have an answer phone, this should be friendly but professional, and followed up promptly. It should be updated with relevant information if you are away; the same applies to email responses.

If you have given up a job to work privately, the initial flow of referrals may be dispiriting, but is likely to increase with time. It is important that you either have enough capital to see you through this difficult early stage, or that you go into private work more gradually so that lack of capital would be less of a problem.

Once your referrals start to arrive, you will be involved in some administration, and it will be necessary to put systems in place.

What business/professional administration will I need?

It is unlikely that you will employ an administrator at an early stage, so consider how to minimize your administrative load. The probable minimum requirements are shown in Table 14.5. In addition, if you want to monitor how long patients waited for treatment, etc., you could collect information on date of referral, initial assessment, start of therapy, end of treatment, and the number of sessions in treatment, and so on. If you decide to monitor indices of quality of this kind, then you must ensure that you abide by the principles

Table 14.5 Patient record: minimum requirements.

◆ Name, address, date of birth, telephone numbers, email address
◆ GP name, address, and telephone number
◆ Referrer (if different) name, address, and telephone number
◆ Name and address of payment agency
◆ Source of referral

of the Data Protection Act (2001), which are described on www. Dataprotection. gov.uk.

Letters to referrer/GP

It is important to keep referring agents informed about the progress of your patients, and letters on assessment, at discharge, and at times of clinical change, are the minimum. If patients are self-referred, then their permission to write to their GP should be sought. If they are unwilling for this to happen, it is worth pointing out the advantages of having one key individual who is aware of their complete clinical history. However, if they continue to be unwilling, then you should consider whether you would feel safe treating them without any back up if a crisis occurred. If your patient insists that you do not inform the GP, record in your notes that this was the patient's wish.

Treatment notes/measures

Although therapists differ in the extent to which they write notes during sessions, it is important to keep contemporaneous notes, together with relevant measures, in an individual file which is kept in a secure place, for example, a lockable filing cabinet. You will also need to find time to replenish your stock of psychometric measures and information for patients.

Financial information

As described above, a record must be kept of all money spent (with receipts if they are to be claimed as expenses against tax); and of all income, whether cash, cheque, or credit card, all recorded in a Day Book. An accountant would advise you about what information you need to collect, but if it seems daunting, it may be worthwhile attending a course on bookkeeping. In order to reduce the potential for chaos, and to separate your personal and business financial affairs, it is helpful to have a separate bank or building society account for this purpose. There is a clear description of an administrative system suitable for a small business of this kind in McMahon *et al.* (2005).

Quality standards

Audit

You will want to ensure that your work continues at a high standard, partly by ensuring that you build in time (and budget) for CPD, and partly by monitoring the quality of your work. You will probably want to monitor various aspects of your work such as the gender balance, the age distribution, the number of missed appointments that you have, the source of your referrals, and types of problem, simply so that you know what population you are dealing with. In addition, you may wish to audit some features of your work, to check that it is at a standard that you are happy with.

To conduct an audit, you would need to decide what would constitute a reasonable level for whatever feature you were interested in, which you could either do on *a priori* grounds, or by running an initial exploratory survey. You would then carry out some monitoring to look at whether you were meeting the quality target, and if not, look at the reasons you were falling short, and decide what steps you could take to improve the situation.

Edie realized that it was difficult to proceed with treatment in the absence of a formulation and she felt that one should be present in at least 90% of cases. She decided to conduct a study of her use of formulations and chose the next 40 discharged cases as a sample, looking at how many of them had a written formulation. She also studied the cases without formulations to see what had gone wrong, and to consider what action she might take. She found that in six cases (15%) of her sample, there was no written formulation. On looking at this in more detail, she realized that three of the six had attended only twice, in two cases the assessment had continued over many sessions with only a partial formulation resulting, and in one case the patient's goals had changed half way through treatment, and the formulation had not been revised. Her response was to ensure that a preliminary formulation be agreed with the patient after two sessions, as a prompt for an elaborated one subsequently. She also set a date to review her progress in formulating patient problems.

There are many options for audit, for example you may be interested in how long people were waiting before an initial assessment, in which case you could make a judgement of how long would be a reasonable wait, and then audit the next 40 referrals to see whether your standard was being met. If not, you could look at the reasons why you were falling short, and decide what steps could be taken to improve the situation.

The important point is that by raising questions about the quality of your service, you are likely to continue to improve what you offer to people—and indeed find that there are areas that you would undoubtedly wish to improve. Other indices of the quality of your service reside in your accountability to an accrediting body, via for example, your CPD and supervision records, each of which raises specific difficulties in an independent setting, which we will now consider.

Continuing professional development

As we saw at the beginning of the chapter, your skill and expertise are your main assets, and you cannot afford to let them rust, even though CPD takes up both time and money. Accrediting bodies generally consider CPD to be centrally important, and demand evidence of it when considering whether to continue your accreditation as a therapist. It is more difficult without a manager to objectively consider your professional development, and what steps you might take to continue to develop. You may find it helpful to book a supervision session specifically to deal with such issues, or to find someone to act as a mentor on a very occasional basis. You will also find useful guidance in Chapter 15.

The BABCP offers useful ideas about what activities can be considered as relevant CPD, and you should keep a file of any relevant teaching and training that you provide or receive (together with certificates of attendance, etc.), as well as a record of the journals and books that you have read. These will all alert you to new developments, and it is helpful to keep an ongoing log of areas in which you would like to develop. It is important to then put time aside each year to review these ideas, to decide how much time you can afford to spend on CPD, and to prioritize which ones you will take forward in the coming year. This will help to ensure that you put sufficient time into CPD, which may otherwise slip down the priorities as more urgent tasks grab your attention on a day-to-day basis.

If you are working in relative isolation, attending training events, especially conferences, increases your opportunities for networking and connecting with other cognitive therapists. You can exchange ideas, be abreast of current developments, and be alerted to new ideas to follow up.

The nature of referrals, and the requests for help from patients, differ from year to year, partly as a result of your reputation growing. You should be conservative about taking referrals for problems or patients that may be beyond your competence, but include the skill area in your log of possible topics for CPD. You should be able to say, 'Sorry, I have insufficient experience in that area', and decide whether it is an area that you would like to learn more about. An alternative would be to seek additional supervision specifically for that work, and as this is an area which has general importance for the quality of your work, it is this that we will next turn to.

Supervision

The most important reason for arranging regular supervision is to protect your patients. Supervision gives you the opportunity to question whether you are approaching problems appropriately. As with many other psychological therapies, ongoing supervision is a prerequisite of maintaining your accreditation as a CBT therapist. It is more important if you are working in a setting where the exchange of ideas with other therapists is more difficult to come by than if you are part of a department or team. General issues of supervision are discussed in Chapter 16, and so only the issues pertinent to private working will be considered here.

Individual, peer, or self-supervision

Although individual supervision with a skilled supervisor may appear to be the gold standard, this is not necessarily true if you are working in relative isolation. The opportunity to bounce ideas off a peer or peers, the suggestions of new ways of working prompted by group supervision, can be invaluable if you get little opportunity to meet with other therapists in your everyday work. However, the importance of self-supervision via reflection, reading and reformulation, and including listening to your own treatment tapes, cannot be overstated; this is also discussed in Chapter 16. It allows you to identify issues that you would like to raise in supervision with someone else, but many supervision questions can be answered by careful identification of the issue, and subsequent reflection. There are a number of cognitive therapy rating scales, for example, that developed by Young and Beck (1980), or the revised version of Blackburn *et al.*, (2001), which can be used to monitor your provision of therapy if you record your treatment sessions.

Many therapists find that different modes of supervision meet different needs, and as supervision is expensive (in terms of time and money), it is worthwhile asking yourself which would be the best kind of supervision for different kinds of questions or needs. It may require ingenuity and perseverance to organize peer supervision with another therapist, and even more so with a group of peers, but it is worth the effort, and will make an enormous difference to the quality of your work with patients, both for them, and for your own work experience. You can take advantage of any network that you have, CPD events, and advertising on the Internet to find potential peers—though particularly in the latter case, you should set up a trial period to check out whether the supervision sessions are providing what you need.

Although the apparent cost of supervision can be reduced through peer supervision arrangements, it will take more time as your co-supervisee(s) will also presents questions for consideration. However, you will learn vicariously from the discussion by generalizing to your own experience, and it can be supportive by reminding you that other people find challenges and problems that they cannot deal with by themselves. Peer supervision sessions should be appropriately structured, as described in Chapter 16.

Clearly, there is a place for individual supervision, and you should try and ensure that you choose an experienced supervisor, for example, by checking the BABCP website. It is worthwhile considering telephone, video, or email supervision if you have difficulty finding a good local supervisor. You could supplement any of these with an occasional face-to-face meeting if necessary. A good supervisor can help you identify blind spots in your understanding, possibly those associated with unhelpful beliefs of your own; and help you to become aware of gaps in your skills or knowledge. They can also be invaluable in providing you with support and reassurance if you are dealing with distressing and difficult material. This can be particularly valuable if you work alone, without easy access to other therapists for support.

Getting the best out of supervision

However, if you do work in relative isolation, it is important to acknowledge that some sessions can be more draining than others, and to give yourself space to self-soothe. This may mean leaving sufficient time between patients to allow yourself to absorb what you have been exposed to, before you go on to the next person; leaving time to summarize what you have discovered in the session, and what implication it has for the formulation, and possibly what implications it has for your own beliefs; perhaps leaving the therapy room for a few minutes, even going outside; or using a relaxation strategy of some kind. You can be more flexible about the spacing of sessions if you are working independently, and you should use this constructively for your own good, and the good of the patient.

It is probable that different kinds of supervision will serve different purposes, and that you can sample different kinds to that end. For example, you may welcome the consistency and sparking of ideas that meeting regularly with one or two trusted colleagues gives you, but would still find it helpful to book two sessions with an eating disorder expert, to discuss your high dropout rate in this problem area; and you may feel more comfortable about this if you were receiving regular emotional support from your peer supervision sessions. Although the costs are not irrelevant, you have more freedom in independent practice to set your own priorities, and to determine how much supervision is desirable for you.

Be explicit with your patients about receiving supervision, to reassure them about confidentiality. This is particularly so if you are using recorded information, especially in a small community. You will need to develop your own policy about the use, storage, and disposal of tapes at the end of treatment, part of which should include obtaining consent from the patient. It is important that you raise this in such a way as not to jeopardize your relationship with your patient. This draws attention to the general importance of the therapeutic relationship.

The therapeutic relationship

The quality of the therapeutic relationship in CBT is as crucial to outcome as it is in other treatment modalities, and this is no different in private work. However, the relationship between therapist and patient may reflect the nature of the contract between them—the patients are commissioning the treatment for themselves, and may feel more comfortable about giving critical feedback, negotiating more or fewer sessions, and so on. Nevertheless, the general tone of the relationship remains that of the therapist as a guide or mentor, walking alongside patients as they work out new ways of feeling, thinking, and behaving, with open-minded curiosity and respect about their current position. The private setting presents specific issues related to boundaries within the therapeutic relationship, and they will be considered next.

Boundaries

Treatment boundaries delimit the roles adopted by the therapist and patient, and include such elements as where, when, and at what cost treatment is provided, as well as what happens in the interaction between the therapist and patient. The main guiding principles are that the patients' needs have primacy, and that the gratification of the therapist's personal needs is excluded from the therapeutic setting. Typically, there is marked non-reciprocity in a therapeutic relationship and a patient may seek to redress the balance by attempting to change the boundaries, for example, by offering special deals on reciprocal services like building work or accountancy, or repeatedly asking the therapist about family issues or holidays. Before violating any boundaries, you must evaluate what impact it would have on the patient.

Dual relationships

Also bear in mind the pitfalls inherent in entering dual relationships (Smith and Fitzpatrick, 1995). The usual advice is to avoid dual relationships whenever possible, but this may be difficult in a community where there are few private CBT therapists. If you refuse to take on patients with whom you have another relationship, you may in effect be excluding them from treatment. For example, it may be that health professionals with whom you have had contact or even worked, may prefer to have private treatment for themselves or their families (in order to avoid the minefields of the dual relationships inherent in their using services in which *they* work, or network!). You may also find yourself referred people who are of the same religious, political, gender, or ethnic leaning as yourself, as people tend to choose therapists with similar values to those they themselves hold. Gottleib (1993) suggested that there are three dimensions relevant to the non-therapeutic aspects of a dual relationship—power, duration, and whether there would be a finite end—and that each of these should be considered when deciding whether to take on a patient where there would be a dual relationship. For example, taking on one's ex-employer for therapy may be too far along the power dimension to allow a constructive therapeutic relationship to develop.

Your premises

The location of the therapy may make it more important to maintain firm boundaries. If the therapy is taking place in a hospital or clinic setting, while undesirable in some ways, it at least provides a clear frame for the therapeutic interactions. If on the other hand, you are seeing patients in your own home, or in a setting where there are no other therapists or clinical staff, it is potentially easier to blur boundaries. For example, patients may bring presents for your home, or ask questions or make suggestions about it. It is important that you are mindful of what messages you are giving to the patient; for example, a photograph of you with your children may be read as showing that you are happy to discuss your family relationships. Pictures with a neutral theme may be more appropriate.

It is important to ensure that disturbances and distractions from the therapeutic sessions are minimized, particularly ones related to the therapist's private life. It is difficult to maintain a professional image, and hence, the patient's confidence, if a child is crying at the door, or if an unexpected visitor turns up at the house. This is particularly difficult if there is no receptionist, and the same door is used by family and friends as by patients. You should go to some lengths to let friends know as a general principle that you are not available if you have patients with you.

It is important for your stress levels that you are not available at all times/in all situations to patients. The facilities on telephones to pick up calls while away from your base, as well as mobile phones, increase the risks of that. You should develop rules about when you are willing to be available, and you should then let your patients know about how rapidly they can expect a response to a call to you.

A dedicated line for clinical purposes is desirable, and this is more practicable now that mobile phones are readily available. This provides a clear boundary for you, allows you to prepare yourself for a personal or professional call, to limit your working hours more easily, and makes it easier to maintain confidentiality. At the very least, any answer phone message should be appropriately professional for the purpose—a 4-year old's message may be enchanting to your relatives, less so to a distressed patient.

Physical contact

The issue of non-sexual physical contact is an important one for all therapists, but may be more of an issue for a therapist working privately in relative isolation. Inappropriate behaviour generally develops from a gradual blurring of boundaries, which may be more likely in a non-clinical setting. Furthermore, the sexual violation of boundaries is more common in therapists who are experiencing personal problems, and are professionally isolated (Simon, 1991). While many therapists would never make physical contact with a patient, others may respond to a patient's distress by patting a shoulder. This should always be done in a considered way, taking account of the client's formulation. A reassuring pat may be misconstrued by someone with a history of emotional deprivation, or feel unwelcome and intrusive to someone with issues of trust. It would be useful to be explicit with patients at a time when they are not distressed, by saying, for example:

> *You were obviously very upset when we were talking about your previous admission to hospital. I wonder what you would find most helpful at times like that. Some people find it a relief to express their feelings, and to deal with it themselves. Other people find a pat on the arm comforting. I wonder what you would find the most helpful at times like that?*

If the patient suggested something that you would find unacceptable, then this could be directly addressed.

The maintenance of clear boundaries contributes to your safety, as inappropriate behaviour is less likely to occur when boundaries are clear. Planning for both your physical safety and also the safety of your reputation is paramount if you are working in settings where you may be alone, including on home visits. This is the final clinical issue that will be considered (see also Chapter 3).

Safety

Therapist safety

Establish policies about acceptable referrals. Many patients refer themselves independently of their GPs, so it is possible to see new patients who have not been screened for safety by anyone. You could decide to only accept self-referrals from patients willing for you to contact their GP; or that you would only accept referrals from known referrers who were aware of the setting of your clinic. Alternatively, you could screen on the nature of the problem, for example, by not accepting referrals for anger management or poor impulse control. In any event, think through the issue, taking account of the degree of isolation in which you work, and the help that would be available if you were at risk.

Assess carefully and be alert for any previous history of violence. Although physical harm to therapists is very rare, the risks you could take in a busy medical centre are different from those you could take if working by yourself in an otherwise empty house. If you have any doubt about your safety, it would be wiser to refer on to someone working in a different setting. It is important to maintain your assessment skills, and to be alert to signs that a patient is becoming agitated or angry.

Document your contacts. Have systems in place that make it clear who you have been seeing, and if you do home visits, where you have gone. This can be as simple as a list in a desk diary, possibly with an index of names and addresses of patients. An additional safeguard can be tape-recording sessions on a regular basis: in addition to its clinical uses, it could be helpful for an angry patient to know that the tape recorder is running as usual. If in advance of a session, you are worrying that a patient may be a risk, it would be worth arranging for someone else to be in the building if it is usually empty, and to make the patient aware of that.

Consider location and think carefully about using a room that is in an isolated position; a peaceful, calming rural idyll may be inappropriate. Similarly, it may not be sensible to use a room at the top of a house, as opposed to a ground floor room with ready access to the main door. It is unlikely that you could have a panic button or alarm in your room, but if calming a patient is unsuccessful, you should be willing to leave the room if necessary. This means that it is sensible to position your chair between the patient and the door.

Patient safety

It is possible that your patient may be at risk, particularly of self-harm, and your assessment skills are important in this respect. You need to have procedures worked out in advance, so that you are not trying to work out what to do in a crisis. To begin with, your information sheet about your conditions of working should include a statement about the necessity of breaching confidentiality if the patient (or other) were at risk. If you are concerned that a patient may be at risk of harm, it is important to assess this carefully, and not to underestimate the probability. You should then ensure that you record your assessment in your notes, including your conclusions. If your conclusion is that the person is at risk, you need to decide whether you can deal with this by yourself, for example, by putting in place a plan to reduce the risk (arranging an early appointment, problem-solving to look at other solutions, ensuring that the person will not be socially isolated), but you should in any event inform the patients' GP, even if up to that point they had been unwilling for you to do so. Apart from the safety of the patients themselves, you would need to consider the response of relatives, and even a coroner, if the patients went on to harm themselves, and it transpired that you had not reported the risk. If, on the other hand you feel that the patient needs the back up of mental health services, you should have information about how to access this (which may be via the GP, unless the patient is already in contact with the service). As arrangements for access are highly varied, you should be familiar with local services. Similar principles apply if you are dealing with children, and assess that they are at risk. You should have information in your system which will allow you to readily contact the Child Protection services if necessary.

You might be dealing with someone who presents a chronic but low risk of self-harm, in which case the same principles apply. If in your opinion the risk has increased, you should record your assessment of the risk in the notes, your planned response to this, and you should discuss this with the patient's GP.

You may be in a difficult practical situation if you assess a patient to be at immediate risk, when you have a list of patients to see in the next few hours. Unless you feel that the patient is able to proceed unaccompanied for further assessment, or there is a carer present who is willing to accompany the patient, you will need to find time to arrange the immediate care. This may take some hours, thus flexibility is required and you may need to postpone sessions with other patients.

Key points

- Working in private practice presents particular clinical challenges, as well as the need to acquire new business skills.
- It can however be a satisfying way of providing help, and allow you independence from others' priorities.
- It is important that you plan in advance, and in detail, how you will run your business, even if you are operating as a lone practitioner.
- You are responsible for ensuring that you maintain your clinical skills and knowledge and thus should invest in CPD and supervision.
- You may be at particular risk in independent practice, so ensure that you give thought to maximizing your safety and well-being.

Further reading

British Association of Behavioural and Cognitive Psychotherapists. Available at: www.babcp.com (accessed 29 September 2009).

Butler,G. and Hope, T.(2007). Manage Your Mind. Oxford: Oxford University Press.

Chapter 19 in this book: Promoting and surviving change and developing services.

Data Protection Act (2001). Available at: www.dataprotection.gov.uk (accessed 29 September 2009).

McMahon, G., Palmer, S. and Wilding, C. (2005). *The Essential Skills for Setting up a Counseling and Psychotherapy Practice.* London: Routledge.

Which Guide to planning your retirement. Available at: www.which.co.uk/advice/planning-your-retirement/retirement-countdown/index.jsp (accessed 29 September 2009).

References

Blackburn, I.M., James, I.A., Milne, D.L., Baker, C., Standard, S., Garland, A. and Reichelt, K. (2001). The revised cognitive therapy scale (CTS-R): psychometric properties. *Behavioural and Cognitive Psychotherapy*, **29**, 431–446.

Data Protection Act (2001). Available at: www.dataprotection.gov.uk (accessed 29 September 2009).

Gottlieb, M.C. (1993) Avoiding exploitative dual relationships: a decision-making model. *Psychotherapy*, **30**, 41–48.

McMahon, G., Palmer, S. and Wilding, C. (2005). *The Essential Skills for Setting up a Counseling and Psychotherapy Practice.* London: Routledge.

Simon, R. (1991). Psychological injury caused by boundary violation precursors to therapist-patient sex. *Psychiatric Annals*, **21**, 616–619.

Smith, D. and Fitzpatrick, M. (1995). Patient-boundary issues: an integrative review of theory and research. *Professional Psychology: Research and Practice*, **26**, 499–506.

Wright, J.H. and Davis, D. (1994). The therapeutic relationship in cognitive-behavioural therapy: patient perceptions and therapist responses. *Cognitive and Behavioural Practice*, **1**, 25–45.

Young, J. and Beck, A.T. (1980). *Cognitive Therapy Scale: Rating Manual.* Unpublished Manuscript. Philadelphia, PA: University of Pennsylvania.

Chapter 15

Developing and progressing as a CBT therapist

Freda McManus, Kate Rosen, and
Helen Jenkins

You have invested a huge amount of time, energy and planning into getting qualified as a CBT therapist. But what then? More of the same for the next 40 years?

Introduction

Completion of your training as a CBT therapist is an important milestone. However, it is doubtful whether, in the current climate of rapidly evolving healthcare services, any professional training can equip you with the knowledge and skills to address the complex world of practice as a CBT therapist in a definitive or enduring sense (Corrie *et al.*, 2008). Hence, continuing professional development (CPD) becomes necessary in order to develop and extend the skills acquired in training, to incorporate new developments into your skills, and to learn to apply them to different settings, contexts, and patient groups. As CBT has blossomed in recent years the pace of change within CBT research and therapy services has accelerated, meaning that more CPD is necessary for therapists to keep abreast of developments. Also, CPD had previously been structured into the roles of the professional groups that carried out CBT interventions (e.g. Clinical Psychologist often had one session/week for CPD activities) and it was possible to keep up-to-date by using this time to attend courses/conferences and read journals. However, this is often no longer the case with the increased variety in CBT therapists' professional backgrounds, roles, and settings (e.g. in private work, in training, in National Health Service [NHS] or voluntary organizations) and the rapidly changing professional and economic climate. Hence, there has been an increased emphasis on formal requirements and structures for CPD, and on CPD as a requirement for ongoing professional registration and for accreditation with the British Association for Behavioural and Cognitive Psychotherapies (BABCP).

At a more personal level, the greater diversity in career paths for CBT therapists also means that it makes sense for individual CBT therapists to spend some time thinking about and planning their own development as there is, as yet, no career structure for CBT therapists. This chapter provides a framework for thinking about development and progression as a CBT therapist and gives some hints on areas that you may want to consider. There are three main motivations for considering your career development:

- To meet formal requirements for registration or regulation. For example, the Health Professions Council lays down strict criteria about the CPD needed for maintaining professional registration for the professions that fall under its remit. Something that is relevant for all CBT therapists is the accreditation process laid out by the BABCP. In this chapter, we outline the process and criteria for accreditation by the BABCP.
- To develop your skills as a CBT therapist. As the field develops you will no doubt want to keep up with developments in CBT (e.g. 'third wave' therapies) in order to maximize your effectiveness with patients, develop and refine your repertoire of skills, and maintain interest in the field.
- To progress your career, whether this be in terms of formal or informal status. For example, advancing your career formally by setting your sights on a higher graded job. Or less formal ways such as by making a name for yourself in the field and amassing 'CV points' by developing clinical innovations to enhancing your research or training profile.

These three areas will be covered in turn. We begin by outlining formal processes for development such as accreditation and then go on to look at more personal motivations such as the development of your CBT skills and plans for developing your career.

Formal requirements and accreditation as a CBT therapist

Different professional groups have their own formal requirements for CPD and its documentation, but in the United Kingdom none is specific to CBT other than that of the national association for CBT therapists (BABCP). The BABCP system confers three possible types of accreditation:

- CBT therapist
- CBT supervisor
- CBT trainer

It is necessary to be accredited as a therapist to become accredited as a supervisor or a trainer but neither supervisor nor trainer accreditation is necessary for the other. For accreditation as a CBT therapist you are required to demonstrate CBT knowledge, experience, and skill in several areas. See Boxes 15.1 and 15.2 for more detailed information.

Box 15.1 Criteria for accreditation by BABCP as a CBT therapist

Currently, to be accredited by BABCP as a CBT therapist you must:

- Have a relevant *professional training* (e.g. clinical psychology, nursing, medicine, occupational therapy, social work) and a year's post-qualification experience. For those without a 'core professional training' there is an alternative route in which you complete a supplementary form to evidence that you have acquired the core knowledge, skills, and attitudes relevant to the practice of psychological therapies that would usually be gained through core professional qualification.
- Have been *accountable* for your own professional practice to a senior member of your profession for at least a year since qualifying in your profession. This is typical in NHS jobs but may prove more difficult for those in private practice.
- Provide a satisfactory statement of *training in the theory and practice of CBT* related to designated areas of competence (Roth and Pilling, 2007). The training must be sufficient to provide an understanding of the theoretical basis of CBT and its application across a wide range of problem areas. Some of this may have been provided as part of your core professional training (e.g. as a nurse, counsellor, or clinical psychologist) but it may need to be supplemented through attendance at further training courses. The BABCP requires you to evidence 450 hours training, 200 hours of which should be provided by recognized trainers, and at least 50% of this should/must be skills focused. The remaining 250 hours can be through training providers or can be achieved via private study (e.g. reading). Some people will achieve this through a mix of short courses but others will undertake a Post-graduate Diploma in CBT. Diploma in CBT courses are usually day-release courses that will provide training and supervision in CBT (see http://www.babcp.com/

Box 15.1 Criteria for accreditation by BABCP as a CBT therapist *(continued)*

cbt-training/cbt-training-courses/ for details of diploma courses in CBT). Whichever route you choose it is probably helpful to keep a log of your CBT training, including the number of taught hours/private study, the topics and trainers, and what specific competencies were being focused on.

- Have ongoing CBT *clinical supervision.* You need to have conducted a minimum of 200 hours of supervised assessment and therapy, to have treated a minimum of 8 patients, and for this work to have been on at least three different problem areas (e.g. depression, panic disorder, and eating disorders). The supervision should be from a supervisor who is BABCP accredited as a therapist and at least three cases should have involved 'live' supervision (live observation of therapy skills or reviewing tapes of actual sessions). Four patients should have been written up and assessed (e.g. as case reports). Supervision should be ongoing (minimum 1 hour/month for full time staff) and for the purposes of accreditation it may be helpful to record details of supervised clinical practice and case mix in a log.
- Demonstrate *knowledge and understanding of the therapeutic relationship* and competence in the development, maintenance, and ending of such relationships—this can be demonstrated through references.
- Sign a statement of intent of *sustained commitment* to the theory and practice of CBT which includes ongoing CPD. To evidence your commitment to CBT you are asked to give details of your last year of CBT practice and what proportion of your time you spend in CBT-related activities (e.g. 50% of the time you do clinical work and 50% of that involves CBT), and to show evidence of undertaking CPD in CBT. On an ongoing basis, accredited CBT therapists are expected to engage in 30 hours/year of CBT-related CPD (attendance at or provision of symposia/lectures/workshops/seminars plus reading CBT books/journals).
- Adhere to the *Guidelines for Good Practice* of the BABCP and be willing to be scrutinized in this adherence as required.

Although the above criteria were accurate at the time of going to press, exact details of what is required are likely to change, so it is always wise to check the website www.babcp.com/about-babcp/accreditation/ for the most up-to-date information.

Box 15.2 Criteria for accreditation by BABCP as a supervisor and trainer

Currently, to gain accreditation from BABCP as a supervisor/trainer you must:

- Be BABCP accredited (or eligible for accreditation) as a therapist with a minimum of 3 years CBT practice since achieving eligibility for accreditation as a therapist.
- Have treated a significant number of (at least 50) patients using CBT, across the range of complexity (at least 10 who were severe, chronic, and/or complex cases) drawn from a spectrum of disorders and problem areas.
- Be receiving regular clinical supervision from an expert CBT supervisor and appropriate supervision/support for your CBT supervisory and/or training practice (minimum 1 hour/month full time for both clinical and supervisory/training supervision).
- Show evidence of ongoing CPD in CBT (minimum 30 hours/year) which includes a minimum of 6 hours/year of CPD relating to your professional development as a supervisor or trainer in CBT.
- Be a dedicated CBT practitioner (spend at least 50% of your work time in CBT practice related activities).
- Be providing regular specialist CBT supervision and/or training (40 hours of training or 80 hours of supervision in the previous 2 years).

Although the idea of accreditation has been around for many years, it is only in the last few years that it has gained momentum. If the majority of CBT therapists are not accredited there is little motivation or need for anyone to overcome the hurdles of getting themselves accredited (i.e. filling out a *long* form and writing a cheque to BABCP—significant hurdles!). However, the recent proliferation in CBT training courses and therapists being trained has led to an increased need to provide some form of 'quality control' on the profession. Thus, a formal process of accreditation for CBT therapists, supervisors, trainers, and training courses has been developed. One condition for the accreditation of training courses is that they use only BABCP accredited therapists to provide the training (teaching, marking, and supervision). Hence, anyone who wants to contribute to a BABCP accredited training course needs to be accredited themselves. Once a significant proportion of CBT therapists are accredited, lack of accreditation begins to look suspicious, in the way that a non-chartered accountant would. A particular advantage of accreditation is in private practice where there are few restrictions on the label 'CBT therapist' so BABCP accreditation can provide a means by which patients or other employers can determine whether a therapist has the necessary training and experience to provide CBT.

At the early stages of your CBT career you will be primarily concerned with achieving the criteria required for accreditation as a therapist. And indeed this may be advantageous for some aspect of your employment setting (e.g. contributing to a BABCP accredited training course, or getting your name on BABCP's 'find a therapist website'). However, as your career progresses you may want to consider gaining BABCP accreditation as a CBT supervisor and/or trainer. With the increase in the provision of CBT there is an associated increase in the provision of CBT training and supervision. This has put pressure on CBT therapists to develop skills in training and supervision, and to evidence these skills by gaining BABCP accreditation as a CBT supervisor and/or trainer. See Box 15.2 for more detail on BABCP's criteria for accreditation as a supervisor and/or trainer.

As yet BABCP accreditation as a supervisor or trainer isn't required in order for a CBT therapist to provide training or supervision but it may become so in the future, or you may simply want to formally acknowledge your skills in this area. For those who are interested in developing skills in CBT training and/or supervision both the Oxford and Newcastle cognitive therapy centres offer relevant courses and the BABCP sometimes hosts a 1-day supervision/training conference. Although the empirical literature on CBT training and supervision is sparse, we have listed some further reading at the end of this chapter.

As can be seen from Boxes 15.1 and 15.2, the BABCP's criteria for accreditation are quite comprehensive. However it is also worth noting that, with the exception of references, they relate to the applicant's *quantity* of experience rather than the *quality* of the experience. For example, while Dr N O Good, may have received plenty of CBT training and supervision, he may not have learnt much from it—Dr N O Good may have written up four case reports that were assessed as being very poor, and 'close supervision' of his sessions using the Cognitive Therapy Scale may confirm him to be carrying out sub-standard CBT. In theory these factors would not stop him becoming BABCP accredited as BABCP do not state a minimum quality standard (or even that tapes/case reports must 'pass'). In practice it is unlikely that such an individual would gain accreditation but it is worth noting that BABCP's accreditation criteria relate mainly to quantity of CBT experiences and thus do not guarantee quality. The recent development of CBT competences and supervision competences (Roth and Pilling, 2007) may help to refine accreditation criteria for CBT therapists and supervisors, and similar competences for CBT training would be a welcome addition.

Developing and progressing CBT skills and your CBT career

Developing and progressing as a CBT therapist is important not only because it is linked to pay scales and thus to the most basic of needs (to pay the mortgage!), and to formal processes of accreditation/continued registration as a therapist, but it is also important for personal satisfaction. For some this satisfaction will come from career advancement but for others it will be more to do with skill development and job satisfaction. Satisfaction at work is related to having the optimal level of challenge—not so much that you are stressed by feeling that you don't have the necessary skill to do the job but not so little that you don't feel challenged at all. Most therapists would find simply rolling out the same interventions year in and year out became tedious very quickly. Thus, there is an inherent desire to advance one's skills. In addition because CBT is grounded in the 'scientist-practitioner' tradition, which includes the idea that developments in the evidence-base of CBT will be incorporated into routine clinical practice, this also creates a drive towards developing one's skills in line with developments in the wider field of CBT (Salkovskis, 2002). However, as Waller (2009) points out, there is sometimes a danger of reduced efficacy in CBT when therapists put too much emphasis on skill development—they may abandon standard CBT, for which there is a considerable evidence base attesting to its efficacy, in favour of the latest CBT 'fashion', for which there may be limited evidence of efficacy.

In addition, there is some evidence to suggest that CBT competence is linked to appropriate training and supervision (Brosan *et al.*, 2006), and that in the absence of ongoing skills development and supervision, CBT skills may decline (Mannix *et al.*, 2006). Given that there is much evidence linking higher levels of therapist competence with improved patient outcomes (Kuyken and Tsivrikos, 2009; Davidson *et al.*, 2004; Shaw *et al.*, 1999), it is also for our patients' sake that we strive to continue to develop our CBT skills.

Using CBT skills in the context of your own development and progression as a therapist

In thinking about and planning your development as a CBT therapist it may be possible to utilize your own CBT skills, however fledgling they are. For instance, you would begin CBT with a patient by identifying relevant therapy goals. Thus, you can use these goal setting skills to identify goals and set learning objectives for your own development and progression as a CBT therapist. In the clinical setting, once you have defined goals you would then move on to developing a plan for how to achieve these goals. In identifying your career goals and developing plans to achieve them you may need to give consideration to your 'career anchors' (see section 'Establishing career anchors') and preferred learning style. And as in therapy, it is wise to ask yourself what the possible blocks to implementing your plan may be and problem-solve how you might overcome such blocks to progress. Finally, in any CBT intervention you would also want to specify ways of measuring progress towards these goals and a process and timescale for reviewing progress. The process of applying these skills to your own development as a CBT therapist is outlined in more detail in Table 15.1.

Stage 1: Setting goals and specifying learning objectives for your development

In order to set goals for your career development and progression as a CBT therapist you will need to have some sense of where you want to progress to. What is it that you are hoping to achieve in your job? As a CBT therapist? What skills and/or experiences do you need to obtain in order to have the best chance of getting there? This may include developing skills and/or gaining experience in any or all of the areas described in Table 15.2.

Table 15.1 Using your CBT skills to develop and progress as a therapist.

Stage of treatment	Relevant process in career/skill development
1 Identifying relevant goals for treatment: ◆ Ensuring goals are SMART (see section 'Ensuring success: using SMART goals')	1 Identifying relevant goals and specifying learning objectives for your development: ◆ Ensuring goals are SMART (see section 'Ensuring success: using SMART goals')
2 Formulation of individual's internal rules/motivations and relation to current problems	2 Formulation—assessment of career anchors and learning style and of current options
3 Specifying a treatment plan for how to achieve goals: ◆ Attempt to predict and plan to overcome obstacles	3 Specifying a development plan for achieving goals ◆ Attempt to predict and plan to overcome obstacles
4 Review progress towards goals: ◆ Revise goals and reformulate if necessary	4 Review progress towards goals ◆ Revise goals and reformulate if necessary

Table 15.2 Areas of CBT skill development and examples of relevant goals.

Domain	Example
Specific clinical CBT skills or competencies	Being able to set an agenda for CBT sessions in the first 10 minutes of the session with straightforward primary care patients; being able to identity when agenda setting is not working and collaboratively review this with the patient. To develop a formulation, in collaboration with the patient, that is informed by relevant cognitive model, by session 3 of treatment.
Skills in CBT training or supervision	To be able to provide supervision that is perceived to be helpful to junior members of the team including using the following methods: case discussion, role-play, rating tapes. Or to provide a workshop on basic CBT skills to (target group X) that achieves the aim of increasing their skill in activity scheduling and Socratic questioning.
Skills in working in different settings or with specific patient groups	To be able to carrying out 'low-intensity interventions' or an evidence-based protocol for a particular disorder to a specified standard (e.g. as measured by self-ratings of sessions on the Cognitive Therapy Rating Scale; Young and Beck, 1980).
Skills in managing teams or services or components of the service	Managing the wait list such that all patients are seen within 4 weeks and begin treatment within 18 weeks; developing a forum for sharing knowledge such that at least three members of the team increase their knowledge of a disorder as measured by their self-report and willingness to take on a practice case for treatment.
Developing skills required for promotion to a higher grading	If one of your goals is to progress to the next level in a particular hierarchy (e.g. the NHS's Agenda for Change gradings) then you may want to look at job specifications at that level and set goals that relate to achieving the skills/experiences that will put you in the best position to apply for that level of job. This might involve developing specialist clinical skills; for example, in working with complex cases or in supervising others; or research or management skills such as responsibilities for resources.

Setting goals for your career is not something that most CBT therapists pay a great deal of attention to on a day-to-day basis. However, it may be worth taking some time to think about where you would ideally like your career to go so that you are in the best position to make the most of any opportunities that do happen to come your way. If, like many CBT therapists, your career development is constrained by factors such as location and the availability of jobs, then there may be relatively few opportunities to choose from, making it even more important to make the most of any opportunities that do arise. In addition, many of the experiences that might advance your career are often taken on in addition to your usual duties, so can increase the pressure of work, making it even more necessary to choose wisely. For example, progression to higher grades is often dependent on developing some area of specialism or management so it might be worth thinking about what specialist area needs developing within your team or service? Is there a particular patient group whose needs are not met, or a therapy approach that the team currently lacks? Alternatively, career progression can sometimes be dependent on developing skills in working with complex presentations or for management responsibilities. It might be worth thinking about whether any of your actual interests could fit under one of these umbrellas? Or what opportunities are there for line management or budgetary responsibilities?

Although we may put some thought and planning into career progression, there are also unforeseen opportunities that come along and these can be used not only to follow your interests, but may also progress your career.

One of the editors of this book (DW) early on in his career developed an interest in service evaluation research (see Chapter 18) and did several small audit projects within the psychology department where he worked. He had no particular goal in mind for taking this interest any further, until he happened to notice a newspaper advert for a new M. Phil. course at a nearby University, in "The evaluation of public services". This sparked his interest and after some negotiation with managers he was able to get agreement to his having one day a week free for 2 years to do the course; he applied and was accepted by the course and eventually awarded the M. Phil.

As a result of this course and the discussions it led to with managers, he was subsequently asked to undertake larger scale evaluations within his NHS Trust, and such work became a significant and rewarding part of his job for many years, as well as leading to new training roles in evaluation research.

Establishing career anchors

In trying to work out how you most want to develop and/or progress as a CBT therapist it may be worth giving some consideration to Schein's (1990) concept of 'career anchors'. Schein (1990) proposed that a person's career anchor is his or her self-concept consisting of:

1. Self-perceived talents and abilities (e.g. creativity),
2. Basic values (e.g. a desire to contribute to society), and most important,
3. The evolved sense of motives and needs as they pertain to the career. This will most likely involve thinking about your talents and abilities, and basic values, in the context of where you are in your career/life at present, and where you would like to be. For example, your life stage may mean that a

role that could be done term-time only would be advantageous and you feel that your talents include communication and teaching so although skilled as a therapist, you are equally stimulated by training others. As a consequence you look towards a role in CBT education (e.g. as part of a CBT training course) that makes the most of your skills and fits with where you are in your career/life at present.

Career anchors only evolve as you acquire occupational and life experience. However, once the self-concept has been formed, it functions as a stabilizing force—hence the metaphor of 'anchor'—and can be thought of as the values and motives that the person will not give up if forced to make a choice, as we often are in the face of competing demands on our time. Most of us are not aware of our career anchors until we are forced to make choices pertaining to self-development, family, or career. Yet it is important to become aware of our anchors so that we can choose wisely when choices have to be made. Recognizing your main career anchor may help you to identify and prioritize goals, and to establish the most important focus for your development and progression as a CBT therapist (see Table 15.3).

Table 15.3 Career anchor.

Career anchor	Description
Technical/functional	Enjoy applying and continuing to develop core skills and knowledge in area of expertise; motivated by learning new skills and expanding current knowledge base. Enjoy the exercise of your talent; satisfaction from knowing concepts. If it is not a challenge, you feel bored and/or demeaned. Content of the work is more important to you than the context of the work. Concerned with the actual work rather than the organization or overall mission of the work. Teaching or mentoring may offer you the opportunity to demonstrate expertise. You are happiest when work challenges you in your specialist area (e.g. working with complex patients or developing therapy techniques).
General managerial competence	You see specialization as limiting; primarily want to manage or supervise people; enjoy motivating, training, and directing the work of others; enjoy authority and thrive on responsibility.
Autonomy/ independence	You want a high level of control over work and want to be recognized for achievements; can't tolerate other people's rules or procedures; need to do things your own way. Independent consulting and/or setting up in private practice may be a good fit for you, it could give you the flexibility regarding how and when you work as well as the ability to do it your own way.
Security/stability	You are primarily concerned with employment security, and pay, benefits, work environment will be important to you. Motivated by calmness and consistency of work; don't like to take chances, strive for predictability, safety, structure, and the knowledge that the task has been completed properly. Unused talents may be channelled outside work.

(continued)

Table 15.3 (continued) Career anchor.

Career anchor	Description
Entrepreneurial creativity	You have lots of energy and interests so enjoy the challenge of starting new projects or businesses, and often have multiple projects going at once. Easily bored, and restless, you need the challenge of creating new outlets. Different from autonomy in that the emphasis is on creating new business; often pursuing dreams at early age. May be attracted to developing new techniques or setting up novel services as you enjoy creating an organization on your own initiative.
Service/dedication to a cause	Motivated by core values rather than the work itself. You have a strong desire to make the world a better place and want to achieve something of value such as helping others. The mission statement of the service or organization is likely to be as important to you as the content of the work.
Pure challenge	Strongest desire is overcoming obstacles; conquering, problem-solving; competition; winning; constant self-testing. Tends to be single-minded individuals who enjoy the challenge of solving difficult problems, winning over tough opponents or overcoming difficult obstacles.
Lifestyle/integration	You enjoy work, but balance this with other areas of your life. You 'work to live', rather than 'live to work' and want a career that can be accommodated within your overall life goals including family and other commitments.

So thinking about your 'career anchor' may help you to identify what your priorities are for progressing and developing as a CBT therapist (see Example 15.1).

Example 15.1 Identifying priorities for progressing and developing as a CBT therapist

Jane had recently completed training as a CBT therapist. She worked in a primary care setting which required that she saw people quickly for brief therapy. Given the variety of presenting problems referred to her and the brevity of the therapy she was able to offer, she realized quickly that she needed to consider her development. Being at the start of what she hoped would be a long and satisfying career, she identified her main career anchor to be that of 'technical/functional' meaning that she was most interested in the details of the work she was doing, and was excited by learning and applying new skills successfully. At this time in her career her focus was primarily on working with the variety of patients to the best of her ability thereby consolidating her CBT training and improving her confidence. Having established this, Jane identified her goals as shown in Box 15.3.

Box 15.3 Jane's general goals

1 To improve my confidence in using CBT techniques with specific disorders (obsessive compulsive disorder [OCD] and eating disorders).

2 To improve my efficacy with patients.

3 To develop the confidence and necessary skills to supervise another CBT therapist.

Ensuring success: using SMART goals

Once you have identified your priorities for development and progression, the next step is to turn these aspirations into specific goals, just as you would with a patient who comes to CBT saying he wants 'to feel better' or 'get back to normal'—this needs to be translated into exactly what that would mean. This will involve setting SMART goals (learning objectives) in regard to your own development and progression as a therapist. In order to be SMART, your goals (learning objectives) should be (also see Chapter 17 for an example of SMART goals):

- **S**—Specific. Identify exactly what it is you want to be able to do when this goal is realized.
- **M**—Measurable. Specify how you will know when you are able to do this.
- **A**—Achievable/attainable. It helps to state in active language exactly what you will be able to do (see Chapter 17 for examples of how to do this with regard to training objectives). And to consider whether the goal that you are setting is achievable in your current context (if not, what could you change about the context to mean the goal would be achievable? Or do you need to modify the goal?)
- **R**—Realistic/relevant. Making sure that the goal is something that is worth devoting your time and energy to achieving. And that it is relevant to your development and progression.
- **T**—Time-bound. That the goal you specify takes account of the time available.

In setting learning objectives for your own development and progression it may be worth considering the following questions:

1 What is my present level of skill/standard in this area?

2 What is my desired level of skill/standard in this area?

3 Under what conditions do I want to be able to demonstrate this skill? In what settings/contexts?

4 How will I know if I have achieved it? What would I be able to do differently? How would I feel differently? What would others notice was different about me?

Looking at the 'cat litter' example in Chapter 17 and asking yourself the questions above will enable you to refine the 'SMART'ness of your learning objectives. For example, Jane realized that her goals, while relevant and realistic, were not specific, measurable, or time-bound. By considering these issues, she was able to reframe her original goals as specified in Box 15.4.

Box 15.4 Jane's revised SMART goals

1 Complete targeted training in OCD and eating disorders:
   - Attend a 2-day workshop on each and read at least 3 papers from the reading list.

2 Seek supervision for all cases but prioritize those with OCD and eating disorders by putting them first on the agenda.

3 Prioritize supervision and training events by scheduling 1 day/month for training events or reading. Review attendance at training and reading in supervision once/month.

4 Continue to prioritize CPD in the areas of eating disorders and OCD until I feel confident that I can approach a new patient without having to draw up a detailed agenda before each session.

5 Routinely use patient self-report outcome evaluation forms to assess my efficacy. Make sure that I score them in the session so I can use the data from them for that session.

6 Begin to develop confidence and skills in supervision by:
   - Reviewing some video tapes of my supervisor's supervision sessions.
   - Offering to supervise the medical student attached to the service on an *ad hoc* basis.
   - Seeking supervision of supervision.

Jane then set a time frame for each of these goals with review dates. She discussed them with her line manager and agreed that these goals were achievable and realistic given the demands of the service that she worked in and her relative inexperience. They were able to integrate them into Jane's appraisal process and they became part of her personal development plan.

For Jane the most influential factor in determining her career anchor and goals was the stage of her career—being newly qualified as a CBT therapist and wanting to focus on developing skills and options for progression. Others will have different priorities (see Example 15.2).

Example 15.2 Using career anchors to identify and prioritize career goals

Patsy was returning to work after her third period of maternity leave. While she was ambitious, her current career anchor was, by necessity, more about lifestyle/integration in that she needed to find a job that would fit within the constraints of her current lifestyle. For Patsy this meant having a local job with some flexibility of hours such that she could drop her children at school/childcare before work. After this constraint was met, Patsy's next most important anchor was 'service/dedication to a cause'—she wanted to feel that what she was doing was worthwhile and contributed to the overall good, so she took a role working clinically for a charity working with a marginalized group that she felt were in particular need. Patsy also wanted to prioritize opportunities for career progression as after several years of working part-time she felt that her CPD had been neglected and her career had suffered from 'downward drift'. Hence she looked at what she might be able to get out of her current role that would enhance her CV. Given that she was working in a specialist setting with a specific client group it seemed a good opportunity to develop her research skills and increase her clinical profile by aiming to publish an evaluation of the effectiveness of CBT in this setting. She also managed to get some supervision experience by offering placements to trainees from a local training course.

Stage 2: Developing a plan including consideration of learning style

As with patients' goals, once you have established your career goals or objectives, the more 'SMART' these are, the easier it is to specify a plan to ensure your success in meeting them. The plan should also take account of stages of learning (Kolb, 1984). As mentioned in Chapter 16 (Supervision) and Chapter 17 (Training), Kolb developed a theory of experiential learning which states that in order for successful learning to occur, a cycle of four stages must take place. See Fig. 15.1 for more detail.

While learning can begin at any stage of the learning cycle, all four stages must be undertaken in order to maximize learning as each stage enhances the previous one. These stages are:

- Experience: the concrete experience of doing something.
- Observation: reflective observation of what actually happened.

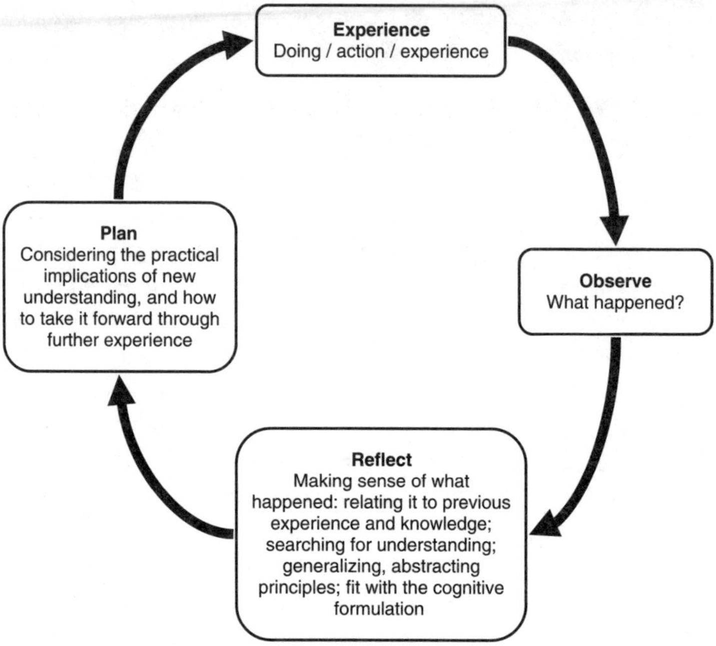

Fig. 15.1 Kolb's (1984) learning cycle.

Kolb, David A. Experimental learning: Experience as a source of learning & development; © 1984, Pg21. Reprinted with the permission of Pearson Education, Inc., Upper Saddle River, NJ.

- Reflection: analysing and making sense of what happened; relating the information to previous knowledge, ideas, and experience; drawing conclusions, generalizing, abstracting principles.
- Planning: considering the practical implications of new learning and planning how to take it forward through new experience.

Put more simply, the stages are those of doing something, reviewing or reflecting on this experience, concluding from these reflections, and planning how to implement or try out what you have learned. In the absence of completing each stage of this cycle, learning may not be consolidated and changes in behaviour as a result of such learning may not occur.

As well as considering Kolb's (1984) stages of learning, personal preferences for learning and individual learning styles need to be taken into account when planning the completion of the various stages of the learning cycle. Honey and Mumford (1986) propose four learning styles which map onto Kolb's stages of the learning cycle:

- **The activist**—you are a 'hands-on' learner who prefers to have a go and learn by being thrown into the deep end. Activists are more likely to engage with experiencing tasks but may neglect planning and active reflection on what they do.

- **The reflector**—the 'tell me' learner who prefers to observe and think about events and to be thoroughly briefed before proceeding. You tend to review thoroughly but may neglect active experimentation and concrete experience.
- **The theorist**—the 'convince me' learner who needs to know the models and concepts before learning takes place. Theorists are good at abstract conceptualization but may need to put more energy into observing and reviewing.
- **The pragmatist**—the 'show me' learner who wants a demonstration from an acknowledged expert and likes to try things out to see the advantage of specific techniques. Pragmatists are more likely to start at the planning stage and may need to push themselves to follow through with experience, observation, and reflecting.

Once you have identified your preferred learning style and methods, you can take this into account when planning how best to learn. Because Jane's learning style was more pragmatic and activist than reflector or theorist, she tended to focus on the planning and experiencing and needed to put particular effort into observation and reflection to ensure learning from theory took place. So she needed to pay particular attention to identifying particular learning points from her CPD activities and consider how she would implement this learning in her clinical practice and thus take herself through the stages of the learning cycle. One way in which she tried to achieve this was to put CPD activities (reading/training event) on the agenda for supervision to focus her on specifying what she had learnt from these events, and what she was going to do differently with patients as a result of this learning. She also committed to keeping clinical sessions to a maximum of 55 minutes so that she had 5 minutes at the end of each session to review the session and reflect on her observations of what had occurred in the session and try to relate it to theory, and to think about changes she could make or directions she could follow in subsequent sessions. She challenged herself to identify one thing she would do differently next time, after each session.

As stated above, it is essential to incorporate all aspects of the learning cycle into your plan for developing skills. Research has demonstrated that teaching theoretical concepts without the rehearsal of skills does not lead to identifiable changes in therapist practice (Bernstein, 1982; Mannix *et al.*, 2006). Although people might report greater knowledge after workshops, their competence in delivering a therapy may not be demonstrably improved (Miller and Mount, 2001). It is therefore important to devise a plan which incorporates a number of training modalities and overt behavioural practice. Suggestions for such CPD activities include:

- Consultation with an expert (in addition to supervision)
- Forming links with a working group
- Peer supervision (to include role-play and use of session recordings)
- Supervising or teaching others
- Joint work or shadowing another colleague
- Reviewing relevant websites regularly
- Accessing e-learning resources (e.g. Oxford Cognitive Therapy Centre [OCTC] online training: www.octc.co.uk)
- Subscribing to email alerts for relevant interests or joining a special interest group or discussion forum (e.g. BABCP listserv)
- Engaging in CBT-related research

Stage 3: Reviewing progress

As in CBT practice, in attempting to achieve your goals for developing and progressing as a CBT therapist, it is important to try to anticipate and problem-solve potential hurdles. Having established goals, it is all too easy to find that weeks or months pass without any progress, regardless of how SMART your goals were at the time of setting them up. For example, issues such as finding time or funding for CPD might halt progress.

Reviewing past goals and plans in order to identify what has stopped you from achieving similar goals in the past might help to identify likely obstacles, just as thinking about how you successfully overcame such hurdles might give you some ideas for how to get round such obstacles (see Example 15.3).

Example 15.3 Putting mechanisms in place to ensure that goals are regularly reviewed and progressed towards them is monitored

Jane was able to reflect that one of the things that had prevented her from developing confidence in her CBT skills previously was always having managed to avoid having any of her actual session tapes listened to in their entirety by supervisors. The block was an understandable fear of criticism. However, Jane could see that if she wanted to develop her CBT skills and to meet her goal of feeling more confident about her CBT practice this was a block that she needed to overcome. Thus she actively sought out a supervisor that she felt would give supportive feedback but also negotiated with the supervisor that she must have whole tapes of sessions rated in spite of her desire to avoid this, and that any procrastination about providing session tapes should rightly be seen as avoidance and addressed in supervision.

Similarly, when Patsy reviewed her past successes and failures in achieving personal development goals at work she identified that one of the things that had prevented her from making progress on such goals in the past was her tendency to prioritize the work that she 'had to' do for other people (patients, colleagues, trainees) and not to prioritize the time for her own career development. In order to prevent her current career goal of writing up an evaluation of the service from being squeezed out by tasks that were more urgent, but not necessarily more important, Patsy diaried monthly time for this task to take place away from her normal work base so that this time couldn't be 'ambushed' by more urgent tasks. She also asked a colleague to collaborate on the project and they set deadlines for when different aspects would be completed by so that her desire to 'not let others down' would help her to prioritize this project rather than letting it slip in favour of work that would not contribute as much to her CV and future career options. Both Patsy and Jane found that reviewing where previous plans did and didn't come to fruition, and gaining their manager's support for the current plan helped them to maximize the chances of their goals being met.

Conclusion

While therapists at all stages of their careers need to give some consideration to skills acquisition, it may be especially relevant for those at the beginning and middle of their careers. The transition from novice practitioner to skilled expert has been described as a staged process. Bennett-Levy (2006) proposed a model of therapist skill development which builds on Binder's (1993, 1999) information processing theory and combines it with Schön's (1987) emphasis on reflection to give rise to three interactive systems:

- Declarative knowledge ('knowing that' or factual information),
- Procedural knowledge ('how/when to'), and
- Reflective system.

Bennett-Levy (2006) proposes that the declarative and procedural systems are more in action for novice practitioners than the reflective system. For example, a new therapist may learn the cognitive model for panic (declarative system) and that in order for this knowledge to be useful as a clinical skill it needs to supplemented by procedural knowledge from practice, role-play, or rehearsal. The reflective system, including both reflection-on-action (reviewing a session after it has taken place) and reflection-in-action (thinking about what is happening as it is occurring) is more engaged by expert therapists. This capacity for reflection, that is being able to analyze unexpected information in a session, restructure existing knowledge and test out new hypotheses immediately, may be what develops as therapists move from novice to expert (Skovholt *et al.* 1997; Schön, 1987). Hence, a key element for all CBT therapists will be making time and space for reflection on practice and on your own development needs. Although there is perhaps more focus on the acquisition of new skills at the earlier stages of career development, the need to reflect upon and consider your clinical practice never goes away. This is essential not only because CBT models and techniques are constantly being updated and developed, but also because professional development is essential to prevent stagnation, burn-out, and decay from the profession (Skovholt and Ronnestad, 1995).

As outlined in this chapter, the benefits of directly attending to career development and progression are important for both CBT therapists and the patients they treat. We have outlined the requirements and methods for gaining formal accreditation as a CBT therapist, which constitute a useful framework for thinking about training and the minimum amount of CPD necessary for practice as a CBT therapist, regardless of the environment in which you work. However, as in CBT, a comprehensive formulation-driven approach is recommended over a one-size-fits-all prescriptive approach as it is able to take into account the individual variance as well as the shared variance. Thus, we have stressed the importance of considering your individual goals, learning needs, career anchors, and current circumstances, as well as your preferred learning styles and methods, in order to come up with a successful plan for developing and progressing as a CBT therapist that takes account of your current circumstances and goals.

Key points

- There are personal and professional reasons for developing your skills as a CBT therapist: to make sure your skills are kept up-to-date with the most current evidence base, not only for the benefit of your patients but also to ensure the job stays challenging for you and so that you feel that you are progressing both as a CBT therapist and in your career.
- You may want to think about applying to the BABCP for accreditation as a CBT therapist, supervisor, and/or trainer.

Key points *(cotinued)*

- You can utilize your CBT skills to develop and progress as a CBT therapist:
  - You can set SMART goals for your development and specify plans for achieving these goals.
  - You can anticipate potential obstacles to implementing the plans and use your problem-solving skills to identify possible solutions to them.
  - As in CBT you will want to measure and regularly review your progress towards these goals.
- In specifying goals for your development and making plans for achieving these goals you may want to give some consideration to your career anchor and your optimal learning style.
- Good supervision, which focuses on your skills development as well as case supervision, can be extremely useful in helping you to structure your plans for developing and progressing as a CBT therapist.

Further reading

British Association of Behavioural and Cognitive Psychotherapists website. Available at: www.babcp.com (accessed on 19 February 2010)

Chapters 16 (Supervision) and 17 (Training) in this book.

Oxford Cognitive Therapy Centre website. Available at: www.octc.co.uk (accessed on 19 February 2010)

Newcastle Cognitive Therapy Centre: email: cbttraining@ntw.nhs.uk

Padesky, C.A. (1996). Developing cognitive therapist competency: teaching and supervision models, in Salkovskis, P. (ed.), *Frontiers of Cognitive therapy*. New York, NY: Guilford Press.

References

Bennett-Levy, J. (2006). Therapist skills: a cognitive model of their acquisition and refinement. *Behavioural and Cognitive Psychotherapy*, **34**, 57–78.

Bernstein, G.S. (1982). Training behaviour change agents: a conceptual review. *Behaviour Therapy*, **13**, 1–23.

Binder, J.L. (1993). Is it time to improve psychotherapy training? *Clinical Psychology Review*, **13**, 301–331.

Binder, J.L. (1999). Issues in teaching and learning time-limited psychodynamic psychotherapy. *Clinical Psychology Review*, **19**, 705–719.

Brosan, L., Reynolds, S. and Moore, R.G. (2006). Factors associated with competence in cognitive therapists. *Behavioural and Cognitive Psychotherapy*, **35**, 179–190.

Corrie, S., Hurton, N. and Lane, D. (2008). How to develop your career and organise your continuing professional development, in Palmer, S. and Bor, R. (eds.), *The Practitioner's Handbook: A Guide for Counsellors, Psychotherapists and Counselling Psychologists.* London: Sage, pp. 5–20.

Davidson, K., Scott, J., Schmidt, U., Tata, P., Thornton, S. and Tyrer, P. (2004). Therapist competence and clinical outcome in the Prevention of Parasuicide by Manual Assisted Cognitive Behaviour Therapy Trial: the POPMACT study. *Psychological Medicine*, **34**, 855–863.

Honey, P. and Mumford, A. (1986). *The Manual of Learning Styles.* Peter Honey, 10 Linden Avenue, Maidenhead.

Kuyken, W. and Tsivrikos, D. (2009). Therapist competence, comorbidity and cognitive-behavioral therapy for depression. *Psychotherapy and Psychosomatics*, **78**, 42–48.

Kolb, D.A. (1984). *Experiential Learning.* New Jersey, NJ: Prentice-Hall.

Miller, W.R. and Mount, K.A. (2001). A small study of training in motivational interviewing: does one workshop change clinician and patient behaviour? *Behavioural and Cognitive Psychotherapy*, **29**, 457–471.

Mannix, K.A., Blackburn, I.M., Garland, A., Gracie, J., Moorey, S., Reid, B., Standart, S. and Scott, J. (2006). Effectiveness of brief training in cognitive behaviour therapy techniques for palliative care practitioners. *Palliative Medicine*, **20**, 579–584.

Roth, T. and Pilling, S. (2007). *Centre for Outcomes, Research and Effectiveness: Competence Frameworks.* Available at: www.ucl.ac.uk/clinicalpsychology/CORE/competence_frameworks.htm (retrieved 22nd July 2009).

Salkovskis, P.M. (2002). Empirically grounded clinical interventions: cognitive behaviour therapy progresses through a multi-dimensional approach to clinical science. *Behavioural and Cognitive Psychotherapy*, **30**, 3–9.

Schein, E.H. (1990). *Career Anchors (Discovering your Real Values).* San Francisco, CA: Jossey-Bass/Pfeiffer.

Schön, D. (1987). *Educating the Reflective Practitioner.* San Francisco, CA: Jossey-Bass.

Shaw, B.F., Elkin, I., Yamaguchi, J., Olmsted, M., Vallis, T.M., Dobson, K.S., Lowery, A., Sotsky, S.M., Watkins, J.T. and Imber, S.D. (1999). Therapist competence ratings in relation to clinical outcome in cognitive therapy for depression. *Journal of Consulting and Clinical Psychology*, **67**, 837–846.

Skovholt, T.M. and Ronnestad, M.H. (1995). The Evolving Professional Self: Themes in Counsellor and Therapist Development. New York, NY: Wiley.

Skovholt, T.M., Ronnestad, M.H. and Jennings, L. (1997). Searching for expertise in counseling, psychotherapy, and professional psychology. Educational Psychology Review, **9**, 361–369.

Waller, G. (2009). Evidence based treatment and therapist drift. Behavior, Research and Therapy, **47**, 119–127.

Young, J. and Beck, A.T. (1980). Cognitive Therapy Scale Rating Manual. Unpublished manuscript. Philadelphia, PA: University of Pennsylvania.

Chapter 16

Becoming a supervisor

Helen Kennerley and Sue Clohessy

Twenty minutes into the supervision session, it still lacked focus. It was a pleasant enough exchange and Kate learnt some interesting things about CBT but she did not feel that her supervision needs were being met. Hugh, her supervisor, enjoyed sharing his knowledge and he always found supervision sessions stimulating. He tended to end the session by asking: "How was that—okay?" To which the reserved Kate would answer "Yes".

Introduction

Supervision is regarded as crucial in developing and maintaining adequate standards of cognitive behavioural therapy (CBT). The IAPT (Improving Access to Psychological Therapies, Department of Health [DOH], 2007) initiative requires close supervision of CBT therapists in training while the British Association of Behavioural and Cognitive Psychotherapy (BABCP) will only accredit CBT therapists who receive regular clinical supervision. Therefore, in this chapter we aim to help you become a 'good' supervisor. We will review how you can best prepare yourself, emphasize the core skills of supervision and explore how you can optimize your practice by also considering process issues in supervision and developing the supervisory alliance.

Preparing yourself

Your first step is becoming familiar with the purpose of supervision and guidelines for good practice. It is generally accepted that the role of a clinical supervisor is to facilitate therapeutic competence and CBT is no exception, but only very recently have cognitive therapists been given comprehensive guidelines for good practice of supervision (Pilling and Roth, 2008). Thus far, CBT supervisors' best guide has been lists of generic guidelines for good supervision practice (Scaife, 2009), an appreciation that aspects of CBT practice might transfer to supervision practice (Liese and Beck, 1997; Padesky, 1996) and very few theoretical models, the most comprehensive being that of Freeston and Armstrong (2006). In general, the practice of CBT supervision has been neglected and, at worst, has been carried out on an idiosyncratic 'See one-do one-supervise one' basis. That said, below are summaries of the core skills and competencies which can guide you towards better supervisory practice.

Core skills

Psychotherapy supervisors have, over the years, described 'core skills' of supervision which are now reflected in Pilling and Roth's document (2008) and which are described more fully later in this chapter. There seems to be a general agreement that these include:

- Contracting
- Goal setting
- Structuring the supervision session
- Evaluating both supervisee's and supervisor's performance and skills
- Giving feedback

We would add:

- Developing an effective supervisory relationship (SR) particularly as the first five points are only likely to be effective in promoting good therapy practice and relevant learning if they are embedded within an effective alliance.

Easier to remember than the competencies frameworks (Box 16.1), the above six bullet points provide a useful checklist for a supervisor.

Hugh's supervisory practice would have improved enormously had he simply considered core skills. As it was the session was aimless because he had neglected to negotiate a contract, set goals or impose structure on the session. He had not helped his supervisee clarify her supervision question and he remained ignorant of the fact that he failed to meet her needs because he neglected to ask for feedback and was unappreciative of the value of evaluating his own performance, or her's.

Generic competencies

In 2008, an expert committee led by Pilling and Roth, considered both generic supervision competencies and guiding principles for the supervision of particular psychotherapies. These can now be found on: **www.ucl.ac.uk/CORE/**. The generic competencies are summarized in Box 16.1.

Box 16.1 Summary of Pilling and Roth's generic supervision competencies (2008)

- Gauge supervisee's level of competence
- Use educational principles to enhance learning
- Enable ethical practice
- Foster competence in working with difference
- Adapt supervision to the organizational and governance context
- Form and maintain a supervisory alliance:
  - To structure supervision sessions
  - To help the supervisee present information about clinical work
  - To help the supervisee reflect on his/her work and the usefulness of supervision
  - To use a range of methods to give accurate and constructive feedback
- Reflect (and act on) on limitations in own knowledge and experience

In addition to the above, Pilling and Roth (2008) highlighted the need to:

- Incorporate direct observation into supervision.
- Conduct supervision in group formats.

Chapter 17 in this book addresses ways in which we can enhance learning, ethical practice is considered in Chapter 4, while working with difference is the subject of Chapter 2. The remaining generic competencies are integrated into this chapter with an emphasis on the final point—applying supervision to a specific therapy, namely CBT.

Specific CBT competencies

Pilling and Roth's (2008) competency guidelines for CBT (see Box 16. 2) state that a CBT supervisor should have the sound theoretical knowledge and clinical experience necessary to guide a supervisee towards safe and ethical practice of CBT. This also involves a supervisor being able to identify supervisee's learning needs, communicate and teach effectively, and monitor progress.

Once prepared, you are ready to move on to the practicalities of the supervision session. We assume that you will use supervision sessions as an opportunity to model good CBT practice: agenda setting, using Socratic and didactic methods of teaching, and so on.

Box 16.2 Summary of Pilling and Roth's CBT supervision competencies (2008)

1 An ability to combine sound knowledge of general and specific, theoretical and applied CBT and to use this to recognize and remedy limitations in supervisee practice.

2 An ability to recognize supervisee abilities and learning needs, to promote experiential learning of CBT techniques, to monitor progress, to promote self-reflective practice.

3 An ability to structure supervision sessions in a way which reflects CBT practice using an agenda, so that topics are prioritized, homework and previous practice is reviewed, key issues are discussed, and feedback is exchanged.

4 An ability to impart relevant theoretical knowledge of disorders and their cognitive behavioural conceptualization and to help the supervisee make this personal to the client; to communicate and model necessary cognitive and behavioural skills; to encourage the development of a collaborative alliance; to impart practical guidance for carrying out sessions.

5 Specific supervisory techniques: an ability to use observational and participative methods to develop CBT skills; to use capsule summaries to enhance learning; to elicit feedback; to help the supervisee identify thoughts that interfere with therapy or with supervision.

6 Monitoring the supervisee's work and ability to use recording and direct observation; to use regular measures to guide the supervision agenda; to formally assess supervisee competencies using appropriate instruments.

If we are to be effective as communicators and teachers we need to be familiar with psychological theories and models of communication (Bordin, 1983) and learning (Kolb, 1984). These are covered comprehensively in Chapter 15 and it is worth reading about them as part of your preparation as a supervisor. It is also prudent to prepare your supervisee and there is a useful chapter in Westbrook *et al.* (2007), which is specifically aimed at helping supervisees get the most out of supervision sessions.

Practicalities of 'good' supervision

To begin with, contracting will define the parameters of your supervisory practice with a particular supervisee, then goal setting and structuring will refine this. Within the session, you will also need to attend to the very practical task of note keeping and also the more psychological task of attending to your supervisee's learning needs.

Contracting

A supervision contract defines the parameters of your supervisory alliance or relationship. There are a number of compelling reasons for contracting in supervision: to establish mutual goals and expectations, to provide a context of negotiation and shared planning, to clarify responsibilities, and to establish a context in which mutual feedback can be given. Contracts can be used to create a context of safety as they can define ethical practice, set ground rules for the sessions, and clarify accountability.

Contracts should reflect the needs of the supervisee: a trainee practitioner in weekly supervision might need a very different contract from an experienced therapist seeking bimonthly consultation on a specific case.

Although contracting in supervision does not have an evidence base, it is considered by many as essential to effective supervision (Scaife, 2009).

Had Hugh negotiated a contract with Kate, he would have learnt what her supervision needs were and they would have developed the basis for a collaborative, working relationship. Instead, Hugh worked from his own perspective and assumed that didactic supervision was appropriate.

The BABCP (2005) has developed an extremely useful and detailed example of a CBT supervision agreement which can be downloaded from their website (www.babcp.com) and used as a template for your own contracts (see Appendix 16.1). Below (Box 16.3) is an example of a briefer contract.

Box 16.3 Supervision contract

Supervisor: Jane Bloggs
Supervisee: John Smith
Purpose of supervision: postgraduate skills development, with particular focus on conceptualization
Supervisee is clinically accountable to: Sarah Brown
Commitment: monthly meetings of 90 minutes—for 1 year; one tape submitted each month for evaluation
Responsibilities of supervisor: to review therapy recordings; to provide relevant references; to provide supervisee with feedback on development of skills; and to be open to learning needs and feedback from supervisee

Box 16.3 Supervision contract *(continued)*

Responsibilities of supervisee: to prepare and present a formulation per client, and to identify supervision question(s) prior to the meeting; to provide recordings for discussion; to be open to feedback from supervisor; and to actively engage in supervision
Crisis contact: if Jane not available, contact Sarah Brown
Confidentiality: client details will be disguised and client will be informed of supervision. Supervisee details will be disguised if discussed in supervisor's supervision
Feedback and review: feedback will be invited at the end of each supervision session, and formally reviewed after 6 sessions.

The agenda for each session can be seen as a 'mini-contract' with which we are all familiar. An example agenda is shown in Box 16.4.

This agenda would be ambitious for an hour-long session and you are reminded that you need to prioritize items and allocate time realistically just as you would in a therapy session.

Box 16.4 Agenda

Bridge from previous session

Feedback on assignment(s)

Main item: Supervision question 1

John has a diagnosis of mild Asperger's syndrome: how do I need to modify CBT?

Secondary item: Supervision question 2

How do I formulate Angela's eating disorder?

Third item: Supervision question 3

How do I use the continuum technique?

Feedback on session and summary of learning points with plan for implementing learning.

Structuring

Agenda setting and structuring are closely linked, and done properly will ensure the best use of the time available. Session structure will be influenced by what is agreed to be appropriate given the various requirements of supervision, such as the level of supervision required (e.g. basic skills training for a novice therapist or peer supervision with an experienced colleague), the focus of supervision (e.g. patient-centred or supervisee focused), and the setting of the supervision (e.g. group, peer, telephone).

Kate was a relatively novice CBT therapist who was insecure about her ability to carry out a behavioural experiment with a patient who had a phobia. Her supervision sessions were always one-to-one with an experienced CBT therapist, Hugh. Had he encouraged her to define her needs, Hugh would have appreciated that the sessions needed to be structured to accommodate time for both very practical patient-focused work (discussing how to optimize the behavioural experiment, role playing how to share a rationale with the patient, observing and giving feedback on Kate's therapeutic skills and so on) and a therapist-focused discussion of Kate's reservations and anxieties. Had he facilitated an agenda which reflected this, Kate would have been more confident that her needs (and the needs of her patient) would be met. She would have been more enthusiastic about her sessions.

The structure of a session should be considered afresh at each meeting, and should be overt and flexible, with opportunity for the supervisee to contribute—shared agenda setting will help achieve this.

Goal setting

In supervision, as in therapy, we need to set general goals which span the course of supervision and in-session goals which define the remit of a particular meeting. Goals should be regularly reviewed and should always be SMART (see Chapter 15 for a definition). For example:

- To be able to formulate patients' eating disorders.
- To learn to use the continuum technique.

These do have the potential to be good goals but they are not SMART. The following are more specific:

- To develop maintenance formulations for patients with bulimia nervosa. These will be evaluated by my supervisor and I will get feedback from my patients. My progress will be reviewed in four weeks' time.
- To be able to use the continuum technique to help patients challenge dichotomous thinking. I will role-play and produce recordings for my supervisor to evaluate and will review this goal in six weeks' time.

As well as general supervision goals, supervisees should be encouraged to identify in-session goals in the form of supervision questions. These questions should be prepared in advance of the session to optimize the use of time, and to encourage supervisees to focus on what they need and be an active participant in supervision. For example:

- How do I construct a developmental conceptualization of this patient's anorexia nervosa which will be 'user-friendly'?
- How do I use the continuum technique with a patient with borderline personality disorder (BPD) when trying to help her manage her fears of trusting others?

Goals should, of course, reflect the supervisee's clinical and professional needs and also take into account their developmental and learning needs (see later section 'Attending to learning style and needs').

Note keeping

Both supervisor and supervisee must keep a written record of what is discussed and agreed in supervision. These notes can serve a number of purposes:

- Provide a record of the frequency of meeting and of the clinical work carried out by the supervisee (information which can be required for continuing professional development (CPD) and for accreditation by the BABCP).
- Record supervisory decisions.
- Document the learning needs and progress of the supervisee.
- Record feedback given and received.
- Can record personal reactions to supervision or areas in which supervisory practice could improve.

It is important to remember that your supervision notes can be regarded as public record, and access can be requested, so they must be in a form that is accessible and readable. Individual National Health Service (NHS) Trusts and professional organizations may have their own requirements for note keeping, and we suggest that you refer to this guidance.

Attending to learning style and needs

Adult learning is reviewed in Chapters 15 and 17 and the theory emphasizes the importance of *experiential learning* and the value of *reflection* upon experience and forward planning. Thus, you must keep in mind the need to prompt reflection and planning and the need to complement didactic and Socratic teaching with experiential learning opportunities such as role-play.

We each have strengths and preferences as learners and it is necessary for you, as a supervisor, to be aware of your own and sensitive to the preferences and needs of your supervisee. This will avoid biases towards a certain learning style. For example, if the supervisor and supervisee are both quite reflective there might be the danger that sessions comprise enjoyably theoretical discussion but little problem-solving and planning is achieved and experiential learning is minimal. Awareness of learning style preferences can also stop you slipping into an unproductive supervision style when you and your supervisee have different learning styles.

Hugh's preference was for reflecting and hypothesizing—he was an "armchair supervisor" and he was not sensitive to the fact that Kate preferred to learn through "doing" rather than discussing. Thus Kate frequently felt frustrated with the supervision, she feared that she was not learning enough and her anxieties about being a good therapist increased. This was particularly unfortunate because Hugh's style of reflecting and theorizing could have so easily complimented Kate's learning style and helped her develop better reflective and planning skills. This in turn could have enhanced her practice and her confidence as a therapist.

Stress levels also affect adult learning, with high- and low-levels impairing performance (Yerkes and Dodson, 1908). Thus, your task is also to create an environment that stretches and stimulates your supervisee while avoiding overarousal. You can monitor your supervisee's stress levels by being sensitive to non-verbal signs of over- or underarousal and by eliciting frequent feedback on how your supervisee is finding the session.

Supervision in context

By now it is clear that providing 'good' supervision is challenging and it is further complicated by it being used in different settings with different remits. For example, it can be individual or group; 'expert' led or peer; case management or developmentally focused. You have a range of approaches in your supervision armory: case discussion; video/audio/live observation; role-play/demonstration; didactic and Socratic approaches and your decision to use different approaches will be determined by an appreciation of the function and format of the session as well as an awareness of the wider, systemic implications of the supervision case—'the bigger picture'. Clearly, the basics of good practice apply but you will need to reflect on the particular considerations necessary to ensure that you maintain good practice despite having to accommodate different functions, different foci, or when you supervise using different formats.

Differing functions, foci, and formats

Padesky (1996) developed a useful grid summarizing her ideas about the context of supervision which you could adapt to your own use. Table 16.1 is an

Table 16.1 Supervision options grid.

Focus of supervision session	**Method used in supervision**				
	Case discussion	**Video/audio/ live observation**	**Role-play/ demonstration**	**Discussion of supervisee/ supervisor issue**	**Tutorial**
Improving key knowledge					
Mastery of CBT methods					
Case conceptualization					
Patient-therapist relationship					
Therapist reactions					
Supervisory processes					

adaptation of Padesky's idea. These sorts of grids are useful in planning—when considering the ideal focus and format of your session, in reviewing where you directed attention in a particular session and for reviewing your general approach to supervision so that you can see if you have biases which may need to be addressed.

Given Kate's needs and strengths, several aspects of supervision needed to be considered:

- Improving her appreciation of the rationale and methods of behavioural experiments.
- Formulating her patient's fears so that the approach could be personalized to the patient's needs.
- Reviewing her insecurities.

Had Hugh been more aware of the supervisory process, he would have realized that this too needed to be addressed. Table 16.2 summarizes this and also illustrates the diversity of supervision methods available to Hugh and Kate. Hugh might not have used all these methods within one session but he would have been more aware of the scope of supervision and the teaching options available. As it was, he ignored therapist's reactions and the supervisory process and limited himself to case discussion and the tutorial approach (and even then omitted Socratic methods!).

A further consideration is whether the supervision is face-to-face or distance supervision—perhaps via telephone or email. This type of CBT supervision is

Table 16.2 Hugh and Kate's ideal supervision grid.

Focus of supervision session	Method used in supervision				
	Case discussion	Video/audio/ live observation	Role-play/ demonstration	Discussion of supervisee/ supervisor issue	Tutorial (didactic and Socratic methods)
Improving key knowledge	✓		✓	✓	✓
Mastery of CBT methods	✓	✓	✓	✓	✓
Case conceptua-lization	✓	✓	✓	✓	✓
Therapist reactions	✓	✓	✓	✓	
Supervisory processes				✓	

relatively new, has not been systematically studied, and so there are no specific guidelines for its use. So you will have to scrutinize your practice to ensure your supervisee(s) benefits from the experience. There are obstacles to overcome, for example, the challenges of limited role-play, the lack of a white board to communicate and share ideas, difficulties in listening to or watching recordings in the session. Some of the difficulties are not insurmountable, for example, it can be helpful to use email and fax to share formulations and other written/typed materials while on-line supervision enables real time conversation and permits relatively easy sharing of some information. These unusual circumstances will need to be reflected in your contract.

The 'bigger context'

This refers to the wider brief of supervision: the relevant world outside the supervisee-supervisor-client triad. Patients are embedded within systems (home, work, culture) which impact on them and which they, in turn might influence; patients have children and partners with whom they have a reciprocal role; therapists (and supervisors) similarly exist in settings that can influence their moods, assumptions, and behaviours (Hawkins and Shohet, 2000). Thus, you need to be able to stand back and review this bigger picture from time to time in order to appreciate when factors, external to the 'triad' play a role. This means considering questions such as: '...and when this patient leaves therapy, what is the impact of the workplace and the domineering boss?', '...are their children at risk?', '...I have problems in my relationship at present, am I imposing some of my fears in this supervision session?' Considering the complexities of the 'bigger picture' necessarily involves being sensitive to aspects of the SR.

Supervisory relationship

A good SR is fundamental to good supervision. It is neither a therapeutic relationship nor a friendship. The relationship between supervisor and supervisee has been described as a working alliance—a collaboration for change that involves mutual agreement and understanding between both parties about the goals and tasks of supervision, and the development of an emotional bond between them (Bordin, 1983). Its development is influenced by a number of factors including the working contexts of the supervisor and supervisee (e.g. the service, the training course if the supervisee is in training) and the individual factors that supervisor and supervisee bring to the relationship (such as, their previous experience of supervision, or personal stressors).

What makes a supervisory relationship effective?

Beinart (2004) suggests that an effective relationship between supervisor and supervisee is characterized by:

- **Safety**: your supervisee needs to talk about his/her clinical work without fear of being judged negatively or undermined and in a setting which is emotionally containing.
- **Trust**: your supervisee needs to know that you will behave professionally, maintain professional boundaries and help them, while you need to be confident that your supervisee will follow-up on suggestions, behave ethically and professionally with patients and colleagues.
- **Support**: you need to check that your supervisee feels emotionally supported, understood, and helped with both clinical work and professional development.
- **Collaboration**: both of you should be working together on shared, agreed goals.
- **Sensitivity to the needs of the supervisee**: be aware of, and respond to, the learning needs of your supervisee. For example, if your supervisee needs to develop confidence in agenda-setting, or keeping to time during the session—schedule time to focus on these needs.
- **Openness and honesty**: your supervisee needs to be honest about difficulties with his/her work, or supervision. Similarly, you need to be open and honest if you have reservations about your supervisee's practice or the SR.

- **Boundaries**: supervision time should be well-organized, structured, and free of interruptions and relevant to your supervisee's professional development. Although there may be some similarities with the therapeutic relationship, your relationship with your supervisee is primarily educative and should not stray into the realms of therapy.

Developing such a relationship requires you to achieve a milieu which balances safety and support with challenge, and one which enables your supervisees to reach their potential.

Hugh and Kate's supervisory relationship lacked many of the characteristics of an effective SR. Kate did not feel that Hugh was sensitive to her learning needs, and did not feel safe and trusting enough to be open and honest about her difficulties with her clinical work, and her dissatisfaction with supervision. How could Hugh have encouraged the development of an effective supervisory relationship with Kate?

- *Spending time getting to know Kate, clarifying what she wanted to learn, and what was the best way of enabling her to do this; what she found challenging or difficult in her work; what she enjoyed; what had been helpful or unhelpful in her past experience of supervision. These discussions could have helped them develop a meaningful supervision contract.*
- *Exploring how Kate would like to be given feedback on her skills, and ensuring that this was done regularly and constructively. Hugh also needed to be open to feedback himself and should have asked Kate how she could let him know if she wasn't happy with supervision—this should have been addressed when they were developing their contract. He should also have regularly reviewed how she was finding supervision, whether it was meeting her needs. By inviting feedback, Hugh could help to cultivate a relationship with Kate which was open, and in which she felt that her learning needs and preferences were important.*
- *Encouraging Kate to be an active participant in supervision. Their mutual expectations could be discussed at the contracting phase, and Kate encouraged to think about her learning needs to prepare for supervision. She could then have taken a lead in agenda setting and been an active participant in, rather than a passive recipient of supervision. To some extent this may have depended on Kate's developmental level as a therapist, her learning preferences and on her previous experience of supervision.*

Problems in the supervisory relationship

As in any relationship, problems may arise between you and your supervisee. There may be times when you are distracted by personal stresses which make it difficult to focus on your supervisee's needs; maybe your supervisee does not feel safe enough to talk honestly about the difficulties in her clinical work; perhaps you have a dual relationship as a supervisor and manager, or as a supervisor and a friend which impedes openness and honesty.

Whatever the difficulty, problems in the SR must be attended to as they can interfere with the supervisee's use of supervision and can compromise patient care (Ladany *et al.*, 1996). You can increase your sensitivity to problems in the relationship by:

- **Attending to the relationship**. How do you feel in supervision? How does your supervisee seem to feel? Is supervision characterized by discomfort, frustration, anxiety, or hopelessness? Pay attention to your behaviour in supervision. Do you seem to be doing all of the work? Are you overpreparing for your supervision session? What about your supervisee? Does she seem defensive or avoidant when certain topics are raised?
- **Formulating the problem.** You may need to gather more information, by tentatively checking things out with the supervisee, or using your own supervision to reflect on the problem and develop some initial hypotheses. Taking into account your own cognitions and beliefs, as well as those of the supervisee will be an important part of the process. Your formulation will, of course, guide your subsequent action.

Had Hugh attended to his relationship with Kate, he might have noticed her becoming increasingly withdrawn and contributing less to their discussions. He may have noticed her frustration, and that he was doing most of the talking in supervision. Had he developed an effective contract with Kate, these difficulties may not have arisen in the first place because he would have known her supervision goals, her learning preferences, would have discussed with her how she could give him feedback on supervision, and he would have actively sought this feedback. However, he could still have used his own supervision to think about the strain in his alliance with Kate, and whether supervision was meeting her needs. He could have considered his own cognitions regarding his role as supervisor, particularly his belief that to be a good supervisor he must provide the answers for his supervisee. And finally, he could have raised the issue with Kate, to help develop his formulation:

Hugh: Kate, I wonder if we could take some time today to talk about how supervision is going? Would that be ok?

Kate: I guess so.

Hugh: I've noticed that when we talk about setting up behavioural experiments, you become quiet, and a bit withdrawn. I've been wondering what's going on for you at those times.

Kate: Well, I guess I feel pretty anxious about setting them up, I worry I won't do it well.

Hugh: Ok, that's helpful to know. We can think about that some more. I've been wondering whether supervision has been helping you with this enough. What do you think would help you develop your confidence in this area?

Kate: Well……maybe if I can practice a bit? Or if you could show me how I might explain it to my patient…

Hugh: So it sounds like it would be useful if we did some role-play, perhaps with me as therapist initially, and then give you the chance to practice too? Is that right?

Kate: Yeah, yeah I think that would help.

Hugh: That's really useful to know, Kate. Are there any other ways our supervision could change to help you develop as a therapist?

In this way Hugh could explore Kate's preferences, and demonstrate sensitivity to her needs in supervision. Had he not raised the issue, and given her permission to discuss her preferences, the strain in their alliance would have continued, Kate's learning needs would have remained unmet and she may have continued to struggle in developing skills and confidence in setting up behavioural experiments with her patients.

Raising a difficult issue with your supervisee often takes courage, and may not always be easy. Maintaining a sensitive, positive, non-blaming, collaborative stance is crucial and using problem-solving strategies with your supervisee can be helpful in exploring together what needs to change to make supervision work more effectively.

Giving feedback to the supervisee

The content of feedback will vary according to the context of your supervision and the needs of your supervisee. However it should always be justifiable and relevant, just as withholding feedback must be justifiable. It is best given in a way that is sensitive to your supervisory alliance and which engages your supervisee as your approach in giving feedback can be crucial to maintaining an effective working relationship. It is advisable, therefore, to negotiate the process of giving and receiving feedback, making it predictable and respectful and ensuring that the supervisee feels 'safe' receiving it. This needs to be done as part of contract setting and as a prelude to giving a particular piece of feedback. For example:

Supervisor: I have listened to your therapy tape and there are aspects of it which strike me as being very good and I would like to spend some time talking about them. I also have some suggestions for improvement and there is one thing that concerns me which we need to discuss. How would you prefer the feedback to be organized?

Supervisee: Give me the bad news first and then let's end on a positive note.

This would appear to lead the way for a very direct approach to commenting on performance:

Supervisor: Okay, I'll just be blunt about this: where was your formulation? You were not obviously guided by one, which is going to disadvantage both you and your patient. In addition, you simply assigned the homework without any apparent justification: you need a rationale and the task must overtly link with the patient's difficulties or new perspectives. There were some aspects of the session which were quite well done, though.

This statement immediately highlights the problems that need to be addressed, it is unambiguous and it offers direction, but it has a very negative bias and does not draw the supervisee into a dialogue. This approach risks not engaging the recipient.

There are more helpful ways of giving feedback. A useful acronym for remembering the important aspects of this interaction is CORBS (Hawkins and Shohet, 2000). Hawkins and Shohet suggest that we make feedback:

- **C**lear: if your supervisee cannot interpret what you are saying, s/he cannot act on it.
- **O**wned: your comments should be framed as your opinion not 'truth'.
- **R**egular: and frequent enough for it to be practically useful. We would add a further 'r', namely
- **R**eviewed: supervisors need to encourage learning by checking that feedback has been put into action, prompting a review of its impact and encouraging supervisees to develop further plans based on their findings.
- **B**alanced: feedback should reflect strengths and achievements and be as affirming as possible. Remember challenge and support are equally important in enhancing learning and good practice.
- **S**pecific: use examples to illustrate your supervision points.

As we have indicated in bullet point 4, we would also add that feedback should promote an action plan. Your supervisee should be prompted to consider: 'What have I learnt and how will I take this forward? How will I put this learning into action?'

Below is an example of feedback which is more in line with COR(R)BS. You will see that it is not just a matter of making a statement as the feedback balances praise and criticism and involves didactic and Socratic dialogue.

Supervisor: The aspect of your practice which concerned me was an apparent lack of a shared overview. Technically there were many good aspects to your practice but I did not get a sense that you and your patient were working together from a formulation. It was particularly evident towards the end when you assigned the homework. What did you feel was going on?

The supervisee had an opportunity to explain that he did have a formulation which guided his work but that he did not share it with his patient.

Supervisor: Looking at it, I can see that this is a perfectly reasonable formulation but what do you think might be the disadvantages of not sharing it with your patient?

This Socratic approach helped the supervisee to identify many of the advantages of a shared formulation and the supervisor added an extra suggestion that the supervisee had not recognized. The supervisee was then prompted to reflect on the feedback.

Supervisor: How might this awareness change your practice?

Supervisee: I will try to build a formulation <u>with</u> my patient. We will both have a copy so that we can both refer to it during the session. That way, neither of us will forget that it is central to our work.

Supervisor: Good. Now, how will we know whether or not you have been successful in doing so and whether or not it makes a difference?

Supervisee: I can bring in another recording for you to listen to and I will also ask my patient for her reactions to my sharing the formulation.

Sometimes giving negative feedback could upset your supervisee, for example, when you have to fail an assignment. Thus it is much better to start, rather than end your supervision with the feedback so that there is enough time to deal with your supervisee's reaction. If your supervisee does not agree with your appraisal, acknowledge this perspective and be prepared to engage in a dialogue. If you do not, you may simply reach an immediate impasse. Be clear about your views and the reasons behind the feedback, explore what additional support may be helpful for the supervisee, and be prepared to offer additional time in supervision if necessary.

Formats of supervision

Group supervision

Group supervision can be an extremely productive and engaging mode of supervision but it can be complex. In addition to considering several contracts, several SRs, developmental needs of a number of supervisees, the 'bigger picture', and the tasks of the session, you will also have to consider how to handle group dynamics. Since the 1960s, psychotherapists have suggested that there are helpful processes occurring within groups (e.g. the instillation of hope and peer guidance), unhelpful processes (e.g. dependency and splitting) and that there are commonly stages of disharmony as well as cooperation as a group develops. It is your task to both recognize and to manage these dynamics, minimizing the unhelpful and distracting aspects of group interaction while maximizing the benefits of the setting.

There are, potentially, many ways of running groups but Proctor and Inskipp (2001) have defined four common styles of approaching group supervision, namely:

- **Authoritative**: whereby the supervisor supervises while other group members observe.
- **Participative**: where the supervisor supervises and teaches *and* encourages members to participate.
- **Cooperative**: where the supervisor facilitates group members sharing responsibility for the tasks of group supervision.
- **Peer**: where all group members share responsibility for all the group tasks and there is no distinct 'leader'.

The different styles will suit groups with different developmental and task requirements. For example, the authoritative style might best suit a novice group who would benefit from observing the supervision process or a brief case management meeting, while peer supervision would be more beneficial to those already experienced in supervision and who would benefit from honing their supervision skills. As a supervisor you will need to assess the needs of your particular set of supervisees and respond to their feedback.

Peer supervision

Peer supervision can offer an opportunity for mutual learning in an atmosphere of safety and trust (Proctor and Inskipp, 2001). It provides an opportunity for two or more peers to supervise each other. Responsibilities and roles of supervision are shared, and supervision provides an opportunity to learn from each other. As with all supervision formats, contracting and agreeing how supervision will operate is important, as is agreeing a focus, so that the peer meeting does not become a social one, or dominated by the needs of a single member.

Self-supervision

Although professional guidelines quite properly require cognitive therapists to secure supervision for themselves, it is not always possible to receive supervision on all our patients or just at the time we need it. We can then supplement our supervision by self-supervising—but once more there exist few guidelines to help us.

The minimum requirement is probably the allocation of time to review one's clinical practice, but this can be elaborated to gain more from the self-supervision process. At present the onus is on us as therapists to devise the best means of self-supervision. To do this it can be useful to:

- **Keep a self-reflection diary of clinical sessions.** Allocate time following each clinical session, or a number of clinical sessions, so that a review journal or diary can be compiled. The content of the diary will reflect your needs as a practitioner and so there is scope for variation. You might log all clinical contacts to ensure that targets are met or that your caseload is sufficiently varied, or you might summarize difficult sessions in order to better review them. You could keep a thought record relating to your own difficulties in therapy, and so on. It is helpful to review these for themes which indicate your strengths and needs as a clinician.
- **Self-rate your performance.** Use the Cognitive Therapy Scale (CTS; Young and Beck, 1980) or similar evaluation tool to review and rate your session (this was very likely routine practice during your training, but have you continued to do it?). This provides the opportunity for in-depth reflection on practice and a quantitative appraisal of your performance against which to measure subsequent performance. Of course, you can also ask colleagues or your own supervisor to rate your recorded sessions.
- **Use a self-supervision framework.** This is likely to be an idiosyncratic exercise which reflects your particular needs. However, some of you might find Padesky's Clinical Supervision Consultation Worksheet (1996) or an adaptation of it (see Box 16.5) very relevant. The worksheet was devised as a preliminary exercise to prepare a supervisee for the supervision session. The intention was that aspects of a clinical problem that could be resolved by the supervisee would be prompted by the questions in the worksheet and only issues that needed external supervision would be brought to the supervisor.

Not only does the worksheet guide self-supervision, but also serves as a screening tool which means that unnecessary questions are not taken to supervision. Thus, it facilitates both self- and other supervision.

Evaluating supervision

There is evidence that supervision contributes to good CBT practice in therapists. Beck (1986) found that therapists who did not receive supervision following training in cognitive therapy showed deterioration in skills to pre-training levels. In a more recent study of CBT training and supervision (Mannix *et al.*, 2006), established that those who continued to receive supervision gained in skills and confidence whereas skills deteriorated in those who discontinued supervision.

Box 16.5 Padesky's clinical supervision consultation worksheet

Consultation worksheet

My consultation question:______________________________

1 Have you and your client constructed a conceptualization model for understanding and treating this issue? If so, write or draw it here. If not, collaborate with client to construct it.

2 Do you have a treatment plan which fits the conceptualization? If so, write it here. If not, consider what evidence-based interventions might apply and summarize them here.

3 Is therapy following the conceptualization and treatment plan? If not, is there a good reason? Would an alternative conceptualization or treatment plan be better? Why? Does the client agree?

4 Do you have the knowledge and skill to properly implement the CT treatment? If not, ask for help with these skills and this knowledge.

5 Is the therapeutic response following expected patterns? If not, formulate hypotheses about why client response is different from expected. Consider client beliefs, skill deficits, emotional responses, interpersonal patterns, life circumstances, and developmental history. Also consider the factors in #6 below.

6 What else might be interfering with success? Include hypotheses about:

The therapist (beliefs, skill deficits, emotional responses, interpersonal patterns, life circumstances, developmental history):

The therapy relationship (e.g. is it positive and collaborative?):

The cognitive conceptualization (e.g. is something missing or inaccurate?):

The treatment plan (e.g. are there additional approaches which might help?):

Source: Adapted from Padesky, C.A. (1996). Developing cognitive therapist competency: teaching and supervision models, in Salkoskis, P. (ed.), *Frontiers of Cognitive Therapy*. New York, NY: Guilford Press. Available at: www.padesky.com

As an empirical practitioner you need to ask if *your* supervision is effective. As yet, there is no research to indicate the most valid focus for supervision evaluation and you will need to decide what is the most relevant feedback for your practice. The various sources of information available to you are explored below.

Getting feedback from the supervisee

Formal feedback from supervisees is now part of the BABCP's standard evaluation of competence to supervise. As the consumers of supervision, their feedback is important. In addition to formal feedback, you can elicit informal feedback during the supervision session itself, in the same way as you elicit it from a patient in a therapy session. Ask questions such as: How was supervision for you today? What are the main points you'll take away? Is there anything that has bothered you/you're not clear about? You must be mindful of the possibility that your supervisee will not readily give frank feedback, so it is crucial that you discuss the importance of this, preferably when you develop your supervision contract. It goes without saying that you need to be prepared to consider the feedback and act on it appropriately. This process of supervisors reflecting on their practice leads us into the next section.

Self-reflective practice

You are also a source of feedback and this should be routine practice rather than a response to the crisis of having no other means of feedback. Self-reflective practice has been promoted in the general supervision literature for several years (e.g. Hawkins and Shohet, 2000). Often a preliminary to self-supervision, self-reflection requires you to regularly make time to stand back and review aspects of your supervisory practice, such as:

- What went well and what did not go so well in the supervision session: what needs to be changed and what can be further developed?
- How did you feel in the supervision session and what can be learnt from this?
- What are the blocks to effective supervision and how might these be managed?
- What support/supervision is required for necessary change to occur?
- With hindsight what would you do differently and how will you make this more likely next time?

Such reflections can be used to question, shape, and improve your practice and can also be invaluable in preparing you for your own supervision of supervision sessions. It can be helpful to keep a reflective log or journal of your supervisory practice as this will prompt thorough reflection and provide a reference for review.

Structured feedback on supervisory competence

Formal feedback on supervisory competence can usefully come from an 'expert', a peer, or a supervisee. As yet there are no systematically evaluated comprehensive assessments of CBT supervisory practice. There are several psychometrically sound measures which focus on particular aspects of practice, such as the Supervisory Relationship Questionnaire (SRQ; Palomo *et al.*, 2009) and there are CBT assessments which are still being refined, such as Milne's Teacher's Process Evaluation of Training and Supervision (Teacher's PETS), Supervision Adherence and Guidance Evaluation (SAGE) (Milne, 2008), and the Oxford Cognitive Therapy Centre's Supervisor Competency Scale (SCS) which can be found in Appendix 16.2.

Although not specific to CBT supervision, there exist several questionnaires designed to evaluate supervisor performance (see Scaife, 2009 for a review) and you might consider using these as they as they can provide a self-rating against which to assess your development as a supervisor.

Patient outcome and change

Whatever the agreed function of supervision, be it skills development, case management, process focus, etc.—the patient's experience is central. It might be argued that good supervision is more likely to lead to good outcome for the patients (e.g. Schoenwald *et al.*, 2009), but in general the research is sparse. Nonetheless, monitoring patient progress has to be essential practice and it could contribute to evaluating the supervisor's performance.

Therapist competence

Another possibility is that 'good' supervision will positively correlate with therapist competence. Evaluation of therapist competence is commonly carried out in CBT and the most widely used assessment tool is the CTS (Young and Beck, 1980) which was devised specifically to assess cognitive therapist competency. It covers general interview procedures, interpersonal effectiveness, and specific cognitive behavioural techniques and evaluations are made using live, audio-, or video-taped therapy sessions. There is some support for the validity of the CTS as a measure of therapist competence (Dobson *et al.*, 1985) but there is also dissatisfaction with the scale and revised schedules have been developed (e.g. Blackburn *et al.*, 2001 developed the CTS-R). These aim to compensate for the perceived shortcomings of the CTS, such as the lack of opportunity to evaluate therapist competence in managing process issues and provide us with a broader and perhaps more relevant basis for measuring therapist ability. Nonetheless, the original CTS still neatly summarizes what have been seen to be the main skills and qualities of a cognitive therapist. As such, it also constitutes a useful checklist to focus the supervisor.

Feedback from patients might also provide a further source of information on perceived therapist ability.

Developing as a supervisor

In addition to accrediting CBT practitioners, the BABCP now offer supervisor and trainer accreditation, which requires set minimum hours of supervisory practice as well as feedback from supervisees and attendance at relevant training events. This reflects the increased recognition that supervisors should be experienced and competent and in order to gain experience and maintain competence, supervisors will need to seek out training and their own supervision (see also Chapter 15).

Supervision training

Supervision is a complex activity, and training in supervision is therefore appropriate, and becomingly increasingly available. It is important not to assume that the skills required to become a good therapist will be the same as those required to become a good supervisor. Training in the core skills of supervision—for example, in establishing and maintaining good SRs, in facilitating constructive feedback, and ensuring supervisee skill development—is important. Reflecting on those aspects of supervision which are more challenging for us, and embarking on training to help develop these skills is essential in developing as a supervisor.

Supervision of supervision

Using our own supervision to reflect on our supervisory practice provides another opportunity to develop as a supervisor. This offers a chance to consider and formulate problems we may be having in supervision, as well as ensuring that we are providing appropriate guidance and learning opportunities for the supervisee. Consulting with others is important in trying to resolve problems in the SR—doing so helps formulate such problems and consider possible strategies for intervention.

Difficulties arising in supervision

Many difficulties arising in supervision can be averted or managed by carefully developing a contract which is kept under review. Difficulties such as supervisor and supervisee having different expectations of the sessions, the supervisors' role being ambiguous, or the supervisee sharing limited information (perhaps only what went well or only what has gone badly in their sessions) need not arise if the contract is well thought through and is subject to review.

However, difficulties might arise despite you having invested in your contract:

- **Supervisee not carrying out agreed tasks such as bringing along recording for evaluation or carrying out certain clinical strategies**: Discover what is handicapping the supervisee. Use guided discovery to help you unpack the reason(s). Perhaps your supervisee lacks appreciation of the usefulness of recorded sessions or particular interventions and you will need to revisit your rationale. Perhaps your supervisee has performance anxiety, in which case you may need to work on this in your sessions. Just as you would with your patients, take time to understand the impasse.
- **Supervisee uses the sessions for personal therapy**: Establish if this is appropriate. If your supervisee's issue impacted on therapy then it would be acceptable to address this in the supervision session—in so far as it related to therapy. If the issue is wholly personal, discover why the supervisee is bringing it along. Perhaps the supervisee does not realize that asking for personal therapy is inappropriate and the boundaries and contract of supervision need to be reviewed.
- **Workshop attendee or colleague seeks brief supervision**: On occasion a clinician will ask for brief supervision and we would urge caution. As we have indicated in this chapter, good supervision takes time. Sessions need to be prepared, the supervisor needs to be clear about roles and responsibilities and be familiar with the patient-supervisee relationship in order to work competently. This cannot be rushed.

Key points

- Supervision needs preparation: as a supervisor you need to familiarize yourself with the principles of good practice, core skills, and consider the optimum format of your sessions.
- Supervision contracts will define the parameters of your practice and ensure clarity of role, content, and purpose of the sessions. Within the session, agenda setting and structuring will further focus your work.
- The SR is fundamental. You need to attend to this in order to maximize the potential of both the sessions and your supervisee.
- You should strive to evaluate your supervisory practice.

Further reading

BABCP website. Available at: www.babcp.co.uk (for information about supervisor contracts, accreditation, and training). (Last accessed on 1 March 2010.)

King's College London, Strand, London WC2R 2LS, UK. Tel +44(0)207836 5454 for information about supervisor training.

Oxford Cognitive Therapy Centre website. Available at: www.octc.co.uk. Warneford Hospital, Oxford, OX3 7JX, UK. Tel +44 (0)1865 223986 for information about supervisor training. (Last accessed on 1 March 2010.)

Pilling, S. and Roth, A. (2008). *A Competence Framework for the Supervision of Psychological Therapies.* Available at: www.ucl.ac.uk/CORE/supervision_competencies

Westbrook, D., Kennerley, H. and Kirk, J. (2007). *An Introduction to Cognitive Behaviour Therapy; Skills and Applications.* London: Sage.

References

Beck, A.T. (1986). Cognitive therapy: a sign of retrogression or progress. *Behavior Therapist*, **9**, 2–3.

Beinart, H. (2004). Models of supervision and the supervisory relationship and their evidence base, in Fleming, I. and Steen, L. (eds.), *Supervision and Clinical Psychology.* Hove: Brunner-Routledge.

Blackburn, I.M., James, I.A., Milne, D.L., Baker, C., Standart, S., Garland, A. and Reichelt, K. (2001). The revised cognitive therapy scale (CTS-R): psychometric properties. *Behavioural and Cognitive Psychotherapy*, **29**, 431–446.

Bordin, E.S. (1983). A working alliance model of supervision. *Counselling Psychologist*, **11**, 35–42.

Department of Health (2007). *Commissioning a Brighter Future: Improving Access to Psychological Therapies.* London: The Stationery Office.

Dobson, K., Shaw, B. and Vallis, T. (1985). Reliability of a measure of the quality of cognitive therapy. *British Journal of Clinical Psychology*, **24**, 295–300.

Freeston, M. and Armstong, P. (2006). *Conceptualising and formulating cognitive therapy supervision*, in Tarrier, N. (ed.), *Case Formulation in Cognitive Behaviour Therapy.* London: Routledge.

Hawkins, P. and Shohet, R. (2000). *Supervision in the Helping Professions. Milton Keynes*: Open University Press.

Kolb, D.A. (1984). *Experiential Learning.* New Jersey, NJ: Prentice-Hall.

Ladany, N., Hill, C.E., Corbett, M.M. and Nutt, E.A. (1996). Nature, extent and importance of what psychotherapy trainees do not disclose to their supervisors. *Journal of Counselling Psychology*, **43**, 10–24.

Liese, B. and Beck, J. (1997). Cognitive therapy supervision, in Watkins, E. (ed.), *Handbook of Psychotherapy Supervision.* New York, NY: Wiley.

Mannix, K.A., Blackburn, I.M., Garland, A., Gracie, J., Moorey, S., Reid, B., Standart, S. and Scott, J. (2006). Effectiveness of brief training in cognitive behaviour therapy techniques for palliative care practitioners. *Palliative Medicine*, **20**, 579–584.

Milne, D.L. (2008). *Evidence-based Clinical Supervision.* Chichester: Wiley-Blackwell.

Padesky, C.A. (1996). Developing cognitive therapist competency: teaching and supervision models, in Salkoskis, P. (ed.), *Frontiers of Cognitive Therapy.* New York, NY: Guilford Press.

Palomo, M., Beinart, H. and Cooper, M.J. (in press). Development and validation of the Supervisory Relationship Questionnaire (SRQ) in UK trainee clinical psychologists. *British Journal of Clinical Psychology.*

Proctor, B. and Inskipp, F. (2001). Groups supervision, in Scaife, J. (ed.), *Supervision in the Mental Health Professions: A Practitioner's Guide.* Hove: Brunner-Routledge.

Scaife, J. (2009). *Supervision in Clinical Practice.* Hove: Brunner-Routledge.

Schoenwald, S.K., Sheidow, A.J. and Chapman, J.E. (2009). Clinical supervision in treatment transport: effects on adherence and outcomes. *Journal of Consulting and Clinical Psychology*, **77**(30), 410–421.

Yerkes, R.M. and Dodson, J.D. (1908). The relation of strength of stimulus to rapidity of habit-formation. *Journal of Comparative Neurology and Psychology*, **18**, 459–482.

Young, J. and Beck, A.T. (1980). *Cognitive Therapy Scale.* University of Pennsylvania, PA: Centre for Cognitive Therapy.

Appendices

Appendix 16.1

Example supervision agreement from the British Association for Behavioural and Cognitive Psychotherapy (BABCP, 2005)

Supervision agreement between .... and ....

Confidentiality

- All professional and clinical issues discussed are confidential and are not to be discussed outside the supervision session. The exceptions to this are where professional malpractice may be evident, or if requested to release information by a Court of Law, Coroners Office, or Professional Body.
- All cases or professionals discussed during supervision must be made anonymous.
- Where tape recording of sessions takes place this must be agreed with and have the informed consent of the service user, carer, or professional. Arrangements must also be made to destroy/wipe any recordings. The supervisee is responsible for ensuring this process is followed.

Comments

Content of supervision

- Content of supervision will focus on the acquisition of knowledge, conceptualization, and clinical skills within a cognitive behavioural model(s).
- Associated issues will also be discussed when it is relevant to do so, for example, medication, hospitalization, case management.
- Identification (and collaborative change of these if appropriate) of supervisee thoughts, attitudes, beliefs, and values and the impact of these on therapeutic and professional behaviour.

- Discussion and working through relationship and process aspects of supervision.

There will be an equal split between the time spend on each of the above in the time available.

Comments

Practicalities

- One session each ………………… for …………….. hours/minutes
- The venue the session(s) will take place at is …………………………..
- The person responsible for booking the accommodation is ………………..
- Fees for supervision are …………………………………..
- Cancellation arrangements …………………………………

Supervision methods and content

- Discussion of therapeutic relationship and engagement issues
- Case conceptualization/formulation
- Rehearsal of therapeutic techniques (e.g. simulation, role-play)
- Discussion about therapeutic strategies
- Case presentations
- Homework
- Review of audio and videotapes (at least one per month)
- Direct observation of practice—at least once in a month per supervisee
- Identification of supervisee thoughts, attitudes, beliefs with exploration of the impact of these on therapeutic and professional behaviour
- Review of risk and therapist/service user safety
- Review of clinical guidelines/manuals
- Review of psychoeducational material
- Experiential exercises
- Other strategies as agreed

Comments

Aims of supervision

The primary focus of supervision is the welfare of the client through the supervisee's learning process, in terms of knowledge attainment, attitude refinement, and skills development.

Goals for supervision:

1.
2.
3.
4.

Comments

Anti-discriminatory practice

Practice will follow the policy of ....
[employer/professional body]

Comments

Steps in the event of a breakdown in the arrangements for clinical CBT supervision

In the event of inappropriate behaviour by the supervisor/supervisee this should be discussed together initially.......................

If this is unsuccessful or the behaviour is of a serious and immediate nature then .... should be informed IMMEDIATELY.

In the unlikely event that the relationship between the supervisee and supervisor deteriorates, each person is responsible for attempting to work together to resolve the problem.

Comments

Changes to this agreement and timescale

Changes to this agreement can be negotiated at any time.

This agreement covers the period ....

Signed ____________Supervisor ______________Date _____________

Signed ____________Supervisee ______________Date _____________

With thanks to Michael Townend

Please feel free to circulate and edit the document as you wish.

Appendix 16.2

The Oxford Cognitive Therapy Centre Supervisor Competency Scale (2009): guidelines when using the SCS

The purpose of supervision is to foster good practice, as defined by professional guidelines, so as to meet client/patient needs. This rating form has been devised to structure the process of evaluating supervision competency, making use of both specific and general items. It reflects the 2008 supervision competencies of Pilling and Roth, and general guidelines for good supervision practice (see Kennerley and Clohessy, 2010 for a review) while striving to be as short and simple as possible.

It aims to:

1 Enable raters to communicate a standard of practice.

2 To help supervisors reflect on and develop their practice.

3 To indicate the degree to which a particular supervision session fulfils the purpose outlined above.

It can be used both as an instrument to give detailed feedback and/or an evaluation tool for deciding whether or not supervisee performance is adequate.

It comprises three sections:

- **Section I**: The scale used by raters to evaluate a supervisor's performance. This addresses six areas of practice: structuring of sessions; enhancing learning; the supervisory relationship; other process issues; professional and ethical practice; reflective practice. Items within each of these areas of practice are rated on a 5-point scale. Raters also comment on the general strengths of the supervisor, make suggestions for improvement, and consider the appropriateness of the supervisor's reflection on supervision (see Section II).
- **Section II**: A reflection on supervision form to be completed by the supervisor. This encourages self-reflective practice and enables the rater to decide

if the self-reflection is adequate or appropriate and if supervisee's feedback (see Section III) has been considered.

- **Section III**: As recipients of supervision, supervisees' feedback is valuable, if properly attended to by the supervisor. Thus, supervisees are asked to give their supervisors feedback on the session and this should be submitted with the session recording. If the supervisor wishes to s/he can specify the details of feedback and the assessor can comment upon the appropriateness of the supervisor's choice of questions.

Supervisor Competency Scale contributors: Helen Kennerley, Gillian Butler, and Sue Clohessy (OCTC)

Instructions to raters

As a rater, you are expected to use your professional judgement in completing this form and to comment (briefly) on your ratings. If possible, illustrate the basis for more general judgements, so as to clarify your decision and enable the student learn from the evaluation. There are 7 parts to the SCS: within each there is scope for rating particular items, such as contracting use of time, promoting reflective practice, being respectful, etc. Items in Parts 1–5 are rated using the following scale:

Rate supervisor's performance on the following scale:

1	2	3	4	5
Absence of feature or highly incompetent or major problems evident	Evidence of competence, but many problems and/or lack of consistency	Competent, but some problems and/or inconsistencies	Good features, minor problems, and/or inconsistencies	Expert performance or very good even in the face of difficulties

Items within Part 6 are rated using a simple 5-point scale, while items in Part 7 concern general feedback and require written statements.

This is intended to form the basis of detailed feedback which will help the supervisee improve her/his practice. Not all of the items within Parts 1–6 will be applicable for the recording under scrutiny and it is acceptable to rate these as 'not applicable' (N/A). For example, addressing problems within the supervisory relationship might not be relevant in the session which is being assessed.

At the end of end of Parts 1–6, raters are asked to judge whether or not the supervisee has shown competent practice (see level 3 on the above rating scale). This does not necessarily reflect an average score for that part of the SCS (as some items will have been deemed not applicable) but rather the rater's overall view of performance in that particular aspect of supervision. For overall performance in a particular area to be considered competent, none of the scored items should fall below '2' and the majority should score '3' or above. If the SCS is being used as an assessment tool, supervisors have to be deemed competent in all six areas in order to 'pass'.

Notes for raters

Part 1: Structuring the session

1 Contracts use of time: this should be done collaboratively. Time allocation should reflect the demands of supervision and time available.

Supervisors should ensure time is allocated to review the past session and current session as appropriate.

2 Adheres to agreed agenda: the supervisor is expected to pace the session appropriately, remain focused on the agenda and only digress following discussion and renegotiation of the agenda with the supervisee.

3 Selects specific and appropriate topics/goals for session: the topics and goals should be arrived at collaboratively, should reflect both the needs of the supervisee and of the client(s) and should reflect the supervision contract which will have been drawn up prior to beginning the course of supervision.

4 Paces session (i) appropriate to the needs of the supervisee, and (ii) uses time efficiently.

Part 2: Enhancing learning

1 Gathers information to illustrate supervisee's clinical practice using Socratic methods, 'live' supervision, role–play, and case discussion.

2 Uses a variety of methods to appraise and evaluate the skills and knowledge of the supervisee: for example, through role-play or by rating therapy tapes.

3 Shows sensitivity to the learning needs of the supervisee: is aware of the developmental needs and optimum learning style of the supervisee and is able to create a stimulating learning environment that does not over stress the supervisee.

4 Balances use of methods likely to foster supervisee learning (e.g. Socratic method, use of recordings, information giving, experiential methods, etc.) throughout the session and uses learning approaches appropriately. For example, experiential approaches to skills development.

5 Makes available relevant and appropriate materials (e.g. references, measures, recordings, etc.).

6 Gives feedback to supervisee which is sensitive and constructive. Feedback should be clear, specific, framed as the supervisor's opinion and should both challenge and support the supervisee. Feedback should be given frequently enough to be useful and the supervisee should be prompted to reflect on it in the session. Supervisee's feedback should be elicited at the end of each session.

7 Makes theory-practice links, helping the supervisee combine cognitive theory and psychological principles with sound clinical work.

8 Promotes reflective practice by regularly prompting the supervisees to critically appraise and learn from their work, and by encouraging supervisees to record and review their therapy sessions.

9 In a *group setting* facilitates group learning by attending to the input of all group members and by encouraging vicarious learning.

Part 3: Supervisory relationship

1 Collaborative and engaging: there should be evidence of 'team work' on shared, agreed goals.

2 Respectful, supportive, sensitive: the supervisor's practice should communicate a respectful awareness of the learning needs of the supervisee.

3 Creates safe environment for supervisee to be open: the supervisor should create a setting which is supportive, emotionally containing, and which is non-judgemental of the person.

4 Boundaried: the SR reflects a working alliance not a friendship or therapy. Supervision is primarily educative. It should be relevant and free of interruption and unnecessary digression.

5 Open: honest mutual feedback should be exchanged regularly to ensure that there is shared understanding, that clinical goals are being met, that agreed tasks are being carried out, that practice is ethical and that learning needs are met. Supervisors should express reservations in a timely and respectful fashion.

6 Problems within the SR are addressed if this is necessary. Supervisors should be open and honest if they have concerns about the SR and if problems arise the supervisor should address them in a timely and respectful fashion.

Part 4: Other process issues

To score highly in this section the supervisor must:

- Create a setting which facilitates the exploration of process issues. Even though there will be times when detailed attention to process issues is not necessary, it is crucial to make exploration possible. The supervisor will be given credit for creating a setting which allows for this possibility.
- Show an awareness and appreciation of a systemic perspective of the supervision process which embraces not only therapist, supervisor, and client but also the relevant systems within which they operate (e.g. domestic, occupational, and institutional).
- Target key areas if they need to be addressed.

The relevance of process issues might need to be inferred by the rater if the issue is not identified and discussed by the supervisor—in which case the reasons for this inference should be clearly noted under general comments.

Supervisees will be penalized for failing to appreciate key process issues or if process issues are recognized but not addressed properly. The key areas for consideration are:

1 IP issues within the therapeutic relationship
2 IP issues between the supervisor and client or wider system
3 Process issues within the client's wider system
4 Process issues within the supervisee's wider system
5 In a *group setting* the supervisor should recognize and manage group processes appropriately: this means using helpful group processes (e.g. de-stigmatizing, the instillation of hope, and peer guidance) to augment the supervision experience while minimizing unhelpful group processes (e.g. scapegoating, dependency, splitting).

Part 5: Professional and ethical practice

1 Practices within limits of own knowledge and skill: supervisors should restrict their supervisory practice to their areas of knowledge and expertise and be open about the limitations of their skill and awareness.
2 Fosters competence in working with difference: the supervisor should encourage a non-judgemental and sensitive approach, which is enabling of clients from a broad range of backgrounds. This may have to be inferred from the supervisor's attitude towards the patient under discussion and the supervisee(s) in the session. If this is the case, the reasons for the inference should be clearly noted under general comments.
3 Respects confidentiality: the supervisor should protect patient confidentiality and ensure that supervisees do the same. Encouraging or permitting supervisees to disclose the full name of a patient will result in this item being failed.
4 Promotes safe CBT practice (including risk assessment where appropriate). Risk awareness is *crucial* to good supervision and ethical practice. Supervisors should also ensure that supervisees create appropriate therapy boundaries and practice ethically (e.g. fostering *appropriate* therapist-patient alliance, etc.).
5 Encourages realistic and safe case management such that the supervisee is neither overloaded nor understimulated. The supervisor should ensure that the supervisee practices within the limits of his/her knowledge and skill. The supervisor should also support the supervisee in recognizing and bridging gaps in his/her practice.

Part 6: Reflective practice

These items are rated on a 5-point rating scale: scores of 3 and more are acceptable for competent practice.

1 Supervisor elicited appropriate feedback: this reflects the feedback gathered verbally at the end of the supervision session and the written feedback collected from the supervisee(s). The purpose of the feedback is to inform the supervisor's practice and to give information which will improve the supervision experience for the supervisee.

2 Responses to supervisee's feedback were appropriate: the supervisor should show that s/he has properly reviewed and considered supervisee's feedback and has identified learning opportunities.

3 Supervisor's next supervision goal(s) is appropriate: the supervisor should build on reflection by translating new ideas/insights into action in the form of supervision goals, which should be 'SMART'. These might involve seeking supervision of supervision, organizing further CPD, and modifying performance in supervision sessions. Whatever the goals, they should reflect the learning opportunities of the recorded session.

Part 7: General feedback

In this section, raters should give a summary of:

1 The supervisor's main strength (as demonstrated in the submitted recording) along with,

2 Suggestions for improvement of supervisory practice.

Comments should be constructive, specific, and where possible readily translated into tasks which can be reviewed.

Section I

Supervisor Competency Scale (OCTC, 2009)

Supervisor:………………………….. Date of session: ……….......

Rater: ……………………………….. Date of rating: ……………..

Supervision format (e.g. group, peer, etc.): ……………………………………

Items submitted for rating

1 One recording Yes No

2 Feedback from recipient(s) of supervision Yes No

3 Completed reflection on supervision form Yes No

Rate supervisor's performance on the following scale:

1	2	3	4	5
Absence of feature or highly incompetent or major problems evident	Evidence of competence, but many problems and/or lack of consistency	Competent, but some problems and/or inconsistencies	Good features, minor problems, and/ or inconsistencies	Expert performance or very good even in the face of difficulties

Part 1: Structuring the session

1 Contracts use of time …

2 Adheres to agreed agenda …

3 Selects specific and appropriate topics/goals for session …

4 Paces session (i) appropriate to the needs of the supervisee(s) …

(ii) uses time efficiently …

General comments:

Part 1: Considered competent: Yes No

Part 2: Enhancing learning

1 Gathers information to illustrate supervisee's clinical practice ...

2 Uses a variety of methods to appraise and evaluate the skills and knowledge of the supervisee ...

3 Shows sensitivity to the learning needs of the supervisee ...

4 Balances use of methods likely to foster supervisee learning (e.g. Socratic method, use of recordings, information giving, experiential methods, etc.) ...

5 Makes available relevant and appropriate materials (e.g. references, measures, recordings, etc.) ...

6 Gives feedback to supervisee which is sensitive and constructive ...

7 Makes theory-practice links ...

8 Promotes reflective practice ...

9 In a *group setting* facilitates group learning ...

General comments:

Part 2: Considered competent: Yes No

Part 3: Supervisory relationship

1 Collaborative and engaging ....
2 Respectful, supportive, sensitive ...
3 Creates safe environment for supervisee to be open ...
4 Boundaried: the SR reflects a working alliance not a friendship or therapy ...
5 Open: honest mutual feedback ...
6 Problems within the SR are addressed ...

General comments:

Part 3: Considered competent: Yes No

Part 4: Other process issues

1 Shows sensitivity to IP issues within the therapeutic relationship ...

2 Shows sensitivity to IP issues between the supervisor and client or wider system ...

3 Shows sensitivity to process issues within the client's wider system ...

4 Shows sensitivity to process issues within the supervisee's wider system ...

5 In a *group setting* recognizes and manages group processes appropriately ...

General comments:

Part 4: Considered competent: Yes No

Part 5: Professional and ethical practice

1 Practices within limits of own knowledge and skill ...

2 Fosters competence in working with difference ...

3 Respects confidentiality ...

4 Promotes safe CBT practice (including risk assessment where appropriate) ...

5 Encourages appropriate case management ...

General comments:

Part 5: Considered competent: Yes No

Part 6: Reflective practice

	Not at all			Absolutely
1. Supervisor elicited appropriate feedback	1____2_____3_____4____5			
2. Responses to supervisee's feedback were appropriate	1____2_____3_____4____5			
3. Supervisor's next supervision goal is appropriate	1____2_____3_____4____5			

General comments:

Part 6: Considered competent: Yes No

Part 7: General feedback

1 Supervisor's main strength as demonstrated in this recording

2 Suggestions for improvement

Section II

Reflection on supervision form

1 Background information

Give a brief description of the supervisee(s), their level of experience, the number of times you have met, etc.

2 General reflection

(i) Comment on what you are pleased with and less pleased with in this session: consider content, procedure, and process. You might also want to consider your assumptions, shared responsibilities, and shared expertise.

(ii) What is your response to the feedback from your supervisee(s)?

(iii) In the light of (i) and (ii), what is your next goal(s) as a supervisor?

(iv) Does this session reflect your usual practice? Was there anything unusual about this session—if so, how did you manage this?

Section III

Supervisees' feedback*

Supervisor:...............   Date of session: ……….......

As a supervisee, what did you find particularly helpful or less helpful about this session? What, if anything, would suggest to improve the session?

*Supervisors may request more detailed feedback.

Chapter 1 /

Training skills

Melanie Fennell

You have just started the second term of a one year CBT Diploma course. You feel you are just about getting the hang of it, and beginning to have the sense that, by the end of the year, you will be able to do "proper" CBT with your patients—at least the relatively straightforward ones. One day an email arrives from your employers. Since they have invested all this money in training you, they would like a return. You are asked to organize and run a CBT training course for 85 CMHT clinicians with a range of different professional backgrounds. The proposal must be finalized within two weeks, and the course itself must begin at the very beginning of the financial year, just 2½ months away.

You have been a CBT trainer for many years. You usually get very good feedback, and enjoy seeing your participants grow and develop. You yourself have never received training in training skills, but you have made the most of opportunities to learn from trainers whose workshops you have attended and enjoyed. Now you are beginning to feel that your work is becoming a bit repetitive, stale—you could do with time to reflect and opportunities to replenish your resources. In particular, you want to make your training more interactive, and to explore the principles behind what works and what does not work so well.

Introduction

Once you have become a competent CBT (cognitive behavioural therapy) therapist (even before that), you may encounter expectations that—without any further input—you will be able to pass on what you have learned to others. It is as if knowing how to do CBT automatically sets you up to train others. This assumption also means that even highly experienced trainers may never have received training in training skills, and is reflected in relative scarcity of literature on the principles and practice of teaching CBT. Even in the United Kingdom's current initiative to increase patient access to CBT, no training competencies have been defined (Roth and Pilling, 2007). This gap presents challenges to anyone who wants to develop as a trainer. What knowledge and skills are needed? How do you acquire them?

This chapter is intended to help to bridge this gap. It describes:

1 An overview of **the training process**

2 How to identify shortfalls in knowledge and skills (**performance gaps**), and associated **training needs**

3 How to identify specific **learning objectives**, so that your training has focus and direction and is directly relevant to participants' needs

4 How to **design** interactive training which encourages learning, maximizes retention, and facilitates the transfer of learning to the workplace

5 How to **deliver** training in such a way that your participants do much of the work themselves, rather than relying on you to feed them information or tell them what to do

6 How to **evaluate** your training, at the time and in the longer term

7 How to handle common problems.

8 How to **continue to develop** your training skills

Four key points

1. Opportunities to explore new territory

Becoming a trainer means venturing beyond the familiar territory of CBT into new lands—adult learning and education, human resources, and management development. This offers opportunities to develop transferable competencies above and beyond what is involved in becoming a CBT therapist. Unless you work in higher education, these ideas may be unfamiliar. If so, here is a chance to experiment with something new. Alternatively, you may recognize knowledge and skills you already use—intuitively, or because you have successfully transferred the collaborative style of CBT into your training practice, or because this is how you learned to do CBT and you enjoyed it and saw how well it worked. If your knowledge is mainly based on experience rather than formal learning, then this chapter may illuminate the 'grammar' of interactive training—the learning principles that underlie it.

2. You know more than you think

Even if you are a complete beginner as a trainer, you will discover that this approach to training has a great advantage for CBT therapists: it closely matches CBT's collaborative style. So, even if the training literature is foreign territory to you, you already have a sketch-map and the beginnings of a useful kitbag. For example, you will be used to agreeing goals with your patients, creating a respectful working alliance, using experiential learning (behavioural experiments), evaluating progress, and so forth. Thus, even beginner CBT trainers do not in fact start from square one.

3. The ideal—and the realistic

The chapter outlines how you might ideally approach training, given all the resources needed to analyze training needs with care, define associated goals, design and deliver training, and fully evaluate the results. Of course, in real life, the ideal is not always possible. Deadlines may be tight, and resources short. If so, be realistic: do what you can, given the constraints. When circumstances do not allow you thoroughly to analyze training needs, or to evaluate long-term impact, you need not be hard on yourself—or give up, thinking that if you cannot 'do it properly' you might as well not bother at all. The ideal offers possibilities, something to aim toward. Use it to help you identify what you would do under more favourable circumstances, and to encourage you to stretch as far as you can toward it.

4. Making the most of the chapter

In order to get the most from this chapter, we recommend that, before you read any further, you identify a specific training project to which you can apply what you learn. This may be long or short, it may be something forthcoming, or something you have already taught a number of times but would like to rethink and refresh, or even something that you would like to teach but as yet have had no opportunity. Select something that will be of direct practical use to you, so that reading the chapter is more than just an academic exercise. Pause after each section and consider: How does this apply to *my* training project?

What do trainers do? The training process

Imagine shadowing a trainer, observing what he/she does. What most readily comes to mind? Probably an image of the person actually delivering the training—standing at the front of a class, with flipcharts and PowerPoint and so forth in the background. Yet training delivery is only one element of a more complex process, much of which is invisible to participants and to training purchasers. As you will see, this means that *training takes time*, especially in advance—substantially more time than the hour or day of the event itself.

The training process can be encapsulated as a sequence of activities. Each builds on what has gone before, and prepares the ground for what follows. The sequence (illustrated in Fig. 17.1) is adapted from literature on generic training

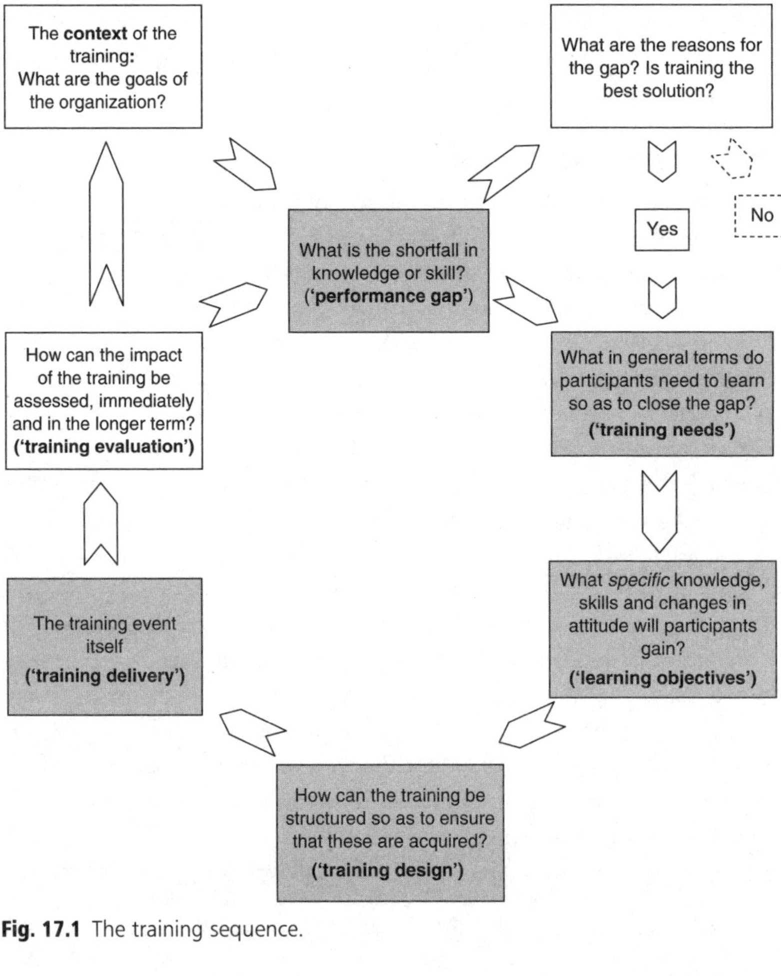

Fig. 17.1 The training sequence.

skills (Bee and Bee, 1994, p. 22), *not* from CBT. Consequently, it can be applied to almost any training:

- How to ice a cake
- How to be an effective telephone sales person
- How to deliver a baby
- How to manage a team
- How to make a burglar alarm

  even

- How to become an effective trainer

Notice the practical 'how to' flavour to this list. 'Training' does not simply mean lectures or PowerPoint presentations. It means interactively teaching an integration of knowledge and practical skills which can be applied in the real world. Training sessions may well include presentations by the trainer but, as you will see below, that is far from the whole story.

We shall now follow the training sequence through, considering each element in turn.

Identifying performance gaps and training needs

Any training initiative starts with identifying a 'gap in performance' (i.e. a discrepancy between actual and desired performance, defined in relation to organizational goals) and an associated training need (i.e. recognition that the gap is caused by deficits in knowledge or skill, and would be closed by appropriate training). Here a disparity between the ideal and the realistic may first emerge. Thorough assessment of performance gaps and training needs creates a solid foundation for training design. In practice, neither the time nor the resources for thoroughness may be available. We shall return to this point later.

The fundamental questions at this stage are:

- What must I know about participants and their work contexts, in order to determine what (if any) training they need in order to do their jobs effectively?
- How can I best gather this information?

Before addressing these questions, let us consider two important issues relating to the training context.

Two contextual issues

1. Is training the best solution?

Shortfalls in performance do not necessarily result from deficits in knowledge or skill which training will remedy. The reason for a performance gap might be systemic—for example, a stressful working environment with high staff turnover, job dissatisfaction, and failure to utilize existing skills. Equally, formal training is only one development option: the gap might be better closed by, for example, clinical supervision, on-the-job coaching, or access to expert consultation.

2. Is there a good fit between the training and the goals of the commissioning organization?

The success of any training initiative depends on fit with the goals of the commissioning organization (e.g. to meet NICE [National Institute for Clinical Excellence] guidelines for offering evidence-based psychological treatment). A good fit encourages management buy-in and support, and makes it more likely that the resources necessary for longer-term impact (e.g. ongoing supervision) will be put in place.

In the interests of ensuring your training is relevant and *seen to be so* by your sponsoring organization, it can be helpful to consult supporting documents (you will find some examples in Table 17.1). You will need to decide which are most pertinent to your particular circumstances. Being familiar with them will allow you to argue that your training is congruent with relevant local and national priorities (see also Chapter 19 on service development).

Measuring performance gaps and training needs: what method for whom?

What measures are most useful (informative, efficient) depends on factors such as the number of people potentially requiring training, and the time and resources available.

Large numbers: quantitative methods

If the number of potential participants is large, the most effective method might be to gather statistical data on current levels of knowledge, skill, previous relevant training, opportunities for ongoing supervision, etc. Possible methods include: self-assessment questionnaires (e.g. competency checklists), surveys (often most conveniently done by email), and documents relating to current and future workforce requirements (e.g. local, national, and professional strategy documents).

Small numbers: qualitative methods

If the number of people is relatively small (e.g. the members of a single community mental health team [CMHT]), then more intensive qualitative methods become feasible. Possible methods include: individual interviews (with staff, line managers, patients); team meetings or discussions, designed to

Table 17.1 Creating a good fit between training and organizational goals: sources of supporting information for training initiatives.

Information sources	Examples
External influences on decision-makers	◆ Government documents (e.g. NICE guidelines) ◆ New UK and EEC legislation (e.g. Mental Health Acts, Equal Opportunities) ◆ Financial developments (e.g. purchasing patterns of PCTs) ◆ National service targets (e.g. ease of access to services, especially for disadvantaged groups) ◆ Changing client base (e.g. ageing population) ◆ Professional standards (e.g. CPD requirements) ◆ New findings from clinical and training research
Internal influences (the priorities of the decision-makers themselves)	◆ Training commissioner's policy documents (e.g. vision statements, business plans) ◆ HR issues (e.g. staff recruitment and retention) ◆ Culture of commissioning organization (e.g. opinions of CBT held by management and by potential participants) ◆ Financial constraints (e.g. training budget, likely cuts) ◆ Feedback from staff and stakeholders (e.g. patients, referral agencies, voluntary sector) ◆ Measures of service quality (e.g. outcome data, complaints/commendations per × patients, re-referrals)

Abbreviations: EEC, European Economic Community; PCTs, Primary Care Trusts; CPD, continuing professional development.

identify recurrent themes; critical incident review (What exactly went wrong? Was it the result of deficits in knowledge and skills?); direct observation (e.g. rating live or recorded therapy sessions). These methods may be more time-consuming, but often yield rich data and can help to engage staff in the training: they will have met you and feel that their voices have been heard.

Combining quantitative and qualitative methods

Quantitative and qualitative methods can usefully be combined. For example, a widely distributed survey or questionnaire could be followed by discussion groups or one-to-one meetings with selected staff, line managers, and/or patients. Equally, preliminary qualitative data from a small number of one-to-one contacts could be used to generate a relevant survey or questionnaire for a larger group.

Data gathering takes time and effort. Why should I bother?

Precision and relevance

Carefully assessing performance gaps and training needs means that your training can be precisely focused. Conversely, inaccurate information can result in training which inadvertently aims too high or too low or is off-target, to the frustration of trainer and participants.

Demonstrating the impact of training

Measuring pre-training performance allows you to evaluate the impact of your intervention against a known baseline. This provides more useful information than a post-course assessment, which could be influenced by many factors—including the disconcerting possibility that everyone was already performing well before the training. Pre-post measures are helpful to you, the trainer, and also to participants and their employers, who can easily see:

- Whether the performance gap has closed or further input is needed.
- Whether the training delivered what it promised (including value for money).
- Whether initial objectives have been met.

Developing a training proposal

Identified performance gaps and training needs can form the basis for a formal training proposal, the purpose of which may be to 'sell' the training to stakeholders (e.g. those who determine service priorities, those who hold the purse strings, those likely to receive the training, their line managers, etc.). A guiding framework for a proposal can be found in Table 17.2. Even if you do not need a formal proposal, you may still find it helpful to use this framework when you embark on training, as it suggests factors you might usefully take into account.

Taking account of the culture of the commissioning organisation

How does whoever commissioned the work view training? As punishment for poor performance, so that people might be reluctant to admit need? Or as a reward, so that people want it whether they need it or not? As irrelevant, unnecessary, expensive, and time-consuming? Purely a means of ticking boxes? Or—the ideal—essential to consistent high quality performance? Whatever the quality and value of the training itself, success can depend on a proposal which speaks the language of the decision-makers and finance managers (what the popular 'buzz' words are in your particular management culture?), and takes account of organizational perspectives.

Table 17.2 A guiding framework for preparing a training proposal.

Background

- What led to the proposal?
- The performance gap, how it was detected and measured, its impact on the capacity of the service to meet user needs. Why training is the best way of closing the gap.
- Relevant future developments/current trends.

Target population

- Who is the training for (profession, work setting, level of seniority, existing levels of knowledge and skill, organization/group/individual)?
- Numbers?
- Special needs?

Aim of training

- Desired outcome. What level of competence is required?

Benefits of supporting training *(the more these match the needs of decision-makers, and are supported by evidence, the greater the chance of success)*

- For example, government targets for access to effective psychological treatment met; improved patient care and outcome, both short term and long term; reduced use of NHS resources (fewer patients hospitalized, reduced use of medication); improved staff morale, reduced staff turnover, and improved recruitment; users and referral agents reassured about service quality.

Costs of not supporting training *(the more these match the needs of decision-makers, and are supported by evidence, the greater the chance of success)*

- For example, government targets not met; poor performance in external service audit; loss of experienced staff; patient dissatisfaction; organization's vision, values, objectives not realized.

Learning objectives

- What knowledge, skills, and attitudes will participants acquire (specific, measurable)?
- What will they know and be able to do, to what standard, and under what conditions?

Delivery system *(selected to match participants' work patterns and service demands)*

- Format (e.g. course, interactive workshop, skills sharing, coaching, supervision)?
- On or off the job?
- Between session continuity, follow-up, etc.?

Trainer skills *(what makes you the best person to do the job?)*

- Qualifications, reputation, references.
- Prior experience of training in the area and of training similar groups.
- Outcome data.

Methods of evaluation

- How will the trainer/participants/organization know if the objectives have been met?
- What changes in knowledge, skill, attitude will be assessed?
- How will transfer of learning to the workplace, and impact on patient care, be evaluated?

(continued)

Table 17.2 (continued) A guiding framework for preparing a training proposal.

Timing

- When will the training take place?
- Urgency? Constraints?
- Special conditions (e.g. staff on split shifts, part-time workers)?
- Follow-up (learning transfer)?

Venue

- Where will the training be carried out?
- Space necessary (e.g. room size, number of breakout rooms)?
- Special needs (e.g. access for those with reduced mobility)?

Resources required

- Equipment, materials, Internet access, publications.
- Special needs (e.g. visual or auditory impairment)?

Costs *(including a formal cost-benefit analysis and budget if appropriate)*

- Costs of training itself (trainer(s), equipment, materials, hire of venue).
- Additional costs of attendance (subsistence, travel, staff cover).
- Administration costs; overheads.

Preparatory work for participants

- Self-assessment (e.g. questionnaires, self-monitoring, personal goal setting).
- Ensuring funding and commitment from line managers.
- Preparatory reading.

What if the context does not support thorough analysis of training needs?

CBT therapists often find themselves in a training role through no choice of their own—you may have little say in what you are expected to deliver. If you find yourself in this unenviable position, it can still be worth asserting the importance of a solid analysis: how else will you provide significant learning experiences, which can be effectively transferred to the workplace and have the desired results for participants and (the bottom line) their patients? Again, it is important to argue this, not from your own perspective, but rather from the perspective of the organization. What are the benefits to them? And what are the costs of failing to do so? A possible line of argument might be something like:

- You (the organization) are eager for this training to go ahead, as am I.
- Equally, you will be keen to ensure value for money, given the outlay of funds and staff time involved.

- I have two serious concerns about this:
  1. Without information about current levels of knowledge and skill, it will be difficult to ensure that the training is relevant, precisely targeted, and at the right level.
  2. What people learn needs to be applied in the workplace, with patients. This means line managers need to be committed to ensure that the training is used and supported by ongoing supervision. Otherwise, lasting performance gains, improved staff morale, and enhanced patient outcome/throughput will not be achieved.
- I recommend:
  - Preliminary assessment of existing CBT knowledge and skill—as a minimum, an email survey.
  - A letter from you keeping line managers in the picture, and asking them to ensure its implementation.
  - Monthly follow-up supervision, to be provided by myself/colleagues.
- With these in place, I am confident that the training will deliver the desired results.

Arguing for thorough assessment and follow-up can be daunting, especially if your management culture is strongly 'top down', and if the deadline for delivery is short. However, acquiring at least basic pre-training information will lead to a much more effectively targeted intervention, more acceptable to participants, and thus ultimately more effective and of greater benefit to all stakeholders—including patients.

'By the end of the training, participants will be able to ...'

Defining learning objectives

When you plan a training session, how do you decide on the content? Often, the first thing to come to mind is 'what I should include'—that is, the training *aims.* Aims state the general intention or direction of the training *from the perspective of the trainer/organization.* This is very different from defining *learning objectives*, which means thinking in terms of specific, concrete desired outcomes *from the perspective of participants.* Objectives require you to put yourself in participants' shoes, to move:

From:	*'What do I (the trainer) want to do?'*	**To:**	*'What will participants go away with?'*

Objectives, defined in terms of observable behaviours, state the desired end point of the training—the destination. From them, everything else follows—design, delivery (e.g. emphasis on systematic skills practice), and evaluation (what and when). Clear objectives, related to identified training needs, also contribute to engaging and motivating participants, clarifying what they can expect take away in their therapeutic kitbags.

Elements of objectives

Objectives can include three elements:

- **Desired performance**: *What* participants will be able to do, for example, conduct a session of CBT.
- **Conditions**: *How and under what circumstances* they will be able to do it, for example, with a moderately depressed patient.
- **Standards of performance**: *How well/to what criterion* they will be able to do it, for example, scoring at least 2 on all items of the revised Cognitive Therapy Rating Scale (CTS-R; Blackburn *et al.*, 2001).

In academic contexts, or where a particular performance criterion is required, it is customary to include conditions and standards; elsewhere, often only desired performance is defined. Table 17.3 offers an example, which goes beyond the remit of CBT but may ring bells for some readers.

What is competence?

Competence is a product of integrating **knowledge, skills, and attitudes** in meaningful and useful ways, and using them flexibly in response to new situations (generalization). Objectives can address any or all of these:

- **Knowledge** refers to information stored in memory, and includes: theory (e.g. cognitive behavioural models for particular disorders); facts, data (e.g. research findings); and methods (e.g. how in principle to develop a formulation).
- **Skill** refers to the ability to apply knowledge in practice. Skills are usually acquired over time, through rehearsal and feedback. Initially performance may be conscious and effortful; with practice it becomes automatic. Knowledge and skill are not necessarily correlated: you can know how to do something in theory without being able to do it in practice (e.g. drive a car), especially if you learned through reading, listening to someone describe it, or watching them do it without trying it yourself, learning from feedback, and trying again.

Table 17.3 Defining training objectives: an example.

- By the end of the training, participants will be able to:
  - Empty the dirty cat litter tray into a strong black rubbish sack, using the shovel provided, and collecting all liquids and solids including those hiding in corners and/or stuck to the tray.
  - Clean and deodorize the tray, using the spray and powder provided.
  - Replace the litter with fresh litter from the bag provided to a depth of 6 cm.
  - Smooth the surface, using the flat of the shovel, so that the depth of litter is consistent throughout the tray.
  - Clean and clear the surrounding area, sweeping up fallen litter and placing it in the black rubbish sack, and wiping the floor with a disposable cloth using lemon scented disinfectant fluid.
  - Tie the mouth of the black rubbish sack, and place it in the rubbish bin outside the house.
- At the end of the Basic Course, participants will be able to complete the above steps only in the absence of the cat.
- At the end of the Intermediate Course, participants will be able to complete the above steps in the presence of the cat, providing the cat is good-humoured (as evidenced by purring, rubbing against the legs, etc.) and is not actually attempting to use the litter tray.
- At the end of the Advanced Course, participants will be able to complete the above steps in the presence of the cat, even if the latter is irate, armed, and ready to fire.

- **Attitude** refers to beliefs, values, assumptions, expectations, and prejudices. CBT therapists are used to working with these in therapy, but may take less account of them in training—unless something goes wrong. Attitude may come into sharp focus, for example, when training clinicians from other psychotherapeutic orientations who have serious doubts about the value of CBT. Pre-existing attitudes can impact on willingness to be open to new ideas, to perform in front of others, to share experiences, to be creative and flexible, to be evaluated, to relate straightforwardly to the trainer. The aim in training is to create a learning culture very similar to that which characterizes CBT: a culture of curiosity, willingness to experiment, and respectful collaboration. Participants' attitudes can make this difficult—and so can trainers' (e.g. 'Unless I have 4,000 PowerPoint slides, referencing 7,000 empirical studies, I have no credibility as a trainer'). Unless tackled (see section 'Helpful hints for handling common problems'), such attitudes can poison the atmosphere and create barriers to learning.

Operationalize your objectives

Objectives need to be 'SMART' (see Chapter 15, pp. 313–315)—simply expressed, measurable, congruent with participants' learning needs, realistic, and likely to be achieved in the time available. You will capture what is needed by completing the following sentence:

> *'By the end of the training,* ***participants will be able to …***'

The aim is to use the language of *action*, overt behaviours rather than internal processes which cannot be seen or assessed ('understand', 'appreciate', 'grasp', 'know', etc.). Understanding, appreciation, etc. are indeed legitimate aims, but the question to ask when defining objectives is:

> *'How will I* ***know?***'

Because unless participants can *demonstrate* that they understand, appreciate, etc., there is no way of ensuring that learning objectives are met.

So:

Not: 'Participants *will appreciate* the role of cognition in emotional disorder'
But: 'Participants *will be able to describe* the role …'

Not: 'Participants *will understand* Clark's cognitive model of panic disorder'
But: 'Participants *will be able to formulate* a case of panic disorder using Clark's model'

Helpful action words include:

List	Plan	Outline	Demonstrate knowledge of
Use	Explain	Investigate	Design
State	Assess	Identify	Describe the application of
Carry out	Implement	Conduct	Demonstrate
Structure	Analyze	Summarize	Create

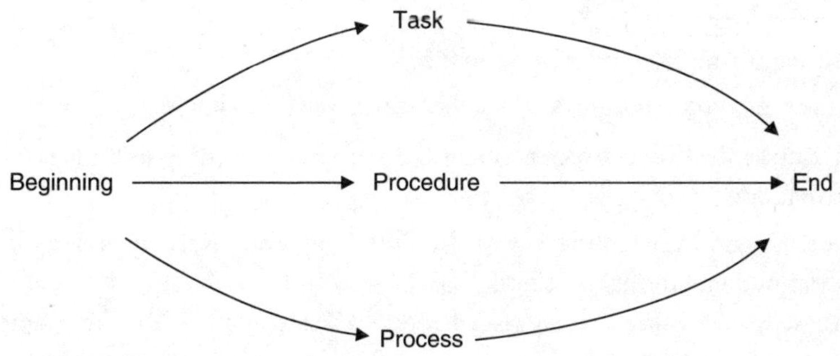

Fig. 17.2 The 3-dimensional model of meetings.

Designing training

Clear objectives, reflecting identified training needs, make training design easier. Objectives signpost where the session is headed, and the design phase then works out how precisely to reach the destination.

In this section, we introduce two frameworks that help to shape the design process:

1 A **'3-dimensional model'** derived from management development (Whitmore, 1994), and

2 A **'learning circle'** derived from adult education (Kolb, 1984; Bennett-Levy *et al.*, 2004).

The 3-dimensional model

This model (illustrated in Fig. 17.2) suggests that, in order for any encounter to be successfully concluded, those involved must bear in mind three dimensions: **Task, Procedure, and Process.**

Task

'Task' involves elaborating your objectives, detailing the content of the training session. If the objective is the destination, Task is the route map. Which roads will you take? What points of interest will you include on the journey? When and where will you refuel (refreshment breaks)? Where might there be roadworks, traffic jams, extreme weather? How much time should you allow for interesting diversions?

Task answers the question:

> *'Given that my objective is x,*
> *what do I need to include in order to ensure that the objective is met?'*

Imagine, for example, that you are planning a 2 hour training session for CBT beginners. The objectives might be:

By the end of this training session, participants will be able to:

1. Describe the link between thoughts and feelings according to Beck's cognitive model.
2. Identify and record their own thoughts and feelings, using a 3-column dysfunctional thoughts record (DTR).

These specific objectives suggest what might be included (Task). For example:

- The nature of thoughts and emotions.
- How to distinguish between them.
- The impact of thoughts on emotions, and of emotions on thoughts.
- Specific relationships between thought content and emotion (e.g. danger/anxiety).
- Exercises, for example, giving participants mixed lists of different thoughts and emotions, and asking them to make matching pairs. (This also allows you to check whether they are meeting the first objective.)
- In-session opportunities for self-observation, such as saying 'In a moment, I'm going to pick someone to come up here and summarize what we've covered so far for everyone'. This usually produces a variety of responses (which can be noted and discussed), ranging from performance anxiety, to amusement in those who realize the real intention of the statement—purely to trigger thoughts and emotions.
- An introduction to the DTR.
- A self-monitoring homework assignment. (Additionally, asking participants to explain the DTR to one another allows you to check whether the second objective is being met.)
- Feedback on learning and on reactions to the session.

Procedure

'Procedure' refers to the nuts and bolts of how the Task will be achieved, including:

- Session timing and structure.
- The space where the training will be carried out (e.g. the size, shape, and layout of the main training room; the number, size, and location of breakout rooms; environmental influences (e.g. lighting, ventilation, temperature control, noise); backup services (e.g. number/location of toilets, outdoor space, refreshment facilities, disabled access).

- Equipment (e.g. audio and video equipment; computer and data projector; flipcharts, whiteboard, pens; stationery; pre-recorded snippets of treatment sessions).
- Participants' documents and learning materials (e.g. pre-course questionnaires; handouts, worksheets, and reference lists; feedback sheets).

Whenever possible, organize Procedure in advance. Specify the nature of the space you require, decide what layout you want (U-shape? rows?), ensure you get the equipment you need, that it works, that you know how to work it, and that technical support is available if necessary. This means visiting the venue before the event or, at the very least, forming a good relationship with whoever is in charge and arriving early on the day. Even if you cannot improve inadequate facilities, you will know what to expect and can adapt and compensate as necessary.

Procedure is the dimension to which trainers commonly pay least attention. For those working in public service, this probably results from having to use whatever facilities are available, however basic or grim. Procedure elements may also appear rather trivial; indeed, if they are as they should be, participants will take them for granted. If not, however (e.g. the room is too hot or ferociously air conditioned, noisy or crowded, the coffee is terrible) this can radically color participants' experience of the training and reduce their capacity to learn. If you are conducting a 'one-off' training session there may be little you can do. If you repeatedly use a single venue, especially if you are paying for it, make your views felt and back them up with participants' comments.

Process

'Process' refers to the nature of the encounter between the people involved, and includes, for example:

- The nature of audience.
- The relationships between trainer and participants, and between the participants themselves.
- How rapport is established and maintained.
- How questions and discussions are handled.
- How difficulties and hiccups are managed (see section 'Helpful hints for handling common problems' for suggestions).

Keeping all three balls in the air

The 3-dimensional model suggests that losing track of any dimension can compromise the success of the training encounter. For example, focussing on Task at the expense of Process may lead you to miss important interpersonal issues. Conversely, focusing on Process at the expense of Task may mean 'feel-good' training that lacks direction and structure. And focussing on Procedure (inevitable when equipment fails to function) can not only interrupt the training session (Task) but also bore or alienate participants (Process). In short: **keep all three balls in the air.**

Kolb's learning circle

Kolb's learning circle describes a 4-step process of experiential learning, in which each element grows naturally out of what precedes it and forms a foundation for what follows (for a fuller explanation, see Chapter 15, pp. 315-316).

In order for effective learning and retention to occur, each step is necessary:

- ***Experience*** (action, doing) takes learning out of the academic sphere and makes it vivid, concrete, and specific. If Experience is omitted, learning remains abstract, theoretical. Imagine, for example, learning to ski by reading about it rather than by taking lessons and practicing.
- ***Observation*** means conscious awareness of what happens during the experience. What do we notice (thoughts, feelings, body sensations, behaviour, others' behaviour, etc.)? Observation is purely descriptive, not analytical. If it is omitted, experience may be wasted because we do not know what happened. This leaves space for pre-existing ideas, biases, and expectations to operate freely.
- ***Reflection*** means formulating the meaning of what has been observed. How can it be understood? What are the underlying principles? Omitting Reflection makes it hard to make sense of observed experience, to link it to other experiences and concepts, to generalize. Experiences remain isolated incidents, with no particular significance.
- ***Planning*** means working out how to carry new understanding forward. What are its practical implications? What's the next step? If Planning is omitted, then fresh perspectives derived from observed experience may remain abstractions, and fail to be consolidated and developed through future experiences.

Omitting any element of the circle aborts the learning process. In contrast, using the circle to structure training events maximizes the chances that new learning will be multi-sensory, vivid, personally relevant, well-retained, and carried back into the work environment. It fosters learning via different systems (Bennett-Levy, 2006): declarative (knowledge), procedural (skill), and reflective (learning from specific experiences). It takes advantage of a robust finding in memory research: that actions performed are more deeply processed and better recalled than actions either read, heard about, or seen (Engelkamp, 1998). As Mark Twain observed, *A man who carries a cat by the tail learns something that can be learned in no other way.* Or *Learning is not a spectator sport* (anon.).

Practical implications

Session structure

The circle (which can be entered at any point) can be used to shape training sessions, in whole or in part (for an example, see Fig. 17.3).

Choosing training methods

Understanding the circle helps you select training methods so as to ensure activity in each quadrant of the circle and appeal to a range of learning styles. Table 17.4 shows some examples of methods, grouped according to where on the circle they predominantly fit.

Which methods you choose at each point depends on your session's learning objectives. Is the intention of the session (or this part of it) knowledge transmission, or skills acquisition, or shaping of attitude? Is this a good point for a short presentation (Reflection), to be followed by a Planning question ('So, what might be the implications of this for our work with patients?'), and then a practical exercise (Experience)? Or would it be better to start this session with

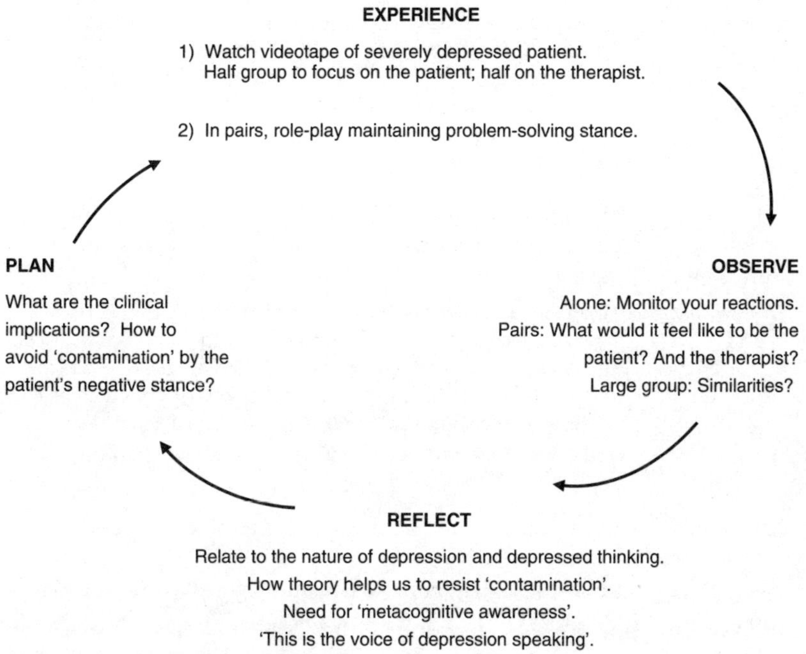

Fig. 17.3 Kolb's learning circle: example.

Table 17.4 The learning circle and training methods.

Where on the circle?	Examples of training methods	Enhance impact by using:
Experience (foundation for accurate observation)	Direct experience; client contact; role-plays; case studies; brainstorming; games, energisers, icebreakers; debate; supervision; self-practice; participant observation	Log books noting immediate experience; training in self-observation, mindful awareness; active listening; focus on thoughts, feelings, body state, others, the environment
Observation (foundation for meaningful reflection)	Self-observation, self-monitoring, self-reflection; observing video/audiotapes of own performance; reflecting on experiential exercises; reflecting on self-practice; reviewing objectives, progress toward personal goals; learning review, learning summaries, learning diaries/logs; peer/ supervisor/trainer feedback	Guided discovery; checklists, questionnaires (e.g. CTS-R, Consultation Worksheet); reviews; structured discussions (pairs, 3s/4s, large group); debriefing; reciprocal interviewing and feedback
Reflection (foundation for effective planning)	Lectures, presentations ('chalk and talk'); reading; written assignments (essays); theory-building, review and analysis; conceptualization exercises; drawing general conclusions from specific experiences; considering how new learning relates to existing knowledge; formulating principles; analysis	Guided discovery; synthesizing questions (e.g. 'What does this mean?', 'How does this relate to …?'); time; exchange of ideas; flowcharts; handouts reading lists
Planning (foundation for effective action)	Learning needs assessment; training needs identification and analysis; learning contracts; defining aims, goals, objectives; training design, planning and preparation; gathering resources; devising interventions, action planning	Observation checklists; questions, instructions (e.g. 'In particular, watch out for ...', 'What do you notice the therapist doing?'); clear outcome criteria ('How will you know when ...?', What will tell you that ...?')

Experience (e.g. an exercise which takes participants to the heart of the matter on a personal, experiential level), followed by Observation questions, discussion designed to highlight meaning (Reflection), closing the circle with 'And what are the practical implications of that?' (Planning).

Delivering training

The learning circle makes it very clear that training should be both active and interactive. Traditionally, educators stood at the front of the class, feeding students information. This may be what your own education was like, with a focus on memorizing facts rather than transmitting skills. Didactic teaching is still common in many educational forums, and for trainers there is a certain security in using PowerPoint slides to tell people things, from the protected space behind the computer and data projector. In therapy, you would never spend sessions 'talking at' patients, with the aid of carefully designed all-singing all-dancing overheads—so why do so in training? Here is a point where well-established therapeutic skills can be transferred into the training context.

Echoes of CBT

CBT's therapeutic style (collaborative, oriented toward curiosity, discovery, and willingness to experiment) closely mirrors the learning culture advocated in adult education (e.g. Knowles, 1990; Knowles *et al.*, 2005). The educator is a facilitator, encouraging inquiry, questioning, and learning through experience. The learner's complementary role is to be independent, active, and self-reliant. Their experience and pre-existing knowledge are respected, valued, and used. The structure of learning is flexible, responsive to learners' questions, problems, and needs. This stylistic congruence means that when you train you can draw on skills you already have, even if you have never trained before.

A rule of thumb

To maximize interactivity, a useful rule of thumb is: never tell people anything they could discover for themselves through an exercise or discussion. The point on the learning circle when you may be most tempted to move into 'teacher' mode is Reflection, because here the specifics of experience are related to theory, general clinical principles, research findings, etc. Certainly, there are times when short presentations are both efficient and helpful, for example, in providing data or syntheses not available elsewhere. However, remember that attention spans are short (never speak for more than 20 minutes). And it may still be more engaging and memorable to derive theory and clinical principle from participants' reflections on what they have observed, rather than from telling (see Examples 17.1 and 17.2 below). This involves trusting them to come up with the goods. When I started training, I always closed workshop sections with one or two detailed overheads on which I gave participants the benefit of *my* wisdom, summarizing the points *I* considered to be most important. I discovered through experience that this is largely unnecessary: if learning (including exercises) is congruent with defined objectives, people are perfectly capable of doing this themselves, gaining real ownership of the material. Not every individual participant is able to identify what is important, but as a collaborative working group they almost always will.

Example 17.1 Teaching theory interactively

In the learning circle example in Fig. 17.3, Reflection could consist of a short lecture on negative automatic thoughts and the negative cognitive triad. Choosing to teach in this way is particularly tempting when time is short—exercises often take longer than telling. Nonetheless, remaining interactive could be worthwhile. For instance, the cognitive model of depression could be elicited using questions like:

- *'So, in the light of what you observed on the video, and your reactions to it, how would you characterize depressed thinking?'*
- *'What are its qualities?'*
- *'And its impact?'*

  If people's observations of the video had been recorded on a whiteboard or flipchart—perhaps in three unlabeled groups ('self', 'world', 'future')—another question might follow:
- *'What do your observations tell you about the content of depressed thinking?'*

The board could be used as a prompt if necessary:

- *'What do you notice about these 3 groups?'*

Two summary overheads would then suffice to underline the theory:

Negative automatic thoughts	*Negative cognitive triad (Self, World, Future)*

Example 17.2 Teaching clinical principle interactively

When introducing novice cognitive therapists to the style of CBT, it may be tempting to tell them about it, with the aid of a closely packed sequence of overheads. Yet everything they need to know would probably emerge from watching an illustrative video or live demonstration (perhaps collaborative agenda-setting) and analysing what they saw the therapist do (questions, capsule summaries, empathic reflections, etc.). Again, one or two concise summary overheads might then suffice to highlight and consolidate, with the option of a more detailed handout or copy of a chapter to be read in participants' own time. (For tips on using PowerPoint effectively, see Table 17.5.)

Table 17.5 Ten top tips for PowerPoint presentations.

1	**PowerPoint is the backup**, not the main attraction. You, the trainer, are the headline act.
2	Ensure that the **specific objectives** of the presentation itself are **clear**. What do you want people to remember? Once you have defined your objectives, stick to the point.
3	Just as in therapy, **don't tell people things they can discover for themselves through experience**. Make use of your audience's knowledge and skill.
4	**LESS IS MORE**. Have no more overheads than you need and can talk to in the time available.
5	Aim to **foster curiosity**, rather than over-catering (too much, too complex).
6	Attention span is short: keep your **presentations** to a **maximum of 20 minutes** before introducing some other activity, however brief.
7	Keep your **overheads clear and simple**: maximum 4–5 bullet points each (typeface: minimum 20 points).
8	If possible, use only **key words or images**, NOT sentences or paragraphs. People will try to read and listen to you at the same time, and their attention will fragment.
9	Let the detail be in what you say, and in **backup handouts** for later reading if you wish.
10	**Rehearse both content and timing**. To work with key words/images and have time to say what you want to say without hurrying or skipping slides, you need to be very familiar with your material.

Source: Thanks to the students of the Oxford Diploma/MSc in Advanced Cognitive Therapy Studies whose reflections contributed to this list.

Beyond PowerPoint

PowerPoint and 3-slides-to-a-page handouts have become standard. Many participants become disquieted if even one slide is omitted from their handouts. It could be interesting to check out whether this format is really necessary. Why not experiment with resisting the lure of technology? Allow yourself to be creative and playful, and experiment with how far you can go *without* PowerPoint (or at least with minimal use of it). Can you help people to find things out for themselves (exercises, questions) instead of feeling obliged to feed them information? The literature on adult education contains a wealth of studies demonstrating that lecturing is no better at conveying information than other methods, such as assigned reading. How much more true this must be of CBT's sophisticated repertoire of technical and interpersonal skills.

The expanding development of online learning (often still mainly information-giving and demonstrations), offers an opportunity to think hard about what 'live' training sessions offer that other methods of delivery may not provide so well, if only as a basis for creatively integrating both delivery methods. Live training may be best placed to provide highly interactive, personally relevant learning, with opportunities for exchange of ideas and experiences with tutors and other learners, for practice and for feedback, as well as opportunities for contact with like-minded colleagues with similar interests and learning needs. However, with increasing technological sophistication and interactivity, this may not remain the case for long.

Evaluating training

Without evaluation, trainers cannot know what impact their training has had, or if it has had any impact at all. Evaluation provides the data commissioning organizations need in order to assess whether training represents value for money. Equally, it will help you to identify your strengths and aspects of your training you want to improve, and to decide on your next training destination.

The gold standard: a 4-level framework

The training literature (e.g. Corrigan and McCracken, 1997) suggests a 4-level framework for evaluating the impact of training:

1 Participant satisfaction
2 Acquisition of knowledge and skills, demonstrated during the training
3 Behaviour changes in the work context
4 The outcome of these changes.

All of these are relevant to CBT training, and some ways of evaluating each are outlined in Table 17.6. The outcome of the evaluation, matched against the original performance gap, organizational goals, and the objectives of the training, creates a sound foundation for the next training sequence.

Once again, be realistic

In practice, the 4-level gold standard is often not achieved (or possible), so it is important to be realistic about what can be done within time and resource constraints. Much training evaluation stops short at Level 1 (satisfaction)—the easiest, least time-consuming, and least costly option. Post-course 'reactionnaires' can provide statistical data (e.g. average ratings of interest, usefulness, the extent to which people would recommend the training to others) which may be useful in terms of public relations, and can form the basis for future training standards (e.g. a minimum of 80% of participants recommend/highly recommend the training). Qualitative data (open comments, such as what people most/least liked, found useful, would recommend be changed), are often more useful to the trainer because (if consistent) they can specify which

Table 17.6 How to evaluate training: the 4-level framework.

1 **Participant satisfaction**

- In-session behaviour (smiling, laughing, attentiveness, coffee time conversation, 'buzz', etc.)
- Written feedback ('reactionnaires'; ratings and open comments)
- Checking in with individuals, groups, course organizers and sponsors—during and after (face-to-face, email, telephone)

2 **Acquisition of knowledge and skills during training event**

Knowledge

- Question and answer sessions, group discussions
- Quizzes, tests, multiple choice questionnaires, examinations
- Essays, dissertations

Skills (also imply knowledge acquisition)

- Role-plays, demonstrations
- Behaviour tests (e.g. role-plays), pre- and post-training (what changes, and to what extent?); assessed live or recorded for later formal evaluation against pre-determined criteria (e.g. competency checklists, CTS-R)

3 **Application of knowledge and skills in the workplace**

Knowledge (skills implied, but self-report only: may not reflect real behaviour)

- Written case reports, showing how knowledge of theory, research, and clinical principle are applied with individual cases (n.b. limitation: self-report)
- Portfolios of work
- Learning diaries (summaries, reflections, key observations, achievements, disappointments, queries). Most useful when opportunities to discuss

Skills (implies knowledge acquisition)

- Observation/evaluation of live performance on the job (n.b. ethical considerations, consent, patient confidentiality)
- Observation/evaluation of video (or audio) recordings of role-played or real performance (if the latter, n.b. ethical considerations again)
- Measurement of performance against agreed criteria (e.g. CTS-R), by self and/or other
- Self-assessment (knowledge, skill, behaviour, outcome in the real world; identifying strengths and weaknesses; identifying ongoing learning goals)
- Follow-up training sessions/supervision (What were the goals? How far were they achieved? What promoted or hindered continued development? How to foster the former and deal with the latter? What's the next step? What support is needed?)

4 **Outcome**

- Before/after treatment results (e.g. changes in patient scores on standard measures)
- Feedback from clients, colleagues, managers (verbal, written). Can include interviews, designed to assess how far new learning is being applied in the workplace, and with what results
- Appraisals, performance reviews

(continued)

Table 17.6 (continued) How to evaluate training: the 4-level framework.

◆ Critical incident analysis (evaluating frequency/nature of outstandingly good or bad occurrences/situations/pieces of work—e.g. suicide attempts in patients of clinician specifically trained to work with suicidal clients; episodes of violence on ward before and after training in defusing anger)
◆ Analysis of logs, records (e.g. patient throughput, re-referrals)
◆ Questionnaires (knowledge, attitudes, reactions, facts, others' perceptions of changes in participant)

aspects of training are effective and which need to be revised. At the other end of the scale, collecting outcome data (e.g. the impact of training on treatment and service delivery) is considerably more resource-intensive, and consequently usually found only in relation to relatively lengthy training courses (e.g. Diplomas, Master's degrees), dissemination research, and specific projects with considerable organizational sponsorship (e.g. Westbrook *et al.*, 2008).

How do I know that people are learning?

Participants' behaviour during the training is a rich and readily available source of data.

Signs that people are NOT learning:

- Looking bored
- Chatting
- 'Nit picking'
- Repeatedly returning to reasons why things will not work in *their* context
- Describing at length how *they* usually do things
- Reluctance to engage in exercises
- Avoiding making mistakes, sticking to what they know
- Demanding certainty and 'right answers'
- Being over-preoccupied with being evaluated.

When you notice these signs, what will be helpful depends on why they are present. The group may be tired, for instance, because the training is at the end of a busy week or an intensive teaching block, or toward the close of the day. If so, make sure you allow generous time for refreshment breaks. It may also be helpful to inject experiential exercises involving movement, or energizers (See Examples 17.3 and 17.4 below).

Example 17.3 Exercise involving movement

Small group discussion, following allocation to new groups. Ask people to line-up from left to right around the room, in a particular order (e.g. date of birthday, time they got up this morning, height). Once the line-up is complete, divide people into groups, again from left to right (e.g. 4's). This involves physical activity, which is immediately energising, plus talking to fellow participants ('Did I get up earlier or later than you?'). The process in itself is entertaining, and the line-up means people get to work with someone fresh.

Example 17.4 Energizer

Ask everyone to stand up and find a space. Lead the group in some simple standing stretches, with appropriate stretching noises. Again, this is likely interactive because people have to take care not to knock each other out. You can finish with a Mexican wave or clapping if you want.

It is important to do this sort of thing with conviction, no matter how daft you feel. If you lead the way, and do so with energy and enthusiasm, the chances are the group will follow and indeed enjoy and learn from the experience.

It could be that lack of learning is more to do with other factors, for example, that participants are there for reasons other than a genuine motivation to learn. We shall explore this difficult situation in the section 'Helpful hints for handling common problems'.

Signs that people ARE learning

- Attentive listening, to the trainer and to each other.
- Comments and questions are directly relevant to the topic, and often elaborate or develop it in interesting ways—looking for possibilities and applications, thinking about further implications and where to go next.
- Good eye contact, alert facial expression, relaxed and attentive body posture.
- 'Buzz', a sense of channelled energy and enjoyment.
- Rapid engagement in experiential exercises.
- Willing to have a go, use trial and error, suck it and see, tolerate ambiguity, be wrong and make mistakes, because these are understood as an essential part of development.
- Unafraid to express half-formed ideas, to guess, envision, and approximate.

A learning continuum

These two categories describe polar extremes; actually, a continuum would better represent what happens. People can move along the continuum according to circumstances and their internal state (e.g. familiarity of the material, hunger). Carefully observing participant behaviour will give you a wealth of information on the 'feel' of the group, responses to specific interventions, and variations across time which you may wish to address (e.g. making sure you get people moving in the early afternoon slot).

Helpful hints for handling common problems

However experienced and skilled you are as a trainer, there will be times when you encounter difficulties—it is part of the territory. In this section, we address some common problems that can arise, and add a couple of points related to running longer courses successfully.

- Your prime task as a trainer is to create a secure learning environment.
- Aim to facilitate a reciprocal adult-to-adult interaction: straightforward, collaborative, and respectful.
- Most people are there to learn, not to make difficulties for the trainer or disrupt the training.
- If you follow the design principles outlined in this chapter, you will short-circuit many difficulties.
- In CBT, you cannot proceed with technical interventions if a process issue gets in the way. The same is true in training.
- However, training is not therapy. You are not working from a clinical formulation, nor 'treating' difficulties through detailed investigation of underlying factors.
- Be aware of your own learning style (*cf.* Chapter 15). Difficulties can arise from a simple mismatch between you and your participants, for example, as an activist, you may feel uncomfortable with the silences and slow responses of reflectors. Be flexible.
- One disruptive person can absorb much time and effort and contaminate others' experience. Don't delay—tackle them right away. Speak to them privately, and if they cannot or will not change, ask them to leave—the event is clearly not meeting their needs.

Invest in 'Managing Difficult Participants' by John Townsend (Management Pocketbooks, 1994). This clever little book provides thumbnail sketches and ingenious tips for dealing with tough situations.

Specific problems

Participants are there because someone has sent them

- CBT is currently 'flavour of the month', and clinicians may be sent for training whether or not they are motivated to learn.

- Address this as soon as you realize it is an issue (see section 'Signs that people are not learning'). Take time out from teaching, and investigate what is happening.
- For example, say that you are wondering if people have not chosen to be there. Is that right? How does it feel? What impact is it having on their experience of the training? Your own willingness to be open about the difficulty is likely to be appreciated.
- Move on to explore how people might make the most of this time. This is an opportunity for learning and development. How can they best use it? What would they like to know? Is it possible something interesting might come of what you are planning to teach? This may create a viable working alliance—though you will need to remain vigilant for signs of disaffection.
- If you will teach the same group again, speak to whoever commissioned the training. To avoid a recurrence, preparatory work needs to be done to engage potential participants.

Participants are deeply sceptical about the value and relevance of CBT

- Us CBT therapists are often enthusiastic about what we do, and eager to share it with others—patients and fellow clinicians. Our enthusiasm is not always shared!
- Clinicians new to CBT often misperceive it as a ragbag of techniques, applied without regard to feelings or to the therapeutic relationship.
- If you know (or think) this is the case, after your introductions try a small-group exercise. Ask participants to brainstorm what they know and have heard about CBT—especially its weaknesses and what put them off using it. If you can, do this with humour and respond without defensiveness, no matter what is said. From the discussion, misapprehensions will emerge. Your training then offers an opportunity to reveal what CBT is *really* like.
- Acknowledge your limits. Focusing on CBT in no way disrespects other approaches. CBT is simply your area of expertise, and that is why you have been asked to teach it.
- You can also use participants' doubts and reservations as a chance neatly to demonstrate the cognitive model:

  So, coming here today, your thoughts were: "Why do I have to do this? I don't want to do CBT. I don't like it and my patients won't like it either". And you were feeling reluctant and rather cross and wanting to turn round and go home again. Is that right? OK, now supposing instead of that you had been thinking: "Well, I don't know, I'm not too keen on this approach from what I've heard, but here's a chance to learn more". Then what would you be feeling? And what might you do?

Different levels of experience

- At the beginning of the event, ask about levels of experience. If numbers are small, you can ask each person. With larger numbers, ask people to raise their hands according to their level of experience (e.g. many years/identify myself as a CBT therapist; use CBT methods as part of a wider repertoire; completely new to it).
- Invite people to choose material to work on that reflects their level of expertise, for example, complex cases for the more experienced, simple cases for the less experienced.
- Offer opportunities for people to work with partners/groups at a similar level of experience (once identified, they can catch one another's eyes across the room, or get together at the coffee break).

'Chatting' during exercises

- Make sure your breaks are long enough for people to talk to one another informally, particularly if you know this is a group that do not often have opportunities to meet.
- People are ultimately responsible for their own learning. Provided your exercises are well-designed, relevant, and have clear objectives, it is not up to you to police what people are doing.
- However, when you hear people chatting, you can approach the pair/group and ask straightforwardly: 'Which of you will be summarizing your learning for everyone in a few minutes?'

Challenging questions and comments

- Respond with courtesy, even if through gritted teeth.
- If you see this is a pattern, don't be afraid to acknowledge ('Thank you') and move on ('Does anyone else have a question or comment at this point?')
- Is this a theorist, whose probing questions feel uncomfortable because you do not share their learning style?
- Beware of being drawn into the 'expert role' (having to have all the answers), rather than helping people to find answers for themselves. Summarize the

question, to check your understanding. Say 'I am happy to answer this, but first of all, I wonder what *you* think?' The questioner may then give their perspective, or they may say they don't know. If so, offer the question to the group (you may already have seen non-verbal signals that someone has something to say). This moves the discussion away from a one-to-one dialogue. If necessary, you can then offer your own view (there may be no need).

- If someone challenges the relevance of what you are doing, check with the rest of the group. Is this a shared view? If yes, then you will need to clarify your rationale or even change your programme. If no, then you have legitimate reason to stick with your agenda.

One person hogs the limelight

- Keep your responses courteous but brief, and move swiftly to asking others for contributions.
- If no one else has anything to say, you may come to be grateful to this person!

People seem stressed, overstretched, and tired

- Successful learning results from a balance between challenge and support. Make sure this balance is working for your participants.
- If they are complacent, then up the challenge.
- If (as if more common) they are doing this training in the midst of busy working lives, nurture them. Give them proper time for relaxing breaks, offer biscuits with the tea, sweets, fruits if you can. Include fun exercises and energisers (as above). Give everyone a nice pen, or a pack of Post Its to take away. Include the cost (which will be minimal) in your fees.

Silence/slow responses to requests to participate

- Is this a group of reflectors, who take their time to speak out? If so, possess your soul in patience.
- Or is this a reflection of a cultural rule, for example, that it would be rude to question a teacher? If so, tell the group how much you would value feedback, because it helps you to meet their needs. Warmly validate any offerings: 'What an interesting point!'
- Or is it fear of making a fool of oneself? If so, people who have difficulty speaking out in the larger group may be willing to talk to one another in pairs, 3's or 4's. In small groups, ask them to elect someone who will report on their findings. Otherwise you will have the same problem at feedback time.

Running longer courses (certificates, diploma, etc.)

- Make sure people have plenty of time to acclimatize and get to know one another. Early on, make sure coffee and lunch breaks are generous.
- Choose a first icebreaker which invites people to talk to as many other participants as possible, and encourage them to keep changing partners during exercises so that by the end of Day 1 they have at least said hello to everyone.
- If possible, organize a social event at the beginning of the course, and perhaps at later 'marker' times (e.g. New Year, the end).
- If you are course director, make sure you are regularly available to discuss how things are going and deal with complaints and uncertainties. Use breaks to chat informally with students.
- If your course is recurrent, have no expectations of what next time will be like. Each run of the course will develop its own 'culture' and present you with different joys and challenges.
- If a culture develops which is not conducive to learning (e.g. a culture of complaint, not taking course requirements seriously, the development of an us/them divide), nip it in the bud. This means speaking with the whole group, sharing your observations of what is happening, and asking for their collaboration in putting things to rights. You may prefer to do this in the company of one or two colleagues, for moral support.

The training journey: 10 tips for fostering your own development as a trainer

This chapter has outlined the sequence of activities encapsulated in the training cycle. Within this relatively limited canvas, it has been possible only to sketch key points and possibilities. If you would like to continue to develop as a trainer, you may wish to follow the following steps:

1. 'Perfect Preparation Prevents Pathetic Performance'. Always ring-fence preparation time well in advance. Be ruthless: other activities will demand the time. Resist.
2. As you train, adopt a 'meta-perspective'. Monitor how things are going, what works well and what not so well, why this might be, what adaptations need to be made now in order to be responsive to participant need, and what adaptations might be helpful next time round. Jot these observations down on your training plan right away. Do so in a form that will stand out

when you reflect and review—perhaps on a brightly colored sticker, or in colored ink, or highlighted.

3 Ruthlessly ring-fence time to review the whole event within 24–48 hours, while it is still fresh in your memory. If you leave it till later, you will forget what you thought, and why. Your review will take longer, and be vaguer and less helpful to you.

4 Use the 'Learning circle' as a framework. The training itself was the experience. What did you observe? What did it mean? What are the practical implications for you (e.g. read, get some more training, find a training supervisor, redesign the session or some part of it)? And so to the next training experience.

5 Get honest feedback from co-trainers, training supervisors, and trusted participants.

6 If possible, video-record sessions and assess your performance.

7 Visit your local bookstore and explore what is available under 'management', 'human resources', and '(higher) education'. It is here, rather than under medicine or psychotherapy, that you will find what you need—including lots of big, fun books full of color, cartoons, and practical tips.

8 Use the Internet. You will find a huge range of websites providing free high quality information on every aspect of training. As an experiment, try putting 'learning styles' into your Internet search engine.

9 You may be fortunate enough to work in an organization that provides good training in teaching and training skills. If not, consider going further afield—much training in training skills is delivered outside health care, and indeed outside public service altogether. There are many commercial companies who offer training skills courses. Quality varies, so *caveat emptor*. The Chartered Institute of Personnel and Development (CIPD; www.cipd.co.uk) is a reputable body which offers a wide range of courses, including distance and online learning. The Higher Education Academy website is also worth consulting (www.heacademy.ac.uk).

10 A final point: however gifted and skilled you are as a trainer, there will always be things about your performance that you could refine, new learning methods to experiment with, challenges to master, and boundaries to push back. One of the joys of CBT is that we never reach the horizon—there remains much to learn. The same is true of developing our capacity to disseminate knowledge and skills. Learning to be the best trainer we can be is potentially a lifelong adventure.

Further reading

Although any of the sources cited in this chapter would make useful further reading you may want to begin with the range of books on training published by the Chartered Institute of Personnel and Development (www.cipd.co.uk) and training texts in the 'Management Pocketbooks' series (www.pocketbook.co.uk). There are also many courses available to develop your skills in adult education generally, or specifically in CBT training. Useful websites include:

- Oxford Cognitive Therapy Centre website. Available at: www.octc.co.uk
- Kings College London website. Available at: www.kcl.ac.uk
- British Association for Behavioural and Cognitive Psychotherapies website. Available at: www.babcp.com
- The Chartered Institute of Personnel and Development (CIPD) website. Available at: www.cipd.co.uk
- The Higher Education Academy website. Available at: www.heacademy.ac.uk
- Despite its unpromising title, a rich resource of ideas about training and learning, including many examples of interactive exercises, is www.businessballs.com

References

Bee, F. and Bee, R. (1994). *Training Needs Analysis and Evaluation.* London: Chartered Institute of Personnel and Development (CIPD).

Bennett-Levy, J. (2006). Therapist skills: a cognitive model of their acquisition and refinement. *Behavioural and Cognitive Psychotherapy*, **34**, 57–78.

Bennett-Levy, J., Butler, G., Fennell, M., Hackmann, A., Mueller, M. and Westbrook, D. (eds.) (2004). *The Oxford Guide to Behavioural Experiments in Cognitive Therapy.* Oxford: Oxford University Press (Chapters 1 and 2).

Blackburn, I.M., James, I.A., Milne, D.L., Baker, C., Standart, S., Garland, A., Reichelt, F.K. (2001). The Revised Cognitive Therapy Scale (CTS-R): psychometric properties. *Behavioural and Cognitive Psychotherapy*, **29**, 431–446.

Corrigan, P.W. and McCracken, S.G. (1997). *Interactive Staff Training: Rehabilitation Teams that Work.* New York, NY: Plenum Press.

Engelkamp, J. (1998). *Memory for Actions.* Hove: Psychology Press.

Knowles, M.S. (1990). *The Adult Learner: A Neglected Species.* London: Gulf Publishing Co.

Knowles, M.S., Holton, E.F. III and Swanson, R.A. (2005). *The Adult Learner: The Definitive Classic in Adult Education.* San Diego, CA: Elsevier.

Kolb, D.A. (1984). *Experiential Learning.* New Jersey, NJ: Prentice-Hall.

Roth, A.D. and Pilling, S. (2007). The competences required to deliver effective cognitive and behavioural therapy for people with depression and anxiety disorders. London: DOH Guidance Document. Crown copyright.

Westbrook, D., Sedgwick-Taylor, A., Bennett-Levy, J., Butler, G. and McManus, F. (2008). A pilot evaluation of a brief CBT training course: Impact on participants' satisfaction, clinical skills and patient outcomes. *Behavioural and Cognitive Psychotherapy*, **36**, 569–579.

Whitmore, J. (1994). *Coaching for Performance: A Practical Guide to Growing Your Own Skills*. London: Nicholas Brealey.

Chapter 18

Research and evaluation

David Westbrook

Although most CBT therapists support CBT's commitment to being based on evidence, it is also true that most do not contribute much toward developing that evidence. They do little or no research once they have fulfilled any requirements from their training and, for clinical and counselling psychologists, the most common number of publications from any individual is zero (Brems *et al.*, 1996). This chapter will therefore aim to:

- Explain why research and evaluation are important in CBT, and increase your enthusiasm for such work by trying to remove some of its mystique.
- Briefly describe some common approaches to 'real world research' and how to plan and carry out a study.
- Guide readers in preparing research findings for conference presentations, or for submission to academic journals.

It would take much more space than we have here to detail all the fine points of research design, analysis, and statistics, so we aim only to map out some of the principles and issues for you to think about. See the 'Further reading' section at the end of this chapter for some good sources of more detailed information.

Introduction

One of the defining characteristics of CBT has always been its commitment to empiricism: the idea that it is not enough just to believe that an idea is true, but that we should try to gather *evidence* that will help to tell us whether it is true or not. This empirical approach is at the heart of CBT, both as a clinical intervention, and as a scientific programme. In therapy, we try to help patients gather data that will help them evaluate the truth (or helpfulness) of their thoughts and beliefs. In the wider world, CBT as a movement aims to improve our understanding of, and ability to intervene with, psychological problems through a process of research, both into underlying psychological processes and also into what is effective in therapy, training, or supervision. Many would agree that this evidence-based approach has been crucial to the success of CBT.

However, CBT research is increasingly dominated by a few university centres, and it is easy for the ordinary clinician to feel that research is something only academics do. In contrast, the 'scientist practitioner' model suggests that clinicians can both be clinical practitioners and also generate useful knowledge through research. It is the spirit of the scientist practitioner that we want to encourage in you in this chapter.

There are many possible reasons to contemplate doing research. Perhaps the most common are:

- Because it is enjoyable and interesting, particularly when it gives you *unexpected* answers that make you think again about your practice.
- Because it will give some important new information that may benefit either your own practice or our knowledge about CBT more generally.
- Because it provides some interesting variation to your job.
- Because research skills may be helpful in your future work.
- At the most basic level, because having a research study or two on your CV can be good for your career!

Thinking about research

The fundamental purpose of any form of research is to answer some question, practical or theoretical, in such a way that we have some reasonable grounds to believe the answer: in other words to generate believable *evidence* that can help answer the question '*Why* should I believe this conclusion?'

Scepticism thus has a central role. If I am thinking about what evidence would help to convince me of any particular claim, an obvious question is to think about why I might *not* believe it. Therefore, one of the crucial tasks in setting about research is to ask yourself in what ways the evidence—your own or anyone else's—is weak or unconvincing. Furthermore, one of the central roles of research design is to eliminate as many as possible of the alternative accounts that might be given by someone who does *not* want to believe your conclusions. Hence, there is a value in taking the kind of attitude attributed to the British TV journalist Jeremy Paxman, who is supposed to have said that in preparing for any interview with a politician he would ask himself: 'Why is this lying bastard lying to me?' In fact, Paxman denies that the motto is his and attributes it to another journalist, but whatever the truth of the story, the motto is a good one for anyone thinking about research, whether their own or anyone else's. Not because it is likely that anyone is *intending* to mislead when it comes to research, but rather in recognition of the fact that one can easily be misled by apparently significant, but actually false, evidence. So we should constantly ask ourselves: 'How are these lying data lying to me?'

Research errors and research design

So how can data 'lie' to us? In research language these questions relate to *validity*, that is, whether an experiment gives us accurate conclusions about our area of interest. There are two broad kinds of questions we may be interested in when thinking about this:

- Are the conclusions well justified within the project's own setting, or are there other plausible ways of explaining the results that have not been satisfactorily ruled out? (These are known as questions of *internal* validity.)
- Can we be reasonably confident about applying the results to therapists/patients/service settings other than those involved in the research, or are there critical differences which might mean that the outcomes of interest will be *different* when applied to my service or my patient? (These are known as questions of *external* validity, or generalizability.)

So broadly speaking, when we find research unconvincing it is usually because either:

1. We think the researchers have not excluded an alternative account of the findings (e.g. they claim that their psychological therapy was effective, but take no account of the fact that many patients improve after initial referral even without any treatment); or
2. Because we think there is some factor that makes their conclusions unlikely to apply to our own setting (e.g. they have shown that their therapy is effective, but the therapists had videotaped supervision twice a week and I doubt that my service, which can't afford that much supervision, will get the same results).

The perfect research design would be both internally and externally valid, but in the real world there is an almost inevitable tension between internal and external validity. The more tightly you control your research so as to ensure internal validity, the less like 'ordinary practice' it becomes, which therefore compromises external validity. For example, in order to make sure that they know exactly what the treatment is that results in any changes for patients, researchers usually define very tightly what is to be done in the treatment, and they provide intensive supervision of therapists to make sure that this plan is adhered to. But by doing that, the treatment and the way it is delivered may become quite different to any ordinary clinical service.

On the other hand, if research is based in ordinary clinical practice, using ordinary therapists, who are allowed to do whatever their clinical judgement suggests, the results of that research may be more easily generalizable to other services, but then we cannot know for sure what it was that *caused* those results—the treatment might have been quite variable from one patient to another.

These tensions are reflected in the distinction often made between *efficacy* research (designed to establish that a particular treatment can, in controlled trials and ideal circumstances, produce benefits) and *effectiveness* research (designed to show that such benefits can be delivered in routine clinical practice). For examples of effectiveness research, and discussion of some of the issues around this debate, see Weisz *et al.* (1995); Shadish *et al.* (1997); Wade *et al.* (1998); Merrill *et al.* (2000); and Westbrook and Kirk (2005). Also see Cook and Campbell (1979) for a classic and comprehensive look at the common threats to validity in research.

Example 18.1 Can brief CBT training be effective?

To illustrate some of the points in this chapter in more concrete form, we will use an example that we will return at various points through the chapter.

The example we have chosen is a study of the effects of CBT training (published as Westbrook et al., 2008). This study was firmly in the effectiveness tradition (see above), in that it involved attempting to evaluate a short teaching programme (the 'Foundation course') that was being run as part of a routine service, not for the purposes of research. The only changes to the programme were extra measures: in all other aspects it was implemented just as it would be in routine practice. As a consequence, it lacked many of the experimental controls one would ideally like to have.

Research versus audit and service evaluation

This chapter is aimed primarily at those who might undertake research within their own service, rather than as part of some multi-centre large research trial. It is therefore likely that you will be doing either *clinical audit* or *service evaluation* research. There are many differences between these and traditional pure research, but perhaps some of the most pertinent are:

- They do not usually involve randomizing patients to different treatments (see 'Ethical review' later).
- They are designed with practical rather than scientific concerns as the main goals: they are about making decisions, not just scientific curiosity. The kind of questions they are concerned with are, for example, 'Does our service meet certain standards?' or 'Do patients prefer this method of assessment or that one?', rather than 'What cognitive processes are important in anxiety?'
- They are concerned with evaluating treatments or services that have already been proposed or planned, not with developing new ones.

The question of whether a particular study is *research* or *audit/service evaluation* is of particular practical importance when it comes to ethical review (see section 'Ethical review').

Getting research ideas

The first step in any research is deciding what to look at. A lot of work will be needed to turn that initial idea into a true research question (see section 'Turning ideas into research questions'), but where do ideas come from in the first place? For the kind of research we are concerned with here, ideas will usually come from your day-to-day working life. In any week at work there are probably several occasions when questions come into your mind that could be turned into research. Tune into these thoughts and perhaps write them down as they occur to you. Then you can come back to them later and see whether they do indeed have the potential to become research projects. For example, some of the research projects the author has been involved with, as investigator or supervisor, arose from precisely this kind of reflection on ordinary working practices:

It seems to me that asking supervisees to do more "experiential" tasks in supervision, like role-play, makes them more anxious than standard case discussion does: is that true?

We feel we need to limit patients to 10 sessions in order to reduce our waiting lists: what impact would that have on patients or on therapists?

I have developd this approach to using CBT formulation as part of a consultation to CMHT or in-patient teams who are having problems with particular patients: is it helpful?

Does training people in CBT impact successfully on their skills or on the outcomes they achieve with patients? (See this chapter's foundation course running example.)

Note that these are all good starting points for a study, but they are not yet true research questions, because they are too vague and unspecific. For example, when we say 'Is CBT consultation helpful?', what exactly do we mean? What does the consultation process in question consist of? Is it helpful in what way? Helpful to staff, or patients, or both? Helpful in the sense that staff feel better, or helpful in the sense that the patient's problems improve? Pursuing these thoughts is the process of turning an idea into a research question.

Example 18.2 Background to the course

The Foundation course questions arose directly from the actual teaching programme and the time at which it was being done. Lord Layard's (2006) proposals for an expansion of CBT therapy were in the air but not yet realized in the form of the Improving Access to Psychological

Therapies (IAPT) programme. There was a perceived need for economical forms of teaching CBT, and therefore when this teaching programme was commissioned it seemed worth trying to use it as an example to look at whether brief CBT training (in this case 10 days) can be effective.

Turning ideas into research questions

In order to turn your initial idea into a research question, you need to focus, clarify, and probably simplify, your initial vague ideas. A good research question will be clear enough to enable you to start thinking constructively about *how* to answer that question. The characteristics of a good research question include:

- It is interesting to you, that is, you really want to know the answer to the question. All research projects contain periods of dull, hard work, and it will be much easier to see it through if you really care about the results.
- The answer to the question will be of some practical or clinical importance. This will again help you to keep going through the difficult times, but will also be important when it comes to getting ethical permission, and successfully submitting your work to journals or conferences: nobody wants to hear about a study if their main response to it is 'So what?'
- The question is clear, unambiguous, and *answerable*: that is, you can work out what kind of data is needed, how you can collect the data within the time and other resources available to you, and what to make of the data when you have gathered it. There are many important questions that are not (practicably) answerable. For example, over 40 years ago, Paul (1967) posed the ultimate question about treatment choice, which every therapist would like answered: 'What treatment, by whom, is most effective for this individual with that specific problem, under which set of circumstances?' However much we would *like* to answer this question, it has proved impossible because of the vast number of possible combinations of patient/therapist/problem/treatment that would need testing.
- The methods needed to answer the question are doable. Almost inevitably, research ends up taking twice as long to answer half of the questions you first thought of. Don't be too ambitious: a completed small study is better than a huge project that is abandoned because it is impractical.

Research questions will often change and develop as you start to think through the practicalities of how the question might be answered, what the relevant theories have to say, and so on. Figure 18.1 shows this process of interaction, which eventually results in a clear research question and the

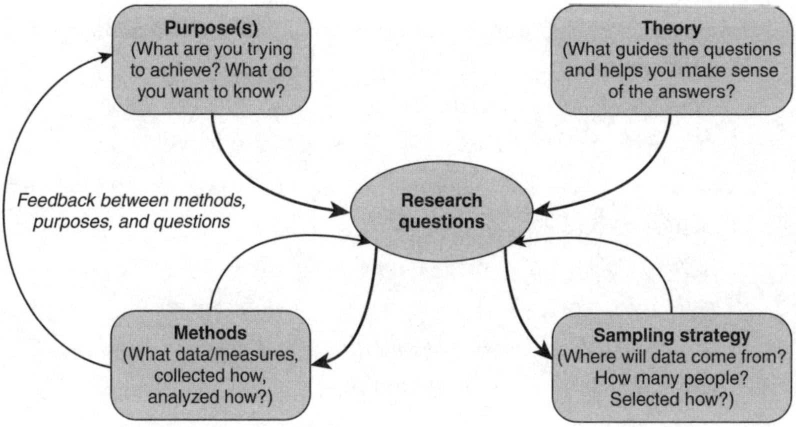

Fig. 18.1 Research questions and research design.

beginnings of a research strategy (or of course, the decision that the question is not answerable by you at this time).

Another useful strategy is to think about how you would interpret the data and explain the findings under all possible outcomes:

- If the data come out as you expect or hope.
- If the data come out the exact opposite of what you expect.
- If there appear to be no significant findings.

An ideal research design would rule out all but one explanation for all possible findings.

Working with others

Finally, a non-technical guideline, perhaps especially important if you are new to research: work together with others. Having partners in research can be absolutely invaluable, for:

- Getting support when things go wrong.
- Increasing creativity and problem-solving when working out how to tackle the research.
- Making sure that you remain resolved and stick to deadlines (it is much harder to make excuses to others for not doing something than to oneself!)

Example 18.3 Research questions

The central design question to be decided in this case was 'What do we mean by "effective" training'—and how much of that could be captured in an evaluation that was very limited in its funding? The final decisions were as follows:

1 *The sample was essentially defined by the topic: it consisted of all the students involved in the course who were willing to take part.*

2 *Four 'levels' of training outcomes are often recognized (Kirkpatrick and Kirkpatrick, 2006):*

   a. *Whether people like it (student satisfaction).*

   b. *Whether they learn something (knowledge gained).*

   c. *Whether what they learn makes a real difference to relevant skills (students' CBT skills in this case).*

   d. *Whether it actually makes a difference to the effectiveness of their job performance (in this case, the outcomes of their treatment of patients).*

In training research, these aspects tend to decrease in frequency in the same order: it is relatively easy to assess satisfaction or knowledge, harder and less common to assess changes in skills, and hardest and least common to assess outcome changes.

At first in the planning of this study, we thought we could only be able to assess satisfaction and skill changes. However, late on in planning the programme it was discovered that the service concerned had recently introduced the routine measurement of patient outcomes. Capitalizing on this coincidental event, we were able to get data on some of the students' patients outcomes before and after the Foundation course, and thus were able to look at whether training affected outcomes in the students' patients.

Research design

Research design often seems a complicated and dry topic, but the basic idea behind it is not really that complicated. The essential point of research design is to make sure that the evidence you gather in your study is as convincing and unambiguous as possible in answering your question. In terms of the motto described earlier, the aim of research design is to stop these lying data from lying to you!

It is therefore not the case, as is sometimes made out, that the only way of doing research is to set up a randomized controlled trial (RCT) using a traditional experimental design. That kind of approach is the best possible way of doing *some* kinds of research, but it is not the only way, and sometimes not even the best way.

Readers are advised to look at Robson (2002) and Cresswell (2008) from the 'Further reading' section of this chapter for more detailed information about different approaches to research design. In this section, we will very briefly survey some of the common approaches.

Quantitative versus qualitative research

There are two main traditions of research. On the one hand there is a tradition of *quantitative* research which, as the name suggests, tends to be focused on the use of numerical measures of some kind: in psychology this kind of research is concerned with scores on questionnaires, numbers of patients seen, rating scales, and the like; and the results are usually analyzed using statistics.

In contrast, the *qualitative* approach usually uses verbal methods—interviews, focus groups, and so on—rather than numerical methods, and is often aimed at describing and understanding people's own experience (of a problem, or a service, or whatever).

These two approaches have sometimes been at war with each other, but increasingly it is being recognized that both approaches may have their advantages for different purposes, and also that they can happily co-exist in the same study, in so-called *mixed method* research. Robson and Cresswell (*op. cit.*) discuss both of these approaches to research.

True experiments

The classic true experimental research is the *randomized controlled trial* (RCT). It involves one or more *experimental* groups, who receive the intervention(s) that we want to study (e.g. treatment or training); and one or more *control* groups, who do not receive that intervention. The control group may get no particular intervention (e.g. a 'waiting list control'); or they may get an intervention designed to contain some non-specific benefits, but not the presumed active ingredient of the treatment we are studying (e.g. a placebo, or 'treatment as usual'). Participants are *randomly assigned* to one group or another, and this is the key strength of this kind of research. The logic is that random assignment will tend, on average and if we have large enough numbers, to even out all the possible random variations between people that we are *not* interested in, so that our treatment is the only difference affecting the results. So, for example, if we are worried about the possible impact on our results of people changing medication, or of people losing or getting new relationships, the process of randomization should mean that those effects apply equally to both groups and therefore any differences we see are due to the difference in treatment.

Quasi-experiments

The problem with true experiments is that they are often difficult, for practical or ethical reasons, to apply in clinical practice (and as noted below, they will always require approval by a Research Ethics Committee [REC]). For these reasons, clinical practice often uses *quasi-experiments*. This means that we are still comparing one or more experimental groups with one or more control groups, but that participants are not randomly assigned to groups. So, for example, we might use *historical controls*, where we compare a group of participants we are seeing now with the same measures for another group seen in the past. Or we might take advantage of different approaches in different areas to compare people referred to one team with people referred to another. Obviously the weakness of such designs is that the lack of randomization means that we cannot be sure that there are no differences between the groups that are not due to our intervention, and which may therefore distort the results. It could be that the people we saw in the past are *different* in important ways to those we are seeing now, or that referrals to Team A are different to referrals to Team B. The art of designing quasi-experiments is to rule out such sources of error as far as possible.

Single case experiments

If we want to study the effects of an intervention, then single case experiments may be particularly suited to clinical practice because, as the name suggests, they can be done with individual patients without much change to routine care (although note that a 'case' in this sense can also be a group, as well as one person). The only absolute requirement for most single case designs is *repeated measurement*. The basic idea is that we take regular measures of some kind (e.g. levels of depression) and collect several measures before introducing our intervention (e.g. CBT for depression). The logic of single case design is that if changes in the measures track changes in the intervention, then we have some grounds for believing that the changes are *because of* the intervention. The initial baseline measures, if reasonably stable, mean that it is relatively unlikely that something other than the intervention happened at exactly the same time as the intervention, so as to cause the changes that we observe. This basic logic is used in many ingenious variations that can be used to study the effects of treatments or treatment components. See Barlow *et al.* (2006) in the 'Further reading' section for a comprehensive account of single case designs.

Non-experimental

The other main variation of quantitative research is the design where there is no actual experiment, in the sense of anything being deliberately manipulated, but rather we want some kind of descriptive or predictive results. Surveys are one common form of such research. For example, we might want to study whether there is any correlation between age and likelihood of dropping out of treatment. In such a study we obviously do not assign people to different age brackets, nor do we decide whether they drop out or not: we just gather data on both variables and see whether they correlate, or co-vary.

One of the difficulties of such an approach may be that it is sometimes impossible to know in which direction, if any, the causal influence is working. For instance, it is often found that patients' ratings of the therapeutic relationship correlate with successful outcomes in treatment. But is that because better relationships cause better outcomes, or because better outcomes make people see the relationship more positively? Or could it even be that some third variable influences both the other two, rather than there being any direct relationship between them? For example, perhaps there is a kind of person who is *both* more likely to form good relationships and more likely to benefit from treatment.

Qualitative research

Qualitative research is less easily definable than quantitative, as there are many different approaches within this broad field. However, there are some features that are shared by most of these approaches. First, they tend to use words rather than numbers as their primary data. Qualitative researchers are typically concerned with what people say (and mean) rather than with their scores on questionnaires or other such measures. Because of this, qualitative data analysis tends to be different as well, often being focused on trying to understand people's experience or concepts, and derive an explanatory model from those, rather than testing a pre-specified hypothesis (although there may be some quantitative aspects to such analysis: e.g. having used qualitative methods to derive the major themes in a series of interviews, you might then count how many of the interviews contained each theme). Second, as a consequence of this, the major tools of qualitative research tend to be recordings or transcripts of interviews or focus groups, and live observation of participants. Finally, qualitative researchers tend not to try to *change* anything about what they're observing, in the way that an experimenter would introduce some intervention, but rather adopt a *naturalistic* approach that aims to study people as they are in their natural settings. See Robson (2002) and Cresswell (2008) for more on qualitative research.

Note that there is sometimes a tendency to see qualitative research as 'not proper research' or as an easy option. Doing good qualitative research is certainly not easy, although the difficulties may come at a different stage of the process. In quantitative work it often takes more time to set up and implement the project, but the analysis is often relatively fast (e.g. with the help of statistical software). In qualitative research, gathering data is often relatively fast (e.g. interviewing half a dozen people) but transcription and analysis is often very time-consuming.

Method and measures

Having decided on your broad approach to the research question, you then need to work out your methodology in more detail. You may need to think about:

- **Sample.** Who will your participants be? How many of them do you need? (For quantitative research you probably need to run a so-called 'power calculation' that tells you how many participants you need in order to get a statistically reliable result—see Robson or Cresswell, *op. cit.*) Also note that it is always wise to plan for approaching more participants than you need, as some will always drop out or get lost in other ways. How will you ensure that your sample is representative rather than biased? Where will you recruit them from? Do you need other people's help? If so, are they willing to help?

  For qualitative work, you still need to think about who your sample will be, but with different criteria. For example, you may want a *purposive* sample rather than a random one (i.e. a sample chosen because they have characteristics that you think will make them useful for exploring your questions). And of course, typically your number of participants will be smaller than in quantitative studies.

- **Measures.** By this stage you should have identified what variables are of interest to you; now you need to decide precisely how to measure them for a quantitative design. Are there already available measures that others have used and validated? If so, use them unless there is some powerful reason not to. If there are no standard measures, you may need to construct *ad hoc* rating scales, that is, ones made up for your specific study (but be aware that this is not as straightforward as it may seem, so it may be wise to pilot any such measures with a few people before your study begins, to get an idea of how well they work in practice). Also consider the burden you are placing on your participants. For example, how long will it take them to complete the questionnaires you want them to do?

  In qualitative studies you will usually not be using 'measures' in the above sense, but similar concerns arise around what questions you will ask your participants, how you will structure interviews, and so on.

- **Procedures.** If your study involves doing something with your participants (treating them, training them, supervising them, etc.), then exactly what will you do and how will it be done? When and how will you take your measures?

Once you have a research protocol, that is, a detailed plan of what is to happen, the next question is to consider ethical approval.

Example 18.4 Measures and experimental design

This was a quantitative study. As noted in Example 18.3, we were able to gather measures on three aspects of the course, as follows:

1. *Student satisfaction. Measured using ad hoc self-report rating scales.*
2. *CBT skills. Measured using two forms of a standard measure of CBT skills, one self-rated by the students and one based on an external rating by supervisor or other therapist of a recorded session between student and patient.*
3. *The outcomes of their treatment with patients. Measured using a widely used questionnaire of patient problems, taken at the start and end of therapy, (a) for a group of patients treated by course students before they did the course and (b) for a similar group of patients treated after the end of the course.*

Experimental design was the weakest part of this study's plan, as it involved what is sometimes called an 'A-B design' (i.e. simply assess the experimental group before and after an intervention—in this case, the training course). The problem with this design is of course that there is no control for the many other reasons why people might change between two time points. In this case, let us suppose (as was in fact the case) that the group shows some positive change between the start and end of the course. Then of course this could be due to our training, but it is impossible to rule out the possibility that something else caused the change. Maybe the simple passage of 3 months meant that they were more experienced and hence more effective therapists; maybe they all went off and read some wonderful textbook in that time and it was that, rather than our training, that increased their skills; or maybe they just tried harder on the second tape than the first! Ideally, we would have a control group to rule out these explanations. In other words, we would have a second group, as similar as possible to the first group, who go through all the assessments in exactly the same way as the experimental groups, except that they do not get the training. Then if the two groups are different at the end of training we can be much more confident that the difference is due to the training, because all other variables should be the same in both groups.

However, it was impossible to have a control group in this study, because we were commissioned to train everyone, not just half of the group; and because we could only run the course once, so we could not have a so-called 'waiting list control' in which half the group get assessed while waiting for the training to happen.

Ethical review

We assume here that you will be doing research in the National Health Service (NHS) in the United Kingdom, and you will therefore need to go through NHS research procedures rather than those for a university or other agency. Procedures in other areas, or other countries, may be very different. Please also bear in mind that your employer may have local requirements that you need to follow.

The distinction between audit/evaluation and research becomes crucial when it comes to one of the most dreaded parts of doing research—applying for ethical approval. Studies defined as research *always* need approval from a Research Ethics Committee (REC), while audit/evaluation studies do not (although you should again consult your own employers to determine whether they require some other ethical procedure). The safest way to determine which heading your study falls under is to approach your local REC and ask them, but some of the differences are outlined in a helpful leaflet downloadable from the NHS's National Research Ethics Service (NRES, 2008), and the key points from this are reproduced in Box 18.1 (see the NRES leaflet for more details).

Box 18.1 Major differences between research and audit/evaluation for ethics

- *Intent:* The primary aim of research is to derive new knowledge; audit and service evaluation measure level of care. Research is to find out what we should be doing; audit is to find out if we are doing it. Nevertheless, a project may have more than one intent; in such a case, a judgement is needed as to what the primary aim is.
- *Treatment:* Neither audit nor service evaluation uses a treatment without a firm basis of support in the clinical community.
- *Allocation:* Neither audit nor service evaluation allocate treatment by protocol. It is by decision of clinician and patient.
- *Randomization:* If randomization is used, it is research.

Source: National Research Ethics Service (2008). Defining Research. Available at: http://www.nres.npsa.nhs.uk/EasySiteWeb/GatewayLink.aspx?alId=355 (accessed 13 September 2008).

Example 18.5 Research or audit?

The Foundation course study was categorized as audit/evaluation:

- *The primary aim was to assess the effectiveness of a routine intervention (i.e. CBT training), not to generate new scientific knowledge.*
- *The 'treatment' (i.e. training people in CBT) was one that is in constant, routine use in the NHS and elsewhere.*
- *The 'treatment' (i.e. training) was administered to people who had applied it for it, not according to some pre-set protocol.*
- *There was no randomization.*

In general, the NRES website at http://www.nres.npsa.nhs.uk/ is a mine of useful information and guidance on NHS research ethics, as well as providing online application facilities, so we will not attempt to reproduce all that information here. Instead, we will focus on some practical tips on REC applications, based on experience—see Box 18.2.

Box 18.2 Practical tips for research ethics applications

- Filling in the REC application form will be aversive, and it will take a significant amount of time. Almost inevitably as you go through the form you will discover questions that you have not yet thought through, so you will need to go off and do some more work before coming back to the form. You will also need to have prepared all the information sheets, questionnaires, consent forms, etc. Don't keep putting it off. Book a good chunk of time—at least half a day at a time—and get started. It is never going to get any easier!
- Remember that research design is an ethical issue as well as a scientific one. No REC will consider it worth subjecting patients or staff to research that cannot possibly give useful information because it is scientifically fundamentally flawed or the question is trivial. Make sure your research has been reviewed by peers before the ethical review and modify the proposal in light of their feedback, and do a power calculation – or get someone else to do it for you! (See the section on 'Sample' above).
- By the time you have added together the time it takes you to prepare the application (including some procrastination) and the time it take the REC to process the application, together with the almost inevitable amendments that will need to be made, the whole process can take a long time: perhaps 6–12 months from start to finish. So start early!

Box 18.2 Practical tips for research ethics applications *(continued)*

- Read all the notes and guidance carefully, both on the NRES website and in the documents available from them, and don't be afraid to contact your local REC to ask questions. The information you need to make a successful application is out there if you look for it.
- It is very rare for any application to succeed at first try: the REC will always raise questions—and furthermore, some of them may seem to you to betray a lack of understanding. Be prepared for this, and respond constructively. Perhaps the most common problem areas are around recruitment, information for participants, and consent.
- Despite the above point, remember also that, unless you have come up with a highly unethical research idea, it very probably will pass eventually, perhaps with some modifications—most proposals do!
- Try to see your study as the committee will. They don't care that you think it is fascinating, or that you need to do it for a course you are doing. They want to know how this research could benefit patients, improve services, or contribute to scientific knowledge.
- A few points about the details of your study:
  - Don't be too detailed in your descriptions. They do not need to know every detail of what you are proposing, and you may end up confusing the picture.
  - RECs usually require that participants must opt in to a research study, not opt out.
  - They will usually require at least 24 hours 'cooling off' time between someone getting the information about your research and their decision about whether to take part.

Gathering your data

So, you have planned your study, and you have been given any necessary ethical permission, and it is now finally time to start putting it into practice. The process of actually gathering your data may sometimes be the easiest part of doing research—but make sure you protect the time you need to do it!

By this stage you should know what to do, and how to do it. The major problems that tend to arise are to do with unexpected events that throw you off course. There is a saying in military circles that: 'No plan of battle survives first contact with the enemy', and the same principle can apply to research. The major trials of this stage are dealing with such unexpected but inevitable problems. The person who was going to be your main service contact goes off sick, or leaves; the type of patient you were looking for, whose prevalence was the original reason for doing the research, suddenly seems to disappear from the face of the planet and you cannot recruit any of them; or you send out 200 questionnaires and only get 3 back. Perseverance and creative problem-solving are the key skills during this phase. The best way of avoiding such problems is to do a *pilot study* if possible, that is, to try out your research methods on a very small sample that are not vital to your plan, and see what problems arise.

Example 18.6 Data collection

Data collection in this case went reasonably smoothly, with the only real problem being the timing of the first CBT skills assessment. The plan was that students would submit one recording for assessment within 4 weeks of the course's starting, and a second one within 4 weeks of the course's ending. The problem was that, through lack of confidence or other reasons, many students did not submit their first tape until 5 or 6 weeks into the course. Bearing in mind that the course only lasted 10 weeks, this mean that the 'start' assessment was sometimes actually halfway through the course. However, this problem was not considered a major threat to the research design because it would most likely lead to underestimating the effect of the course, rather than overestimating it—the lateness of the first tape would be most likely to inflate their 'start' level of skills and thus reduce the change between start and end. Therefore, if we find a significant change between start and end, it is even more likely to be a real effect.

Analysing data

Quantitative studies

If you are doing quantitative research then you are very likely to be faced with doing statistical tests, that is, analysing your data so as to see whether any changes or differences you have found are likely to be real or whether they could plausibly be understood as being merely a result of chance variations. For example, how many times do I have to toss a coin and get heads before I start to think the coin may be biased?

Statistics is a black art to many people and if that includes you, then the best advice is to seek help from someone who does understand the topic. Although modern statistical software such as SPSS, MiniTab, or Statistica has made it much easier to do complex analyses, it still needs some understanding of the principles involved if you are to avoid mistakes. Field (2005) in the 'Further reading' section gives a comprehensive introduction to statistics and to using

SPSS, in as easily readable a form as is possible for such a technical subject—but it is still demanding! Field also has a website with lots of useful resources (Field, 2009); another useful website is 'Which Test?' provided by Canterbury Christ Church University, which helps you in deciding on appropriate statistical tests (Holtum and Blizard, 2003).

If your study involves a clinical treatment of some kind it is also worth thinking about so-called *clinical significance* testing (Jacobson *et al.*, 1999). This approach is designed to respond to the fact that, as clinicians, we want results that are not just significant in a narrow statistical sense but also clinically meaningful. Jacobson and his colleagues have devised an approach that defines a level of individual change that is large enough to be unlikely to be due to chance (known as *reliable change*), and also sets a standard for patients at the end of treatment to be regarded as back in 'normal range' on any measure (set so that someone below the threshold is more likely to be in the 'normal' population than in the clinical population). Only patients who show reliable change and whose final scores are in normal range are regarded as having shown clinically significant change.

Qualitative studies

As noted above, the data in qualitative studies are usually words rather than numbers: for example, the transcribed content of individual or group interviews, or the researcher's field notes of what happened at particular times. Therefore, traditional statistics are irrelevant and the dates have to be analyzed in other ways, usually involving variations on the theme of *content analysis*. Perhaps you might use specific approaches such as *thematic analysis* or *grounded theory*, but in any case the overarching goal is usually to make sense of the mass of data by recoding it into higher-level categories. For example, '*This* sentence by participant 3 and *this* one from participant 5 are both examples of the category "self-critical" statements, and that category is usually found in association with *this* other category…' Although some qualitative researchers would reject the very notion of validity or reliability in such analyses, there is usually some recognition that researchers need to be clear and rigorous in the path they take through the data, with some attempt to be open with the reader about how they arrived at the themes identified.

Disseminating your results

Some research may only be of interest to you and your close colleagues, but in most cases dissemination is just as important as doing the research. Research is only valuable to the extent that people know about it and can therefore learn from it. Even locally based audit or evaluation research will often be of interest to others, because even if their service is not exactly the same as yours, it may be *more* similar to your service than it is to some world-famous university research team.

There are three main methods through which research findings are disseminated: through publication of the findings in academic journals, through presentations at conferences, and through delivering training. Training is covered elsewhere in this volume (see Chapter 17), so we will focus here on the other two. Although writing for publication and presenting at conferences are obviously different activities, there are some common themes that apply to both.

Brevity

Conference presentations will nearly always have a strict time limit, and both convenors and audiences do not like it if you grossly exceed that limit (typically of the order of 15–20 minutes for a symposium presentation). Journal papers do not usually have a fixed length, but editors want papers to be as short as possible because space is at a premium.

Therefore, in both cases you need to trim all the fat out of your study. Think carefully about what is absolutely essential to anyone wanting to understand the study, versus what is interesting but not essential—in most cases you will need to cut out the latter.

Be open about faults

Remember the motto, 'How are these lying data lying to me?' Read your paper as someone hostile to your argument might read it. What criticisms would they have? What alternative interpretations of your data would they come up with? How would they criticize your methods? Whatever those criticisms are, if you have an answer to them then make sure your paper contains that answer.

On the other hand it may well be that on reflection, you feel that the criticism could be valid. If so, do not try to conceal it: acknowledge the problem, provide any evidence you have that mitigates it, and include in your discussion section some ideas for overcoming the problem in future research. In general both journals and conference audiences prefer honesty over trying to pretend your research is perfect. We need to recognize that all research has faults and that by recognizing and identifying these, we can contribute to the gradual growth of knowledge in an area of study.

Avoid excessive claims

One of the commonest errors in reporting one's own research is to be overenthusiastic about the results. Non-significant trends in the results become established facts, and any significant results become world-shaking (even though you have a sample size of seven). In general, it is much better to be modest in what you claim, and realistic about what it might mean.

Statistics

If you use statistics to analyze your results, but are not very expert in using them, then get someone else to check them: faulty or inadequate statistical analysis is a common cause of rejection. One common error is failing to consider the effects of *multiple comparisons*: the fact that the more statistical tests you do on the same set of data, the more likely it is that at least one of those tests will give you a significant result *just by chance*. Appropriate techniques need to be used to minimize such risks.

Example 18.7 Writing up the results

The main points in the writing up of the Foundation course were as follows:

- *In the statistics, one part of the analysis was criticized by the journal's referees, and a more complex analysis requested. The proposed analysis was one that none of the authors was familiar with, so we consulted with a statistical expert.*
- *The flaws in the experimental design were acknowledged, especially the lack of a control group and the fact that the session ratings were not done 'blind', because the raters knew whether the recordings were 'start' or 'end' tapes. Ideally the raters would not know this, because that knowledge might influence their ratings—for example, knowing that this is a second tape might lead the rater to expect it to be better, and therefore to rate it more generously. Unfortunately, we could not hold on to the tapes and rate them all at the same time, so that the task could be done blindly, because feedback on the tapes was part of the training and therefore needed to be done soon after submission; and there was no funding to allow us to re-rate them all blindly after the course had finished.*

Writing for journals

If you are not familiar with writing research reports, make sure you study a few papers in the kind of journals that might publish your paper. Most journals have a standard structure that they require of manuscripts, typically including:

- **Abstract**, a brief description of the major points, which will appear at the top of your paper if published.
- **Introduction**, in which you set the scene for your project and briefly describe and critique previous literature in the field.
- **Method**, in which you describe exactly what you did, with whom, how, with what measures, etc.

- **Results**, in which you present the main findings with, if appropriate, your statistical analysis.
- **Discussion**, in which you explore your findings, their implications, the limitations of your study, and where things might go next.
- **References.**

This structure may be modified when necessary, but the vast majority of empirical papers will use it.

Although the prohibition is not as strict as it once was, most journals still prefer authors to avoid the use of personal pronouns such as 'I' or 'we'. Research papers usually say things like '...patients were treated...' rather than '...I treated the patients...'. This derives from a tradition of focusing on the research rather than the researcher, and attempting to present research as objectively as possible. It is probably safer to stick to this convention.

See Box 18.3 for some tips on preparing a manuscript for submission to a journal.

After submission

For those who are unfamiliar with the process of academic review, papers submitted to journals are typically sent out to a number of referees, or reviewers. These are people who know something about the topic you are writing about, and their job is to scrutinize your paper and make a judgement as to whether it is (a) appropriate for the journal; (b) interesting and/or important enough to take up space in the journal; and (c) up to the journal's standards for writing, research design, data analysis, etc.

After some time (typically 2–6 months) you will get a reply from the editor with the verdict, based on the referees' reports. Possible verdicts are usually:

- Accept straight away, without amendments.
- Accept after amendments (specific revisions are requested, but the article will be accepted if they are made to the editor's satisfaction).
- Revise and resubmit (suggestions for changes are made, and you are invited to resubmit the article after making revisions, but there is *no* commitment that it will necessarily be accepted, even if you make all the revisions; the paper will usually be sent out for review again if resubmitted).
- Straightforward rejection as unsuitable for publication in this journal (note that although this may be because they do not think it is good enough, it may also be simply because it does not fit the journal's brief or because it is interesting but not quite good enough to beat other submissions).

Box 18.3 Preparing for submission to a journal

- Choose an appropriate journal to submit to. Your judgement should be based on:
  - Who you think the journal's main audience is and whether that is the right audience for your paper. Think about which journals usually publish papers in your area of interest.
  - The kind of article they publish and whether yours matches that profile.
  - How hard it is likely to be to get your article accepted. The most prestigious journals naturally tend to have more demanding standards. It may be better to go for a lower-level journal, and have a higher chance of acceptance, than to go for a top-class journal where you are highly unlikely to succeed. However, if you are not in a hurry, a common strategy is to try your luck with a prestigious journal and be prepared to drop your standards if they don't accept it!
- Check with the journal website, or a back issue of the journal, to find the format they require for manuscripts in relation to style, headings, reference style, etc.
- Remember that, although your study's background and scientific context are very familiar to you, they are not necessarily as familiar to the journal's referees and readers. If they cannot read your article easily and cannot understand it, then they may give up and ignore it, or reject it for publication. Keep your language as clear and simple as possible and use jargon without explanation only if you are confident the journal's readers will be familiar with it. A good way to test your article is to ask someone who is *not* familiar with the study to read it.
- Journals are always short of space, so the shorter your article, the more likely you are to succeed. They also try to limit the number of tables and figures, because they are expensive to produce. When you have written a draft, cut it down as far as you can, and ask yourself whether your 11 tables and 17 figures are really necessary!
- Be balanced in your review of previous research: you're allowed to have your own view but you're also expected to show that you have knowledge of, and can respond to, other views, and do so in a manner based on evidence rather than prejudice.
- Have someone else proof-read your manuscript for sense, clarity, grammar, and spelling: reviewers form a bad impression if you can't spell or the manuscript is poorly presented!

To avoid disappointment, be aware that journals will almost *never* accept your first submission without amendment. They will almost always ask you for at least some changes. And also remember that most journal reject most of the papers submitted to them. So if you get as far as 'revise and resubmit' then you are ahead of the game and should be pleased.

Your next task is to decide how to respond. If you have a straightforward rejection then your only real option is to decide whether to try again with a different journal. If it is 'Accept after amendments' then usually you will want to make those amendments (or provide reasons not to—see below) and then submit the amended manuscript. Only in the case of 'Revise and resubmit' is there a real decision to be made. Would it be better to seek publication in a different journal? Are the revisions possible for you to make, or are they beyond your capacity? (e.g. they would need data that you just do not have, or you feel that shortening the paper by the amount requested would destroy its usefulness). Have you still got the time and energy to do some rewriting? In most cases, a 'Revise and resubmit' result is sufficiently encouraging that it will be worth pursuing, but you may sometimes decide it is better to go elsewhere.

In the case of either of the two 'revision' decisions, you will need to do two things in your response: first, make some or all of the requested changes; and second, write a letter to the editor, responding to the referees' comments and either explaining what changes you have made, or explaining your reasons for *not* making the requested changes. In reading the referees' comments, keep in mind that, no matter how much it may seem like it to you, referees are not in fact usually idiots who know nothing about the field and are only trying to advance their own careers—so don't react as if they are. Take some time to digest the feedback and when you respond, do so constructively (even if you think the review was not very constructive). Having said that, you do not have to agree with every point the referees make. The editor wants to know that you have carefully considered the referees' comments, not necessarily that you agree with them all. Reviewers are usually busy people, and they may not have read your paper with the loving care it so obviously deserves! If they have misunderstood something, or they want you to do something that makes no sense to you, then say so—but do it politely and reasonably.

Presenting at conferences

The other main form of disseminating your results is at conference or other meetings. You may be invited by a colleague to join a conference symposium they are organizing on a particular topic (i.e. a grouping of typically three or four papers on a particular theme); you may decide to propose a symposium yourself; or you may submit an 'open paper' (i.e. a presentation that is not part of a specific symposium). If you are submitting a proposal of any kind, be aware that most major conferences require proposals to be submitted many months before the conference—don't leave it too late. Obvious conferences to consider would be the annual British Association for Behavioural and Cognitive Psychotherapies (BABCP) conference or perhaps the European Association for Behavioural and Cognitive Therapy (EABCT) conference. Presenting at a conference for the first time can be exciting but is also inevitably somewhat daunting. The tips in Box 18.4 may be of some help.

Box 18.4 Conference presentations

- Whether one likes it or not, PowerPoint presentation software is now well-nigh universal, so you need to be familiar with it and able to use it confidently.
- For most people it is a bad idea to read your presentation from a script: it nearly always leads to a stilted and uninvolving delivery, and it also means that if something unexpected happens that throws you off the script, you feel lost. Instead of relying on a script, make sure you know your material well and can talk easily about it with prompts from your PowerPoint slides.
- Similarly, don't have slides that contain every word you are going to say, so that you are just reading out what the audience can already see. Use the slides as prompts, summarizing key points that you will talk around.
- Although there are times when complex animations may be useful to make a specific point, don't overdo it: having every slide swooping in or flashing on and off is just a distraction. The audience's focus should be on what you are saying, not on the slides.
- If you are not going to use your own computer, check your presentation on at least one computer that is not your own, especially if you are using any media such as video or audio files inserted in your presentation (playing such media will often depend on their being in a specific place on the computer, which they will not be on a different computer). Similarly, if you are using the very latest version of a software program, it may be better to save it in an older format in case the computer you are given is not up-to-date.
- Rehearse your presentation beforehand in order to check timings (but remember anxiety may make you talk faster).

Box 18.4 Conference presentations *(continued)*

- Approach any question from the audience in a positive frame of mind: see it as 'These are colleagues who are really interested in my results…' rather than 'They are trying to make me look stupid'!
- If you don't know the answer then say so: 'What an interesting question, but I'm afraid I don't know the answer: do you have any thoughts about it?'

Key points

- There is no one 'right' way of doing research: there are many different approaches, any of which may be appropriate depending on your goals (and in many cases multiple methods can be used in one study).
- A key focus is working out a clear research question that is answerable within the constraints you have.
- Design your research so as to eliminate as many possible objections or other interpretations as possible.
- Getting ethical permission can be slow and hard work: start early!
- Research always takes longer to do less than you first thought of: be prepared and allow for unforeseen delays.
- Letting other people know about your findings is an important part of making research useful.
- In presenting your research findings, be open about your study's limitations and cautious in your interpretations of its results.

Further reading

Barlow, D.H., Andrasik, F. and Hersen, M. (2006). *Single Case Experimental Designs.* Third edition. Boston, MA: Allyn and Bacon.

Cook, T.D. and Campbell, D.T. (1979). *Quasi-experimentation: Design and Analysis Issues for Field Settings.* Chicago, IL: Rand McNally.

Cresswell, J. (2008). *Research Design: Qualitative, Quantitative, and Mixed Methods Approaches.* Third edition. London: Sage.

Field, A. (2005). *Discovering Statistics Using SPSS.* London: Sage.

Robson, C. (2002). *Real World Research.* Second edition. Oxford: Blackwell.

References

Brems, C., Johnson, M. and Gallucci, P. (1996). Publication productivity of clinical and counseling psychologists. *Journal of Clinical Psychology*, **52**, 723–725.

Field, A. (2009). *Statistics Hell*. Available at: http://www.statisticshell.com (accessed 11 January 2009).

Holtum, S. and Blizard, B. (2003). *Which Test*? Available at: http://www.whichtest.info/index.html (accessed 18 August 2008).

Jacobson, N.S., Roberts, L.J., Berns, S.B. and McGlinchey, J.B. (1999). Methods for defining and determining the clinical significance of treatment effects: description, application and alternatives. *Journal of Consulting and Clinical Psychology*, **67**, 300–307.

Kirkpatrick, D. and Kirkpatrick, J. (2006). *Evaluating Training Programs: The Four Levels*. Third edition. San Francisco, CA: Berrett-Koehler.

Layard, R. (2006). The case for psychological treatment centres. *British Medical Journal*, **332**, 1030–1032.

Merrill, K.A., Tolbert, V.E. and Wade, W.A. (2000). Effectiveness of cognitive therapy for depression in a community mental health center: a benchmarking study. *Journal of Consulting and Clinical Psychology*, **71**, 404–409.

National Research Ethics Service (2008). *Defining Research*. Available at: http://www.nres.npsa.nhs.uk/EasySiteWeb/GatewayLink.aspx?alId=355 (accessed 13 September 2008).

Paul, G. (1967). Outcome research in psychotherapy. *Journal of Consulting Psychology*, **31**, 109–118.

Shadish, W., Matt, G., Navarro, A., Siegle, G., Crits-Christoph, P., Hazelrigg, M. and Jorm, A.F. (1997). Evidence that therapy works in clinically relevant conditions. *Journal of Consulting and Clinical Psychology*, **65**, 355–365.

Wade, W.A., Treat, T.A. and Stuart, G.L. (1998). Transporting an empirically supported treatment for panic disorder to a service clinic setting: a benchmarking strategy. *Journal of Consulting and Clinical Psychology*, **66**, 231–239.

Weisz, J., Donenberg, G., Han, S. and Weiss, B. (1995). Bridging the gap between laboratory and clinic in child and adolescent psychotherapy. *Journal of Consulting and Clinical Psychology*, **63**, 688–701.

Westbrook, D. and Kirk, J. (2005). The clinical effectiveness of cognitive behaviour therapy: outcome for a large sample of adults treated in routine practice. *Behaviour Research and Therapy*, **43**, 1243–1261.

Westbrook, D., Sedgwick-Taylor, A., Bennett-Levy, J., Butler, G. and McManus, F. (2008). A pilot evaluation of a brief CBT training course: impact on trainees' satisfaction, clinical skills and patient outcomes. *Behavioural and Cognitive Psychotherapy*, **36**, 569–579.

Chapter 19

Service development

June Dent

You return from the annual cognitive behavioural therapy (CBT) conference fired up with enthusiasm to adopt a new way of delivering CBT in your local service. You might want to work with patients who have not previously had a service, or improve the service you provide to your existing patients. You might need to raise money to do this, or your organization might need to make cost savings. You might want to lead the initiative yourself, or work as part of a team. You might envisage a small scale service improvement, or a large scale service redesign. Whatever your ambitions for changing CBT services, this chapter aims to help you achieve them by understanding, managing, and consolidating service change. It helps you:

1 To **build** on core CBT skills;

2 To gain the knowledge, skills, and attitudes necessary to **prepare** to undertake the development;

3 To **make the case** for the development, taking advantage of the current widespread drive for CBT;

4 To **build a change team** and **get senior support;**

5 To devise a realistic **plan** for its implementation;

6 To **take account of opposition to CBT**;

7 To ensure the development is **sustained**, and if possible spread to other services; and

8 To **enjoy and survive** the journey.

Building on core CBT skills

Embarking on the process of service development for the first time may seem a daunting task for which you may feel ill-equipped but remember that *you have knowledge and many relevant and transferable skills* for looking at larger, service-related matters. Within therapy you are already familiar and practised in forming strong collaborative relationships, formulating problems, agreeing goals, measuring progress, and working on the therapeutic tasks until changes take place and are well-established. Compare in Box 19.1 the tasks of CBT with the tasks of change management. The tasks and the process to be followed are broadly the same.

Consider Example 19.1 below and decide what steps you would already be able to undertake. You probably found that you would be able to do many of these steps for a small service development. You might have found that you need to gain some additional knowledge and experience, particularly for innovations or developments that are more complex or contentious. The following sections will help you address what else you need to know, what you need to do, and how to survive. In the meantime perhaps you are beginning to move toward a belief that '*I can do this using my core CBT skills*'.

Example 19.1 Small, bottom-up CBT innovation needing little funding

Ahmed and his colleagues worked with patients who had post-traumatic stress disorder (PTSD) and in the main they achieved good results. He was convinced of the value of introducing week long trauma-based CBT as an alternative to weekly 1- to 2-hour appointments. The emerging research evidence suggested that the same or better clinical outcomes could be achieved in 3- to 4-hour appointments delivered on 5 consecutive

Box 19.1 Therapy compared to change management

Common CBT therapy tasks	Common change management tasks
Forming collaborative relationships Formulating problems Agreeing goals Agreeing a plan for therapy Using behavioural experiments Measuring progress Working on tasks until change takes place Understanding and working with resistance Ensuring change is well-established	Building a change team Assessing willingness and capability to change Agreeing objectives of change Devising a plan to achieve change Running pilot projects Monitoring progress Implementing change Expecting and overcoming resistance Consolidating change

Source: Newton, R. (2007). *Managing Change Step by Step: All You Need to Build a Plan and Make it Happen*. London: Pearson Education.

days rather than 15 1- to 2-hour appointments provided over 15 weeks. Although there had not been a pressing problem to be solved, Ahmed had identified a new goal: to adopt this new approach in the local service. The outcomes he wanted were that patients would have a choice of approach and that those who opted for the intensive programme would improve as much as or more than those on the usual programme—and improve sooner. First he discussed the matter with his managers to express his interest in taking the matter further, and asked one of them to attend a series of development team meetings. Then he provoked the interest of some of the CBT practitioners whom he hoped would join him in doing the work differently. He did this by reporting back on a workshop he had attended and by explicitly asking for interested people to join him in a small pilot project, and for one of them to attend the development meetings. Then he asked patients who took part in the pilot project (and those who did not want to) what they thought of the proposal and, using some of the same measures that had been used in the research project, was able to start to compare the effectiveness of the local service with national evidence. He was able to invite a member of the local users group to join the expanding development team.

Preparation and training: 'be prepared'

You already have an interest in the patient group, an enthusiasm for CBT, and the motivation to improve services for patients within your organization, so what else will you need? The travel analogy is a useful one. In the later sections, we will see the need for an agreed direction of travel and destination; a plan for getting there avoiding pitfalls; and a means for staying there and not drifting off course. But first of all comes the preparation phase. Most survival guides start, for good reasons, with the warning to 'be prepared', and the area of service development is no different.

If you were considering setting out on a trek you might read travel guides, review websites, talk to people who had made the same or similar journeys, employ a guide, and so on. Similarly, you would not start assessing or treating a patient with a particular disorder without reading the literature, talking to more experienced staff, developing some possible options for treatment, and asking for training and supervision. So you should not start a service development without preparation and training. First, you can read service relevant literature, start networking, and visiting other CBT services in order to get the CBT angle. Second, in order to get the organization's angle, you can examine the national picture and local scenario to see what procedures need to be followed, what is likely to succeed, and who is likely to support a development. Third, you can appraise your own strengths and weaknesses in the areas of management of change, business planning, and project management. By undertaking some of the tasks shown in Box 19.2 below you will develop the knowledge and skills necessary for the journey ahead. As you become more informed and competent you will become more confident too. You will be able to bring about improvements in your CBT services by looking for opportunities, by being realistic, creative, and flexible and importantly, by believing you can do it. West (1997) tells us that:

> Innovation is a long path paved with conflict requiring a vision of change, courage in the face of conflict, persistence in the face of resistance, and the wisdom to steer a course through the complex currents of change from the beginning to the end of the process...
>
> West (1997)

The next section addresses how to develop the vision.

Developing the vision/making the case/assessing the currents of change

You need to develop a clear sense of direction and the means of getting there: a vision.

There have never been so many opportunities to improve or develop CBT services. CBT practitioners continue to find new and more effective ways of treating a wider range of patients (see Chapter 10 on 'Working through others' and Chapter 8 on 'Groups' for more information), and CBT researchers continue to provide a robust evidence base for CBT. So it is necessary first, to be clear about your *own* objectives; and second, to understand *other people's* objectives. It is only then that you can develop a vision that is shared and followed.

You might initially have identified a problem in your own service that needs fixing, such as waiting times being too long; or a gap that needs filling, such as insufficient CBT training or supervision. You might have already thought of this in terms of the outcomes you want, such as patients starting treatment within 2 weeks or for unqualified staff to have access to regular training. And you may have already thought of a way to overcome the problems, such as introducing computerized CBT, or running an online training course. Like a journey, it is helpful to be able to express these objectives clearly and succinctly, for example, '*I want us to go north to get to Norway, and I'm thinking of going by schooner*'. After all if you don't know where you would like to be

Box 19.2 Preparation

Knowledge

1 Read CBT, clinical, and popular journals.

2 Read government directives and strategy documents/local directives and strategy documents.

So you can:

- Find out what your patients need (nationally and locally).
- Find out what CBT can and cannot do to meet those needs (nationally and locally).
- Find out what the national strategy and priorities are.
- Find out what your local strategy and priorities are.

3 Talk to people within and outside your service about successful and unsuccessful service developments.

4 Visit successful services.

So you can:

- Find out what sort/size/stage/complexity of development you are involved in.
- Find out what local process you need to follow and when.
- Find out what and who will help you get there.
- Find out what and who will hinder you getting there.

Skills

5 Read management of change/business planning/project management literature.

6 Read business cases, business plans, project plans, and annual reports of successful CBT and other services.

7 Read unsuccessful business cases of CBT and other services.

8 Ask people experienced in developing services if you can shadow them in negotiations, and/or if they will mentor you.

9 Practice negotiation skills (written and verbal) and ask for feedback.

So you can:

- Effectively persuade/negotiate/compromise/collaborate.
- Prepare persuasive and realistic business cases, business plans, and implementation plans.

Box 19.2 Preparation *(continued)*

Attitudes

- Now you are prepared, look for opportunities, be realistic, be creative, be flexible, and believe you can do it.
- 'Maintain a vision, show courage, wisdom, and determination in order to make progress' (West, 1997).
- Show confidence, enthusiasm, and conviction; motivation and hunger for success; risk-taking; determination and tenacity; and self-reliance and self-determination (Lloyd, 2007).

heading, you are going to find it difficult to assess what will help you get there. As the Roman philosopher Seneca said:

> When a man does not know to which port he is heading, no wind is in the right direction.
>
> Seneca (4 BC–65 AD)

There are now many prevailing winds that can help you to drive forward the development of CBT services. Importantly, the UK government's Department of Health has become more directive in stipulating that cost-effective treatments should be provided within the National Health Service (NHS), and the National Institute for Health and Clinical Excellence (NICE) has identified CBT as the current treatment of choice for many patient groups (see http://www.nice.org.uk). The Department of Health has prescribed how commissioning bodies should purchase evidence-based services to meet populations' needs (see http://www.dh.gov.uk/en/Managingyourorganisation/Commissioning/Worldclasscommissioning/index.htm). Since 2008, the Department of Health has provided substantial dedicated funding to provide improved access to psychological therapies (IAPT) for people with common mental health problems (see http://www.iapt.nhs.uk and Chapter 6 of this volume). Users of services also demand greater access to psychological services in general, and to CBT in particular (e.g. Mental Health Foundation, 2006).

These are what are known as *external* drivers, that is, they are coming from outside your organization. You need to understand what impact they are having on the local decision-makers, and also what the local *internal* drivers are. There may, for example, be local cost-cutting targets to meet, or inpatient services to review, so you may need to modify your objectives to make them locally relevant and consistent with local strategy. To use the sailing analogy you will stand a better chance of getting there with others if you revise your provisional direction of travel or method of getting there, for example, *you may still aim to get to Norway but you might be more successful by trimming your sails, or travelling North Easterly, or travelling by ketch.*

When you look for local drivers you will find they range from those initiated low down the organization to those originating high up in the organization. These different drivers may result in quite different forms of service development. Consider the scenarios in Box 19.3, which illustrate different drivers for changing CBT services. They also show the range in size and complexity of service development, and illustrate the different (and slightly overlapping)

Box 19.3 Examples of drivers for development, and examples of stages of development

A. ***Choice***: *Brian returns from the annual CBT conference fired up with enthusiasm to adopt a new way of delivering CBT in the day service where he works. Rather than only treating people individually he wants to persuade his CBT colleagues to introduce a group programme, and thereby offer greater choice.*

As with Ahmed (Box 19.1) this is a relatively modest, internal, and bottom-up innovation. It is driven by the wish to provide choice, but may also gain support from those who wish to see greater throughput, or more evidence-based interventions. It is still in its planning stage and requires mostly bottom-up interventions working with colleagues. (**Preparation and Planning stage**)

B. ***NICE***: *Carla and her colleagues have been working in the field of physical health for some years. NICE guidance stipulates that CBT should be provided for a new patient group with whom they have not previously worked. She will need to persuade managers and/or commissioners to provide new funding and prepare CBT practitioners to work with new patients.*

This is a more significant innovation. The key driver is external, resulting in the need for commissioners and/or providers to conform to NICE guidance. It may also garner support from those who wish to see an expansion of physical health services. It is in its very early stages and requires Carla to persuade people higher up/outside the organization to develop a commissioning plan. (**Planning and Commissioning stage**)

C. ***Programme change***: *Your organization has just been awarded a sizeable contract to deliver CBT services in a Primary Care stepped care model. The new IAPT services will be highly structured and closely monitored. They have*

Box 19.3 Examples of drivers for development, and examples of stages of development

already attracted some local support and some local opposition. Along with others you have been appointed as a CBT therapist and supervisor to deliver the new services alongside existing experienced primary care counsellors.

This represents a significant innovation and service redesign. The key drivers were originally external, but now the contract has been secured there are significant internal pressures to make sure the service meets its targets. It is in its early implementation stages and requires you and your colleagues to quickly introduce new ways of working. (**Commissioning and Implementation stage**)

D. ***Efficiency***: *Davina is a member of an established Psychological Therapy Service which for the last 6 months has been required by her organization to see more patients, more quickly. She and her colleagues had been asked to introduce new ways of working while maintaining the quality of the clinical service. Results are not positive, and staff are mixed in their response.* The driver for this development is internal to the organization and top down. It did not require innovation as much as modifications to existing practice. The development is not so much complex as contentious. It is well into its implementation phase and it's time to review. (**Implementation and Review stage**)

E. ***Replication***: *Eric has been part of a very successful small multidisciplinary team that has been delivering CBT to older people and their carers. He has been asked to help neighboring teams adopt best CBT practice.* The development may be significant in one team which has a long way to develop, but may be relatively straightforward in the other team where the practice is not far from Eric's team. The driver for this development is internal to the organization but external to Eric's team. In aiming to replicate the outcomes and processes to other services this development will inevitably involve some review as well. (**Review and Replication stage**)

stages of the development cycle (*preparation and planning, commissioning and implementation, reviewing and replication*). Broadly, after the thinking comes the detailed definition (commissioning) of the service and then the launch (implementation) to 'make it happen'. When it is up and running there will be need to review to make sure you continue to do what you set out to do, or to modify it or replicate it in the light of new external or internal drivers.

Once you are aware of the drivers for change, you can start to *identify the objectives* of the development. They should be concise so they can be easily communicated to, and understood by, others. As you work with your development team and you exchange ideas with other stakeholders you will be able to refine your aims. They need to be SMART (see Chapter 15). They also need to be accurate, realistic, and achievable. They should refer to the cost, the timescale, and the outcomes. Some examples are given in Box 19.4.

Building a change team and getting senior support

Let's face it, lots of people before you have been determined to implement changes in their own CBT services and had a vision that at the time seemed desirable, reasonable, and achievable. The majority of these aspirations peter out; some become projects, but most of those dwindle over time; a few fail completely. Why?

Perhaps what seemed desirable to the enthusiast did not seem necessary or pressing to local practitioners. Perhaps what seemed reasonable and rational to the convert did not chime with the priorities of patients, managers, or purchasers. Perhaps what seemed easily attainable by the competent therapist did not take sufficient account of the human and financial costs, or give sufficient

Box 19.4 Examples of objectives for service development.

A. Within the same budget and within the next year, to provide patients who have Chronic Fatigue Syndrome with the choice of a Mindfulness CBT group programme as an alternative to the existing individual CBT service. (Choice)

B. Within the next annual business cycle to secure new funding from within the Trust to provide individual CBT to patients with obsessive compulsive disorder (OCD) and body dysmorphic disorder (BDD) according to the NICE implementation advice. (NICE guidance: NICE, 2006)

C. To deliver primary care IAPT services equitably throughout the county according to stepped care model in next 24 months. (New IAPT)

D. Within existing resources, to increase the number of CBT patients seen by 20% in the next 12 months while maintaining a 40–50% improvement rate. (Efficiency drive)

E. For the new CBT service to replicate the original CBT service's output and outcome measures within the next 18 months. (Replication) time for people to change. Lack of support, or even opposition, from within the CBT community, from other psychological therapists, or from patients and sponsors may render a good idea useless or a good project unworkable. So the essence of surviving service development is to *find support* for an agreed direction of travel before you start, *and then maintain it.*

This is a point that cannot be stressed enough to those of us who are used to working largely alone, providing individual CBT. We are most comfortable considering individuals, rather than services. We expect to work autonomously, rather than being interdependent on others. All too often we think service development is something that other people do, and does not concern us. So it can be a big change for some of us even to acknowledge the need to work alongside others, and to aim explicitly to do so. From the outset we need to be good at seeking and maintaining support, first by *building a development team* and second by *securing the sponsorship of senior management.* These points were well made over 30 years ago in a seminal paper by Georgiades and Philimore entitled 'The myth of the hero innovator' (1975). They warned against:

> ...the idea that you can produce, by training, a knight in shining armour who, loins girded with new technology and beliefs, will assault his organizational fortress and institute changes both in himself and others at a stroke. Such a view is ingenuous. The fact of the matter is that organizations such as schools and hospitals will, like dragons, eat hero innovators for breakfast.
>
> Georgiades and Phillimore (1975)

As we will see later, building and maintaining support matters not only at the start of the process but also throughout the development of services.

In a relatively modest service development (such as Ahmed's in Box 19.1 or Brian's in Box 19.3), the development team can be small. It can be led by the CBT enthusiast, as long as it also comprises someone with the authority to sanction changes and provide financial support; and a small team of motivated people to provide support, agree, and implement a plan, and monitor and evaluate progress. In these circumstances, you can be both leader and provider in much the way that a first violin could both lead and play in a string quartet. In larger or more complex service developments the change team needs to be proportionally larger and more diverse in its membership, and it needs to have a distinct leader (like a conductor who leads the orchestra but is not expected to play an instrument). Depending on factors such as the nature of the service development, your experience, and your position within the organization, you may decide to lead yourself or you may ask a senior member of your organization to lead, leaving you to make good use of your technical CBT expertise. Consider this quite different form of service development (see Example 19.2).

Example 19.2 Focused CBT innovation needing funding

Carla, a CBT therapist, worked with a team of psychological therapists in a medical setting. Previous funding from the Cardiac Rehabilitation Unit (CRU) had been discontinued, and although there were regular enquires to their service, the work had to be turned away. Carla had previously used CBT very successfully with patients with chronic heart conditions and wanted to provide a similar service in this setting. The consequences of turning people away were that some remained untreated and distressed by their symptoms; some were referred for expensive and sometimes risky medical procedures; and almost all remained as regular outpatients at the CRU and in primary care. The goal Carla wanted was to secure funding to establish a dedicated CBT service. This would result in the following outcomes:

- *Assessment and treatments would be provided.*
- *Patients' cardiac and emotional symptoms would reduce.*
- *The number of unnecessary medical investigations would fall.*
- *The number of people attending outpatients would fall.*
- *The overall drugs bill would reduce.*

Her first task was to bring together a team of people sufficiently interested in the well-being of CR patients, who were (or could be) persuaded of the benefits of providing CBT, and who had access to money to finance service development. She chose the lead nurse from the CRU, a consultant cardiologist, and a member of the local patients' group. Carla led preliminary meetings but subsequently, as it emerged that external money would have to be sought, the group decided to invite the clinical manager to lead the meetings. The clinical manager was responsible for the overall internal budget and could use his influence to instruct a representative of the finance department to help them work up a detailed business case.

In this example we see how you can develop a supportive team and how, by *not* assuming the lead, you can still continue to work toward the objective of getting the new CBT service developed. You can focus your energies on the details of providing a clinically effective CBT service while others contribute different and valuable skills. Not only that, but you have secured the all important support from senior management.

The reason for doing this is evident when we consider the top three most common causes for project failure identified by the National Audit Office and shown in Box 19.5. By opening communications at the earliest stages with senior staff, colleagues, and stakeholders such as patients, user groups, and

Box 19.5 Common causes of project failure

- Lack of clear link to organization's strategic priorities.
- Lack of clear senior management ownership and leadership.
- Lack of effective engagement with key stakeholders.
- Lack of project management and risk management skills.
- Project development and implementation stages not broken down into manageable steps.
- Evaluation of proposals linked to short-term affordability rather than longer-term value for money.
- Lack of understanding of and contact with suppliers.
- Lack of effective integration between the project team, stakeholder, and supplier.

Source: National Audit Office (2004). *Common Causes of Project Failure*. Available at: http://www.ogc.gov.uk/documents/Project_Failure.pdf.

referrers, you not only start to secure the success of the service development, you also gain invaluable information about the context for your proposed development, and are able to refine the proposal to meet others' needs as well as your own original objectives. With the active participation of the team(s) you have formed you will need to finalize an agreed vision, including agreed *clear objectives that chime with the organization's strategic direction, and an agreed way forward.* This often takes the form of a business case.

Writing the business plan

There are many ways of persuading stakeholders to adopt service developments, including formal and informal meetings, formal and less formal presentations, and written business plans. Even if your development is not sufficiently large or complex to warrant submitting a formal business plan, it is nonetheless helpful for you and your team to have considered the usual topics included in a business plan, for at least four reasons:

- It ensures that you are thorough and have not overlooked key aspects of the proposed change.
- It ensures that your team are using the same language as the key decision-makers and are making it easily understandable to them.
- It can be circulated in draft form for feedback before your plan is finalized.

- It can be summarized to publicize your success when it is adopted.

In the United Kingdom, the Department of Health expects commissioners of services to purchase

> ...the best possible health outcomes (including reduced health inequalities) and the best possible healthcare with the resources made available by the tax payer.
>
> Department of Health (2006)

To do this they follow a commissioning cycle such as one shown in Fig. 19.1.

NHS business cases must fit with the local strategy, local priorities (see section 'Building on core CBT skills') and the local cycle. For example, the Department of Health are looking for improvements in four priority areas:

- The health of the population
- Support to people with long-term conditions
- Access to services
- The patient experience

From this it is clear that you need to get used to talking in terms of outcomes, access, and choice, and value for money. You must learn the language

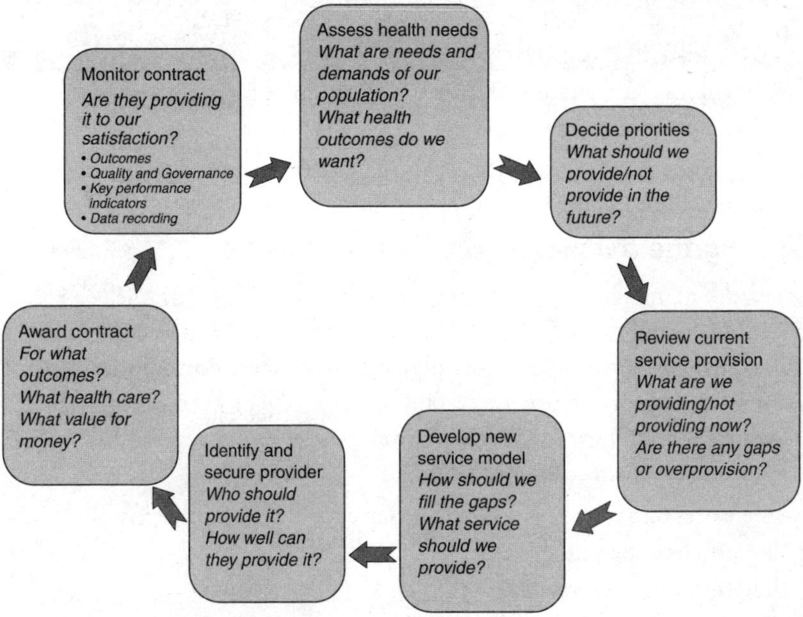

Fig. 19.1 A commissioning cycle.

of change and develop a plan that at a minimum covers: the health outcomes that are required; the rationale for change; and the proposed 'model' to achieve that change. The model should include:

- The strategy, the tactics, and the route map
- Who will deliver the change
- The risks and challenges of making the change, and of not doing so
- The activity required
- The costs that will be incurred
- The timescale over which the change will happen

In essence the business plan must cover the What, the Why, and the How, as well as the Who, the What Ifs, the How Many, the How Much, and the When. The highlights are condensed into the plan's executive summary. These areas are summarized in Box 19.6. There are hundreds of books and *pro formas* available on the Internet to assist you with writing business plans, but remember that yours will be most persuasive when it is presented in the language of the people you are trying to persuade, and at the right time. Remember also that:

Box 19.6 Business plans

Four topics to understand before you write a business plan	**Nine topics for inclusion in a business plan**
Be clear about your goals, strategy, and values (i.e. *what you want*)	The attention grabbing Executive Summary
Be clear about *who* you have to convince and find out their goals, strategy, and values (i.e. *what they want*)	Introduction: What the population needs, what the patients need, now and in future
Be clear about what *written* communication they need (e.g. business case, option appraisal, business plan)	Reasons for change: Why change
Be clear about planning cycle, timescale, and decision-making process	The proposal: How to change
	Delivery: Who
	Risks and how to manage them: What ifs
	Activity: How many
	Financial plan: How much
	Timescale: When

> ...undocumented plans are not worth the paper they are not written on.
>
> Lloyd (2007)

Overcoming resistance

> While the first task of change management is to understand the destination and how to get there, the first task of transition management is to convince people to leave home. You'll save yourself a lot of grief if you remember that.
>
> Bridges, quoted in NHS Institute for Innovation and Improvement (2002)

In our clinical work we know only too well that for patients to achieve the changes they desire, they may need to overcome their own or other people's resistance. In much the same way you will find that in the area of service development you are not able to introduce and maintain change without first understanding and managing resistance to change.

The first blocks may stem from your own lack of skills or confidence to tackle the journey, for example: '*I can't do this, I haven't done this before, what if I try to make a difference and it all goes wrong?*' or from your own reluctance to tackle the task, for example: '*I should not have to do this, my manager should be doing it*'; '*I'd rather stay focused on the clinical work*'.

Some blocks might originate from your own ambivalence about new directions, for example: '*I want to carry on doing CBT the way I was taught; I don't want to learn these new third wave techniques*'; '*I don't think it is right to give CBT away to untrained staff*'.

Another crucial area for resistance comes from other people affected. Much has been written about different groups of people with respect to change (see Fig. 19.2):

- Those who eagerly embrace change ('early adopters');
- Those who follow soon after ('the early majority');
- Those who follow only with persuasion ('the late majority'); and
- Those who resist the change throughout the process (pejoratively known as the 'laggards').

But remember that these categories are not fixed: someone who is a late adopter for one innovation may be an early adopter for another, and vice versa. By understanding what changes they have previously readily embraced you will be better equipped to influence them this time. Just like you, they may resist change in a general sense or they may object to CBT in particular. They may say that they don't have capacity, for example: '*We have too much change going on round here, I am not ready for any more*', or that they want more information, for example: '*I will wait to see what other people do first before I commit*

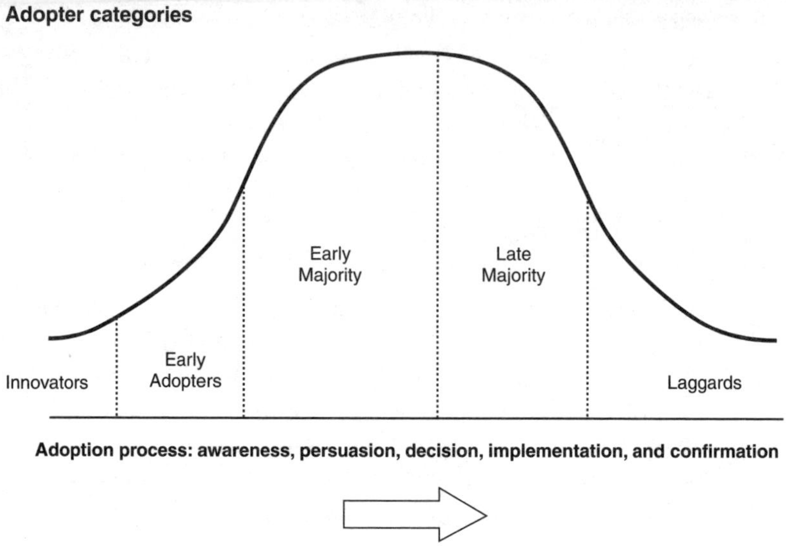

Fig. 19.2 Adopter categories and adoption process.

Source: Rogers, E.(1985). *Diffusion of Innovations*. New York, NY: Free Press.

myself', or that the proposed change does not fit with their experience, for example: '*I have never liked working with that patient group*', '*The last service development fizzled out and this one will be no different*'.

You would not discount patients' reasons for resisting change and you should not ignore these either. Grant *et al.* (2004) give helpful examples of familiar CBT techniques for examining and challenging such thoughts, so that progress can be made in moving people on through the different phases of the adoption process: awareness, persuasion, decision, implementation, and confirmation. As we will see below you may need to take particular care with obstacles that arise concerning CBT itself.

As we saw in section 'Developing the vision/making the case/assessing the currents of change', the prevailing wind in the United Kingdom is in favour of CBT as never before. The evidence base is demonstrable, government money is available, and patient demand is increasing. However, this does not guarantee easy change. As CBT grows, so *opposition* to CBT also grows. And as with a political movement whose success is based partly on fact, partly on opportunity, and partly on popular opinion, there will be many views expressing doubt or outright opposition to the movement. In fact, a well-known management of change technique introduced by Lewin in the 1950s, called Force Field Analysis, asserts that for every driving force there will be an equal and opposing restraining force.

You must therefore anticipate and draw out the opposition to CBT so that you can develop a realistic and sustainable plan for overcoming it. Opponents may challenge the assumptions upon which it is based, for example: '*CBT can't change the underlying causes of disorders*', or its evidence base: '*CBT's evidence base is limited and does not take sufficient account of patient diversity or experience*'. They may oppose the means by which it is being advanced within the NHS: '*CBT is not the only fruit, it is unwarranted to favour it at the expense of other talking therapies*' or the effect that this might have: '*My patients want a choice of approach, not just CBT*'. They may also quote a case example: '*I had a patient who had CBT and it made her worse*'.

It will not be necessary to counter each and every possible objection to the proposed development, but you will need to be aware of the key objectors and objections at any stage so that they can be addressed. For example, in the IAPT programme described above (Example C, Box 19.3), you may come across general practitioners (GPs) who see the new service as a threat to practice-based counselling and who do not want to refer to the new CBT therapists. It may be helpful at the outset to acknowledge their fears, and try to find the means for both services to run alongside each other. If this is possible it may be helpful to highlight the high demand for both sorts of talking therapies, and to differentiate between the two services so that they are not so directly competing for patients. It may also be helpful to provide regular summaries to feedback the benefits of providing the CBT (and counselling) service.

Some objections are based on facts and cannot be altered—but the impact can be minimized. For example, *You are right that the government is providing more money for CBT than counselling. Given that, how can we help you get the best treatments for your patients?* In this example, the intervention uses a collaborative approach, a trial period, and monitoring and review. In Example D, Box 19.3, Davina was part of the review of CBT services where there was a requirement to see more patients within the year. Her colleagues were not happy about the directive and the plan was not working. There was a choice to be made. *Given that we have tried to be more efficient for 6 months without success, what can we do differently that will increase the numbers of patients seen, but still maintain quality of outcomes?* This too uses a collaborative problem-solving approach, and can be the basis for a pilot project. Usually, by keeping the focus on patients (and carers), and by testing out their beliefs, more objectors can be moved along the process a stage further, until there is the 'critical mass' to start the innovation, and eventually a majority of people adopting the new way of doing things.

To return now to the travel analogy you have decided where to head for (section 'Developing the vision/making the case/assessing the currents of change'), who to have in your team (section 'Building a change team and getting senior support'), how to get there (section 'Writing the business plan'), you have also persuaded others to come with you (section 'Overcoming resistance'): how will you get them to stay with you? (section 'Sustaining a service; replicating a service', see below)

Sustaining a service; replicating a service

It is as well to remember that innovations in the NHS are more likely to be adopted and implemented if they have clear, observable advantage(s); are compatible with values and norms; are perceived as simple to use; and also allow intended users to adapt and refine them to suit their own use (Greenhalgh *et al.*, 2004). Successful developments have the features shown in Box 19.7, which importantly includes having systems in place to monitor progress, and by implication to sustain the new ways of doing things. You will want the old ways to be left behind, and the new ways to become the only ways of doing things (see NHS Institute for Innovation and Improvement, 2005 for more information). In clinical work, you know of the importance of having regular supervision to ensure that protocols are followed and that patients receive the best care (see Chapter 16). Likewise in service development work, it is beneficial to find a means to review progress and keep you and the service on track, not just at the outset but throughout the lifetime of the service. This can include mentorship for the leader(s), review meetings for the team(s), and feedback

Box 19.7 Features of successful service developments

- Perception that current situation is intolerable.
- Innovation fits with existing values, norms, and ways of working.
- Has assessed full implication of innovation.
- Supporters outnumber opponents and are more strategically placed.
- Allocated adequate resources.
- Systems in place to monitor and evaluate impact.
- Can therefore respond to expected and unexpected consequences.

reviews for all the stakeholders. You will also want the new service to be able to withstand challenges and variation without reverting back to the old ways, and maybe even to improve (see NHS Institute for Innovation and Improvement, 2002 for more information).

There are three common pitfalls to avoid: believing that the evidence is enough, believing that government guidance is enough, and believing that training is enough. There is a wealth of evidence that CBT is the treatment of choice for particular disorders, and it has been available for many years, but citing the evidence and making a 'rational' argument is not sufficient to persuade decision-makers to adopt this approach.

> *Human institutions and behaviours will always be shaped by processes that are (at least in part) non-rational. In the spirit of both the rational and non-rational, we would do well to reflect on the still germane comments of Cervantes' Don Quixote:* "There have been many who, not knowing how to mingle the useful with the pleasing in the right proportions, have had all their toil and pains for nothing"...
>
> Waddell (2001)

Recently, NICE and other organizations have written guidance stipulating that particular CBT interventions should be provided, but making directives has not been an effective way of sustaining change, and nor is education alone. Drake *et al.* (2003) argue that changes persist over time when you help prepare people for change; you enable them to enact new practice; and you reinforce them to sustain change. This requires greater involvement by stakeholders and is best when it matches the values, needs, and concerns of practitioners.

Although training can enhance CBT knowledge and skills in the short term, there is very little evidence that services improve for patients back in the host services. An important report entitled *Avoiding the Washout* quotes Lipsky (1980):

> Worker training is less important than the nature of working conditions themselves. Without a supportive network of working peer relationships, training to improve service capacity of workers is likely to wash out under pressure of the work context.
>
> Lipsky (1980) quoted in Repper and Brooker (2002)

Repper and Brooker (2002) find that barriers to implementing evidence-based practice include practical ones, such as insufficient resources to support the release of staff; structural ones, such as lack of clarity of purpose of teams where therapists work; and capacity issues such as distraction and uncertainty caused by other significant changes. Fadden (2006) has found that creating sustained change requires time, persistence, and continuity of committed personnel who build and maintain a solid relationship with senior management, and also involve audit and clinical governance departments in monitoring through existing frameworks such as the Care Programme Approach framework. She makes use of a steering group with representation of senior, operational, and middle management as well as user and family representatives; has a detailed implementation plan; and addresses operational issues such as team priorities, out of hours working, caseload size, and management (Fadden, 2006). In the field of CBT training, Milne *et al.* (2002) have suggested the following strategies to enhance sustained training:

- Providing training in context
- Fostering supportive environments
- Making use of 'relapse prevention' which includes heightened awareness of the risk of washout, group problem-solving, and realistic goal setting.

So we find ourselves back at the beginning. As Fadden argues:

> As much if not more attention should be paid to preparing organisations in which the clinicians who are trained work [as to the training itself].
>
> Fadden (2006)

Enjoying and surviving the journey

Preparing and undertaking service development is an exciting, demanding, and rewarding challenge. Its prize is that you will improve CBT services for patients. You might treat more patients, or treat them more efficiently. You might treat new patients who have not received a service before or you might improve their outcomes. You might train more staff or save more money. Whatever your goal, the skills you already have as a CBT practitioner can be used and built upon to make the journey.

Key tips for completing the journey

1. Get prepared: get researching, get a coach, and get determined.
2. Agree your destination and make use of the prevailing winds.
3. Build a crew and get sponsorship.
4. Write a realistic and convincing journey plan.
5. Take account of the opposing forces.
6. Beware of the common pitfalls.
7. Expect more change along the way.

Despite the best laid plans, you will need to be both resilient and flexible to respond when other pressures come to bear, for example, your organization's priorities change, managers leave, and there are tensions between gaining ownership and delivering quickly. Change brings some loss, and opportunities bring some costs (NHS, 2001). You will need to remember that changes can be planned and deliberate or emergent, spontaneous and unplanned, and that organizational level change is not fixed or linear in nature but contains an important emergent element. Accordingly, it is helpful to follow Mintzberg's advice and to be:

> ...like a potter crafting a pot on a wheel: setting out with an intention but making adjustments in response to the way the clay is handling, sometimes making major changes as opportunity arises that wasn't foreseen.
>
> Mintzberg (1989)

Organizations need to accommodate to and experiment with the everyday contingencies, breakdowns, exceptions, opportunities, and unintended consequences that punctuate organizational life; so you will need to be the sailor who trims the sail, steers round the rocky headland, and enjoys the thrill of seeing a school of dolphins on the way.

You will also need to allow for the fact that you and your team will need to be very active throughout the journey and that:

> ...people are not passive recipients of innovations. Rather they seek innovations out, experiment with them, evaluate them, challenge them, complain about them, talk to others about them, modify them to fit particular tasks, and attempt to improve or redesign them.
>
> Greenhalgh *et al.* (2004)

Your development will be all the stronger for that. You may of course get tired or dispirited at times, and that is when you turn to the classic text by Georgiades and Phillimore (1975) who advise you to:

- Choose the path of least organizational resistance.
- Find allies, work with 'critical mass'.
- Work in the healthy part of the organization, don't work with lost causes.
- Work with those with autonomy.
- Get top team support/permission.
- Build team support, and proceed with a realistic timescale.

Good luck!

Further reading

Georgiades, N.J. and Phillimore, L. (1975). The myth of the hero innovator and alternative strategies for organizational change, in Kiernan, C.C. and Woodward, F.P. (eds.), *Behavioural Modification with the Severely Retarded.* London: Associated Scientific Publishers.

The Office of Government Commerce (OGC) is an independent office of HM Treasury, established to help Government deliver best value from its spending. It has useful advice about project management. Available at: http://www.ogc.gov.uk (accessed on 26 Feb 2010)

The National Institute for Health Research Service Delivery and Organisation (NIHR SDO) programme aims to improve health outcomes for people by commissioning research evidence that improves practice in relation to the organization and delivery of health care and by building research capability and capacity amongst those who manage, organize, and deliver. It produces managers' briefing papers on change management. Available at: http://www.sdo.nihr.ac.uk (accessed on 26 Feb 2010)

The NHS Institute for Innovation and Improvement supports the NHS to transform health care for patients and the public by rapidly developing and spreading new ways of working, new technology, and world-class leadership. It has many publications on service transformation. Available at: http://www.institute.nhs.uk

References

Department of Health (2006). *Health Reform in England: Update and Commissioning Framework*. Available at: http://www.dh.gov.uk/en/Publicationsandstatistics/Publications/PublicationsPolicyAndGuidance/DH_4137226 (accessed 16 August 2009).

Drake RE et al (2003) Strategies for implementing evidence-based practices in routine mental health settings. *Evidence-Based Mental Health* **6**, 6-7 available online from http://ebmh.bmjjournals.com (accessed 26 February 2010).

Fadden, G. (2006). Training and disseminating family interventions for schizophrenia: developing family intervention skills with multi-disciplinary groups. *Journal of Family Therapy*, **28**, 23–38.

Georgiades, N.J. and Phillimore, L. (1975). The myth of the hero innovator and alternative strategies for organizational change, in Kiernan, C.C. and Woodward, F.P. (eds.), *Behavioural Modification with the Severely Retarded*. London: Associated Scientific Publishers.

Grant, A., Mills, J., Mulhern, R. and Short, N. (2004). Establishing cognitive behavioural work cultures, in Grant, A., Mills, J., Mulhern, R. and Short, N. (eds.), *Cognitive Behaviour Therapy in Mental Healthcare*. London: Sage.

Greenhalgh, T., Glenn, R. and Bate, P. (2004). *Spreading and Sustaining Innovations in Health Service Delivery and Organisation*. NHS National Institute of Health Research Service Delivery Organisation Programme. Available at: http://www.sdo.nihr.ac.uk/files/project/38-final-report.pdf (accessed 16 August 2009).

Lloyd, D. (2007). *Business Plans*. London: Chartered Institute of Management/Hodder Arnold.

Mental Health Foundation (2006). *We Need to Talk. The Case for Psychological Therapy on the NHS*. Available at: http://www.mentalhealth.org.uk/campaigns/we-need-to-talk/?locale=en (accessed 16 August 2009).

Milne, D., Westerman, C. and Hanner, S. (2002). Can a 'Relapse Prevention' module facilitate the transfer of training? *Behavioural and Cognitive Psychotherapy*, **30**, 361–364.

Mintzberg, H. (1989). *Mintzberg on Management*. New York, NY: Free Press.

National Audit Office (2004). *Common Causes of Project Failure.* Available at: http://www.ogc.gov.uk/documents/Project_Failure.pdf. (accessed 16 August 2009).

NICE (2006). *Obsessive Compulsive Disorder: Core Interventions in the Treatment of Obsessive Compulsive Disorder and Body Dysmorphic Disorder.* National Clinical Practice Guideline Number 31. Available at: http://www.nice.org.uk/nicemedia/pdf/cg031fullguideline.pdf (accessed 16 August 2009).

Newton, R. (2007). *Managing Change Step by Step: All You Need to Build a Plan and Make it Happen.* London: Pearson Education.

NHS Institute for Innovation and Improvement (2001). *Improvement Leaders' Guide to Making Informed Decisions on Change.* Available at: http://www.institute.nhs.uk/option,com_joomcart/Itemid,26/main_page,document_product_info/products_id,309.html (accessed 16 August 2009).

NHS Institute for Innovation and Improvement (2002). *Improvement Leaders' Guide to Sustainability and Spread.* Available at: http://www.institute.nhs.uk/option,com_joomcart/Itemid,26/main_page,document_product_info/products_id,309.html (accessed 16 August 2009).

NHS Institute for Innovation and Improvement (2005). *Improvement Leaders' Guide to Managing the Human Dimensions of Change.* Available at: http://www.institute.nhs.uk/option,com_joomcart/Itemid,26/main_page,document_product_info/products_id,309.html (accessed 16 August 2009).

Repper, D. and Brooker, C. (2002). *Avoiding the Washout: Developing the Organisational Context to Increase the Uptake of Evidence based Practice for Psychosis.* Northern Centre for Mental Health.

Rogers, E. (1985). *Diffusion of Innovations.* New York, NY: Free Press.

Waddell, C. (2001). So much research evidence, so little dissemination and uptake: mixing the useful with the pleasing. *Evidence Based Mental Health*, **4**, 3–5.

West, M.A. (1997). *Developing Creativity in Organizations.* Leicester: British Psychological Society.

Chapter 20

When therapists have problems: what can CBT do for us?

Diana Sanders and James Bennett-Levy

In our training and work, we frequently see how helpful CBT can be for others. At times we may have used the methods on ourselves to look at personal issues or issues which have emerged within our relationships with patients. Sometimes we may find we need more support than can be provided by family and friends. We may want to be more structured in our use of CBT for ourselves, or may want to seek therapy. When the going gets tough, can we turn to CBT for help? In this chapter, we look at how we can use a brief, focused form of CBT to help in our professional and personal development, how to use CBT on ourselves, and whether being CBT therapists is valuable for us as individuals.

Introduction

Early in your cognitive behavioural therapy (CBT) career you will, hopefully, have come across many examples of ways in which CBT can make a difference. You will also be getting a good idea of the limitations of the approach, people whom CBT does and does not suit, and times and situations where the methods are or are not applicable. No doubt the philosophy and method has got under your skin, and maybe you use it in various ways both in your professional life and in your personal life, finding that the methods and approach are as applicable to you as to your patients.

It is only recently in the history of CBT that the role of the therapist has been looked at in any depth (Gilbert and Leahy, 2007). Cognitive models were originally developed for people with relatively short-term focused problems, with the assumption that the therapist is providing at the very least the core conditions of the relationship, and therefore the contribution of the therapist to the relationship was not viewed as of particular importance. In other forms of psychotherapy such as person-centreed and psychodynamic, the relationship is centre stage, and the therapist's issues and process are seen as a central part of the dynamics of change. These differing philosophies are reflected in training requirements. Personal therapy is perceived to be an important, if not essential, requirement for counsellors and psychotherapists (Norcross, 2005; Wilkins, 2006), and therapists rate their time in therapy as an important aspect of their overall clinical development (Macran and Shapiro, 1998; Orlinsky *et al.*, 2001). A minimum of 40 hours of personal therapy is a mandatory requirement for professional membership of the BPS Division of Counselling Psychology, the British Association for Counselling and Psychotherapy (BACP), and the United Kingdom Council for Psychotherapy (UKCP). In countries such as Sweden and Switzerland, CBT therapists need to be registered as psychotherapists in order to practice, and personal therapy is a mandatory requirement for psychotherapy registration.

In the world of cognitive and behavioural therapies, in contrast, personal therapy is not currently seen as an essential, or widely accepted, aspect of training or as necessary for accreditation (EABCT, 2000), The British Association for Behavioural and Cognitive Psychotherapies (BABCP) stipulate, 'Therapists must ensure that they can identify and manage appropriately their personal involvement in the process of cognitive and/or behaviour therapy' and 'Therapists must have developed an ability to recognize when they should seek other professional advice' (BABCP, 2000), and personal therapy is not stipulated as a training requirement within the UK Division of Clinical Psychology. An assumption appears to arise: are we CBT therapists completely well-balanced, sorted people who are able to work with the complexities and sensitivities of other people without being affected by, or affecting, the experience? Are all other therapy schools more suitable to therapists who are themselves in need of personal help? Is the well-being or otherwise of therapists and engagement in personal therapy not relevant to the process of CBT?

Jacqueline Persons (1989) was one of the first to mention the ways in which CBT might be useful for therapists, mainly in the context of improving our therapeutic skills rather than general lives. Many of the key names in cognitive therapy have stressed the importance of trying CBT out for ourselves. 'To fully understand the process of therapy, there is no substitute for using cognitive therapy methods on oneself', wrote Christine Padesky (1996, p. 288). Judith Beck (1995, p. 312) stated, 'to gain experience with basic techniques of cognitive therapy by practicing them on yourself before doing so with patients... and putting yourself in the patient's role affords the opportunity to identify obstacles that interfere with carrying out assignments'.

While such work addresses the issue of using CBT on ourselves to improve our effectiveness as therapists, do we also gain personally as a result of being therapists? Are the methods and approaches useful to us in life in general? Are we better prepared to get through the stresses and difficulties, and hellish times that life can offer?

In this chapter, we consider two central questions about ourselves as therapists. Does personal experience of CBT enhance our understanding and skills as therapists? And second, can we use our training and clinical experience to help us get through the various painful difficulties that can arise in our lives, both from external events and our own issues? The chapter is divided into three sections. In the first section, James Bennett-Levy considers the ways in which personal experience of CBT is used in training, focusing on his work on self-practice/self-reflection (SP/SR). In the second section, Diana Sanders looks at ways in which being a therapist can both help and hinder how we cope with life's difficulties, with illustrations from her own experience of physical illness and disability. In the third section, 'Jess', a CBT therapist, discusses her experience of receiving long-term CBT. She reflects on her struggles as a patient, and the valuable lessons that she learned about being a therapist.

Experiencing CBT for ourselves: the value of self-practice/self-reflection

In 1988, I (James) undertook a 6-month CBT training course at the Institute of Psychiatry, London, the first such training course in the United Kingdom (Moorey *et al.*, 1990). About half way through the course, one of the other trainees 'Susan' and I agreed that we wanted to try out the methods on ourselves. Therefore, we contracted to do four sessions with each other, focusing on a circumscribed problem. Each meeting lasted about 2½ hours: 50-minute sessions each, plus reflection time. At the end of each therapy session, Susan and I reflected on our experience as therapist and client, had a tea break, and then swapped roles. In the following week, we wrote up our reflections and shared any new thoughts at the start of the following session.

At the end of our time together, we both agreed that our work had provided another dimension on being a cognitive therapist. We had integrated our new understandings, and translated them into clinical skills rather better than by simply relying on our learning from clinical experience and supervision, valuable though the latter was. In the client's chair, we had particularly valued the 'non-specific' elements of therapy—the care, empathy, and interest of the other—as well as the opportunity to experience and practice CBT-specific skills. There was no doubt that the sessions had personal value for us as people (not just as therapists), helping us to deal better with the issues on which we had focused in 'therapy'. Those four sessions proved to be, effectively, our first experience of SP/SR in CBT.

SP/SR—developing the model

Ten years later, when teaching my first CBT training program on the clinical psychology course at James Cook University in North Queensland, Australia, and remembering our happy and useful self-therapy experiences, I included a 'personal experiential component' in the course syllabus. Naively in retrospect, I imagined that this innovation would be greeted with enthusiasm by eager-to-experiment trainees. How wrong could I be!

Fortunately, I had the sense to call a meeting before the course started to discuss the experiential component and agree a format and set of procedures. In the words of one trainee, Tina:

> *When I first read that thing about having a reflection assignment, I thought, "Oh god! How stupid!" I was really appalled. It got me offside from the start. It was shocking… It was like, when I'd bump into people who were doing the course, I'd say, "did you read that thing... it's scary isn't it!"*

By the end of the 12-week course, Tina's view had changed radically:

> *I think knowing how to do it for yourself covers all the bases. If you know how to do it… then you can pass that knowledge on to other people. Because you understand it for yourself, rather than having understood it from a book or something. You can then also problem-solve with somebody who does have difficulties with that … put it in your words and explain it to a person, rather than take it from a book and try to explain it from a technical perspective.*

Setting up an SP/SR group

To date, SP/SR groups have been established either in the context of university degree programs (clinical psychology or CBT), or stand-alone professional development courses. However, there is no reason why individuals or pairs may not undertake SP/SR on their own, as Susan and I did. The basic structure is straightforward: the self-practice (SP) part involves trainees practicing CBT techniques on each other, the self-reflection (SR) component has them reflecting on their experience.

We have developed two SP forms: solo and pairs. The 'solo' form of SP (Bennett-Levy *et al.*, 2001) allows trainees to practice CBT techniques on themselves via a purpose-designed SP/SR workbook, which contains weekly structured exercises (e.g. do an activity schedule, thought record, etc.). The second type of SP is a 'co-therapy' form where trainees pair up and offer each other therapy for a few sessions, swapping half way so both have time as 'client' and 'therapist'. Co-therapists are encouraged to focus on a mild-to-moderate, rather than severe, problem, as Susan and I had done during our training (Bennett-Levy *et al.*, 2003).

A key feature of SP/SR is the reflective (SR) component (Bennett-Levy *et al.*, 2009). After both forms of SP, participants write up their session reflections (SR) during the following week. These are collated by the facilitator and emailed—anonymously to preserve confidentiality—to the rest of the group. Participants are encouraged to reflect on their personal experience of CBT techniques, and on its implications for their clinical practice and understanding of cognitive theory. Sharing group reflections provides a rounded context for personal experience; it enables participants to see what kinds of experience may be common to others, and what may be relatively idiosyncratic responses.

SP/SR for personal gains

The rationale for SP/SR has always been founded on its value as a method for developing and enhancing therapist skills (Bennett-Levy *et al.*, 2001). However, of particular relevance for the present chapter is that a significant percentage of people report *personal* as well as professional gains. Interestingly, experienced therapists typically report just as much benefit from SP/SR as novices (Bennett-Levy *et al.*, 2009) and sometimes the changes are dramatic. Jeff, doing a workbook version of SP/SR for experienced therapists, wrote:

> *This whole experience has had so many positive effects, too numerous to detail, but most importantly, what I am now doing is treating myself with compassion—and I really am! I'm managing to sustain it, and of course it is influencing my therapy. I believe that I have pretty much always displayed compassion as a therapist, but there has been a shift within me that has moved it onto a different level.*

Although not everyone who does SP/SR experiences personal and professional shifts of the intensity Jeff describes, almost all trainees report that it impacts on their skills and understanding of CBT (Bennett-Levy *et al.*, 2001). We have also gathered quantitative data which provides harder evidence that practicing CBT on oneself can have personal, as well as professional benefits (Davis *et al.*, 2008). Davis *et al.* (2008) reported that highly experienced SP/SR participants demonstrated significant changes in personal and therapist beliefs, as well as measurable gains in self-reported CBT skills and empathy (Bennett-Levy *et al.*, 2009). Participants were asked at the start of the course to identify one personal belief (e.g. 'I'm a failure') and one therapist belief (e.g. 'I'm an incompetent therapist') that they would like to change. They then used CBT techniques such as positive data logs and behavioural experiments to modify and test out these beliefs. The results showed significant changes in beliefs over the duration of the course for all participants.

The data that have been gathered in the United Kingdom and Australia is supported by a parallel set of studies from Germany, summarized by Laireiter and Willutzki (2003). All these studies suggest that practicing CBT on oneself, either with the support of a 'co-therapist' or on one's own can be valuable both professionally and personally. CBT therapists do not have to have identifiable disorders in order to gain from CBT methods, though like many others, they may also benefit from CBT if they do.

SP/SR: limitations and warnings

During 10 years of research, we have been consistently impressed by the power of SP/SR. Although usually positive, the experience of the client role occasionally causes unexpected levels of emotional distress, at least in the short term. We therefore have several caveats to working effectively with SP/SR.

There is huge variability in the extent to which CBT therapists are willing to engage in personal experiential work and self-reflection. A consistent finding from studies with different groups of novice or experienced therapists is that participants differ considerably in their level of engagement—and degree of engagement with the process of SP/SR is highly correlated with the experience of benefit (Bennett-Levy *et al.*, 2001). Engagement is a function of a variety of factors, the most important of which for the present context are available personal resources and feeling of safety with the process.

Personal resources for SP/SR

SP/SR takes emotional energy and participants need to have time in which to reflect on their experience. We suggest setting aside at least 2 hours a week to do SP/SR. It is one of the ironies of life, both for therapists and clients, that the conditions which best promote reflection—having time, space, and personal resources—are often those most compromised by stressful life events or circumstances. Therefore, we advise prospective participants not to do SP/SR programs at times of high stress or intense work. Even then, 'life' can catch up with people during 10-week programs, and, as in all therapy, some people do dropout (Davis *et al.*, 2008).

Safe practice of SP/SR

Promoting safety within the process is essential. A prerequisite for all SP/SR courses is a clear agreement around boundaries and confidentiality. Typical agreements will include the following:

- All participants' email reflections are circulated anonymously.

- Make clear distinctions between content and process—focus reflections on the *process* of interventions, rather than the personal *content*.
- If you are working in pairs, personal issues discussed stay within the pair unless the person concerned specifically gives his/her permission for it to be discussed in the group.

With groups of professional colleagues working in the same region, our experience is that it is far preferable to go the 'solo workbook' route (rather than pairs), otherwise safety and boundary issues raise their heads. In 'limited co-therapy' SP/SR groups, we always recommend participants to work with people they do not know, even if they already have close confiding friendship with another participant. Prior knowledge of and relationship with another does not mimic therapy and introduces its own complications.

Pandora's box

Some CBT therapists, both novice and experienced, are concerned that if they 'dig', they might unleash something that they are unable to control or deal with in brief SP/SR, and for some this concern is well-grounded. An example is provided by Terry who was doing a responsibility pie chart:

> *I revisited an event from some 16 years ago. I faithfully allocated slices of responsibility … This was when things started to go wrong. I started to feel increasingly depressed about the situation and reassigning slices of responsibility to various contributors only made things worse … Suddenly, I felt even more guilt and shame about my attempts to reconstruct an experience for which I previously took full responsibility. I found myself re-living the whole situation over and over again. Each episode resulted in an increased number of NATs which in turn compelled me to dwell on the events even more … I was so preoccupied with the emotional roller coaster, that I found myself unable to do any meaningful work.*

Although deeply uncomfortable for a couple of weeks, Terry reflected at the end of the course that this had been a pivotal experience which would have a lasting effect on his clinical work.

> *For me personally, it was a chance of self-discovery which unearthed some amazing facets about the way I deal with my problems as well as a true test of the cognitive-behaviour methods of intervention.*

Since that time, we have always insisted that trainees undertaking SP/SR have a 'personal safeguard strategy' in place. We have recommended three levels of safeguards:

1. Discuss your distress or difficulties with another identified member of the group (e.g. co-therapist) if it feels safe to do so.
2. Discuss difficulties with the group facilitator.
3. If the above does not resolve things, seek outside help with a therapist.

In some groups, the SP/SR facilitators have already identified therapists who are prepared to offer their services in the event of significant distress; in others we have asked participants to identify a therapist who they would go to as a condition of acceptance into the program. To our knowledge, only 1 or 2 participants have ever required this kind of outside help.

The strategy above relies to some extent on our ability to make judgements about how our responses and difficulties can be best resolved, and whether we do need personal therapy or outside help. Ironically, we are often least able to make such judgements when we are very low stressed or burnt out ('I should be able to handle this …'). Depression, anxiety, or other 'diagnosable' problems are easier to spot in others than in ourselves. Use of formal measures such as the Beck Depression Inventory II (Beck et al., 1996) or Maslach Burnout Inventory (Schutte et al., 2000) can often be of value in determining level of support needed. High scores might indicate it is time to seek external assistance.

SP/SR: recommendations

To date, SP/SR has only been researched in groups in specific training contexts. We do not know to what extent the results would generalize to, for instance, colleagues setting up an informal SP/SR pairing, as Susan and I did. However, within the parameters of the research to date, we can recommend the following:

1. The vast majority of participants find SP/SR very helpful for their development as therapists (and/or supervisors) and a significant proportion find it helpful in their personal development.
2. Information and choice are central to success of SP/SR. This includes clear information about expectations (time, commitment, emotional resources, potential benefits); pros and cons of different SP/SR methods (e.g. limited co-therapy or workbook); choice of partners (do not work with colleagues or friends); and well-negotiated agreements around safety and confidentiality.
3. Reflection and evaluation are as important in SP/SR as the experiential work. Our experience suggests that written reflections add enormous value, enabling participants to conceptualize and integrate personal experience with professional understanding and clinical skills.
4. A small proportion of participants experience unexpected distress during SP/SR programs. Each participant should have a personal safeguard strategy in place prior to commencement of a program.

Does it help, being a therapist?

I (Diana) was asked the question at 2 in the morning in June 2002. I had just come out of intensive care following a heart and lung transplant, and couldn't get to sleep. My chest was held together with wires, four large drains came out of my abdomen, tubes from my neck and both arms, and I was hallucinating and nauseous from morphine and a cocktail of other medication. I was crying and wanted to go home. It was not the best time for a question about work.

It was a question I revisited several times in my recovery from the operation. Was CBT helpful, or did it in fact get in the way, giving me and my carers expectations that I should be able to cope, given my training? A visit to the website and journal of the BACP gives many examples of therapists writing about their personal experience and how these impact on themselves as people as well as therapists (www.bacp.org.uk). However, there is far less within the CBT literature. For me, although my training and experience of CBT was in some ways enormously helpful, giving me methods such as goal setting, activity scheduling, and reducing negative thinking, to cope with a long period of illness and waiting for a transplant, at other times it felt like a hindrance (Sanders, 2006; Sanders, 2008). For example, I found it very tough to both recognize, and admit, that I had become depressed after the surgery. Although I had worked with many clients with depression, it was extremely difficult to detect and accept the problem in myself. On some level, perhaps not always consciously, I expected to be able to cope better than I felt I did. The expectations came not just from me—medical staff would sometimes treat me differently from other patients, perhaps with the assumption that I would need less psychological support since I could do it myself. Beck and Butler (2005), in a chapter on treating psychotherapists with cognitive therapy made a similar observation, that a high percentage of therapists come to therapy with ideas like 'I shouldn't have these problems' and 'I should be able to handle my problems without help'.

It is possible that many of us in the caring professions find it hard to spot when things are too much, when low mood tips into clinical depression. In a survey of 1,000 therapists (Gilroy *et al.*, 2002), those who had experienced depression reported that their emotional issues gave them more empathy for their clients; however, they also experienced an increased sense of isolation from their colleagues and difficulties in discussing their personal experience.

The issue of whether being CBT therapists is helpful to us, personally, raises important questions which we consider below: do we chose to work in the area of psychology and psychotherapy because of our personal histories and experience of mental health difficulties? How can we use CBT methods on ourselves to help with issues that come up during therapy; and what to do when we, as therapists, need professional help?

Choosing therapy as a profession

Is psychotherapy a profession we choose because of our own experience of mental health issues? Choosing a career is a complex decision, and personal experience of problems may be only part of the reason: however, it makes sense for us to choose a career path which we find personally engaging, for whatever reasons. To our knowledge, there is no study looking specifically at CBT psychotherapists. In one small study, Fussell and Bonney (1990) compared the childhood experiences of 42 psychotherapists and 38 physicists. The psychotherapists reported a comparatively high incidence of childhood trauma and emotional deprivation, suggesting that they were aware of the potential negative impact of the past on their present lives. They felt that their difficulties enhanced, instead of extinguished, their continuing interest in people. It makes sense that our personal experience can help us to understand those with similar backgrounds, and in certain professions may be an almost essential requirement. It is probably the case that some experience of emotional upset, which comes with the simple fact of being human, is an essential requirement for being an effective therapist. But with regard to the question of whether lifelong struggles with mental health issues are essential, or indeed make for good therapists, opinion may be divided. In my own experience, I have a particular interest in working with the cardiac rehabilitation service. I find that I can certainly empathize with my patient's experience of various medical tests and investigations, side effects of medication, and recovery from surgery—but I always have to be wary of comparing my patient's experience to my own, and listen to their stories with no bias from my own. We need to be aware of our own issues and their impact on therapy through careful use of regular supervision, as illustrated below.

When our personal lives affect therapy

Although our patients may like to think of us as towers of granite, unfailingly there for them with unwavering attention, leaving all our 'baggage' on our doorsteps, in reality we are all too human and life takes its toll, as the following personal example illustrates.

> *When my father died, I took two weeks off before returning to work. When I returned, my first patient of the day, Angela, knew why I had taken leave and offered me her condolences. The session then focused on her difficulties coping with her elderly father who had terminal cancer. I was aware as she spoke of my own feelings coming to the surface, which made me want to steer the session away from the emotion in case I started crying. Angela, being a warm and sympathetic*

person, was all too aware of what was going on. Half-way through the session, she stopped, looked aghast at me and said "Listen to me going on about my father. At least I still have him, unlike you. I am so sorry, I've been so selfish".

In this case, it was clear that my own grief around losing my father meant that it almost became unclear who was the patient, and we potentially swapped roles. I was also unclear about how to deal with my own distress. I felt a moment of panic—I am going to start crying. I mustn't cry—and a dilemma about which direction to go in: should I stop the session and say that I am not able to continue? In fact, I pushed down my own feelings, told Angela that the therapy time was for her, not for me, and that she could say whatever she liked to me. She changed the subject and talked instead about her young grand-daughter. We seemed to get back on track, somehow. After the session, I locked myself in the loo and howled.

These moments affect all of us at some stage, and mean that at times of difficulty in our own lives, we need to ask ourselves whether we are sufficiently OK to be working. Sometimes we do not know until a situation such as above arises. In my case, I thought that I was more OK than I actually was, that I could simply put my own feelings on the back burner, which in retrospect was a mistake. It would, perhaps, have been better to stay away from clinical work for a little longer, which is, however, not always possible within a busy NHS (National Health Service) setting. I realize that my patient, Angela, would be fine and understanding if I cancelled sessions; however, other patients find cancellations much more difficult. I also recognized that I needed more time to grieve, and was able to share a very informal SP/SR arrangement with a friend and colleague who had also lost her father recently. We also need to be aware of our own beliefs which impact on how we look after ourselves: for example, 'I should be OK', 'I'm a therapist, I can cope with this' and 'My personal feelings and reactions can be neatly tidied away when necessary' may get in the way of us taking time out when we need it.

When personal beliefs affect treatment

In addition to what is going on in our lives, our own beliefs impact on therapy, and may cause not only one-off but recurrent problems in our therapeutic style or process (Haarhoff, 2006; Persons, 1989; Sanders and Wills, 2006). One study has identified how therapists' beliefs about homework, such as 'it makes me feel like a teacher' and 'I don't like to put pressure on my patients', may cause homework-setting to be rushed or trivialized (Haarhoff and Kazantzis, 2007). Core beliefs about being a caring person, whereas others are needy and vulnerable, may lead us to focus on empathy and allowing the client to talk uninterruptedly, not allowing time for collaboratively worked on interventions. Other beliefs which might affect us include: 'It is wrong to dislike/disagree with/feel attracted to/be angry with my patients'; 'I must cure everyone I see, otherwise I'm a useless therapist'; or 'I'm totally responsible for whether or not my therapy is successful' (Gilbert and Leahy, 2007; Sanders and Wills, 2006). Such rules are likely to interfere with the therapeutic relationship: if you have particular feelings or thoughts that contravene your rules, then they may be ignored or put back on to the patient, rather than be actively used in therapy (Haarhoff, 2006). If, for example, you are feeling annoyed with a patient, which is not an uncommon reaction, but you also believe that you must never show or share this annoyance, you may be more likely to think 'So and so is being irritating: it is his fault: I won't let it affect me', rather than stopping and thinking what exactly is going on to arouse these feelings of annoyance in you—and therefore gain potentially valuable insights. Sometimes our annoyance, anger, or attraction is reflecting whatever is going on for the patient, and needs examining.

A rule of thumb is to first be able to spot when our own beliefs may be getting in the way, and second, find a potential solution. Spotting difficulties can be enormously helped by taking a compassionate and reflective view of our own work. Using thought records and therapy tapes, we can ask ourselves questions such as:

- How did that go?
- Was there a problem?
- How did the patient make me feel?
- What goes through my mind when I think about the patient?
- Are there 'oughts', 'shoulds', or 'musts'?
- What is making it difficult to really understand and empathize with this person?
- Am I making assumptions?
- What does the patient need right now?
- What do I need?

Sometimes finding an image of the patient can be helpful in pointing toward our own feelings: seeing our patients as ever-hungry babies or seeing yourself as a wise owl or a helpful teacher may indicate that we are feeling the need to cure, or teach, or take care of the patients, to a degree which risks losing collaboration. Feeling dragged down into the mud at the thought of seeing our patients means that we may be feeling stuck due to chronic avoidance, by ourselves or the patients. Negative feelings in general toward our patients are useful pointers to issues going on in the therapeutic relationship, and we cannot automatically assume they arise from the patient, but may be pointers that we need to focus on ourselves.

We cannot stress too much the importance of taking supervision in these situations. Self-reflection can take us a certain distance, but our interpersonal styles may have become so ingrained over many years that we may simply not notice what is obvious to the external observer (Bennett-Levy and Thwaites, 2007). Various CBT resources are now available to help therapists work with their beliefs and assumptions (Bennett-Levy and Thwaites, 2007; Davis *et al.*, 2008; Gilbert and Leahy, 2007; Haarhof, 2006). The key is to tackle problems at an early stage and to be prepared to look at the process of the relationship when necessary. This does not mean that the relationship itself needs to be the focus of the therapy, but realizing that, even in short-term focused work, relationship issues can become a problem needing attention.

However good a therapist we are, however compassionate, it is likely that at times unhelpful thoughts and beliefs will be activated. We are after all humans interacting in a human situation, so our own views and experiences are bound to impinge on the relationship. All in all, we feel that we should, as Lao-Tzu advises, in the Tao te ching (Lao-Tzu, 1963) yield to our own fallibility in order to overcome the problems of therapist perfectionism. We should be ready to admit our mistakes, a gesture often appreciated by clients frequently burdened by a sense of their own fallibility.

When we need therapy ourselves

What do we as CBT therapists do when problems in our personal lives become too difficult to tackle on our own, and we need professional help? How do we spot such problems? From our earlier examples, the latter is probably the more difficult: knowing and admitting that we need help. Often it is our close friends and relatives who can identify problems before we are aware of them, and taking their advice is often far more important than listening to our own, inevitably biased, judgements. Knowing our own distress signatures is important: for example, the more stressed I get, the more work I take on, and the more unrealistic my expectations of myself, a condition well-recognized by my husband long before the penny drops for me. I personally feel that colleagues working in a mental health setting have an ethical responsibility to keep an eye open for other colleague's well-being, which may mean a difficult discussion about what he or she needs.

Once we make the decision to undergo formal therapy, we face the same question that our clients ask: what type of therapist and form of therapy is going to be right for me at this time for this particular issue (Wilkins, 2006)?

Where do I find a suitable therapist? Should I choose another CBT therapist or go for another model?

Therapists seek therapy for three main reasons: personal growth, personal problems, and personal training, with personal growth being the most commonly cited reason for undertaking therapy (Orlinsky *et al.*, 2005). Being able to identify what we are looking for helps us choose where to go: is it for specific problems, such as anxiety, panic, or depression, or are we identifying chronic difficulties, suggesting schema issues? Is the problem within our relationship at home, and do we need relationship therapy? As for assessing the needs of our patients, assessing our own can be vital, either alone or within SP/SR arrangement.

Should CBT therapists choose CBT therapists for therapy, or therapists from different orientations? Interestingly, CBT therapists seeking therapy tend to choose orientations other than CBT (Orlinsky *et al.*, 2001). Although choosing a therapist of the same orientation can be affirming and informative, Christine Padesky (1996) stresses the value of using another CBT therapist: 'It is helpful for cognitive therapists to seek cognitive therapy when in need of psychotherapy. Cognitive therapy initiated during a crisis can be extended to include identification and exploration of schema issues that may maintain problem patterns' (p. 288). She goes on to state, however, that it can be difficult to find another local therapist who is not also a colleague or friend (Padesky, 1996). Another potential problem is that being familiar with our therapist's model may mean we are overly aware of technique and therefore miss opportunities to look at things differently: 'I know what you are going to ask me next', or 'why hasn't she asked me the right questions' may get in the way of us being able to 'relax' into the role of patient.

Choosing a therapist working with a different model, such as person-centreed or psychodynamic, has disadvantages as well as advantages. Our commitment to a particular model such as CBT may be a matter of deeply held beliefs, and we may find it difficult to experience therapy coming from different approaches. For example, if you feel strongly that the collaborative and open nature of CBT is an empowering and essential way of working, psychoanalytic traditions may be uncomfortable—which is not to say that a different approach is not valuable. If you know that your problems fall into categories where the evidence falls in favour of CBT over other models, such as depression, then CBT may be your therapy of choice. If, however, you mainly want a chance to talk over difficulties, and find solutions yourself, a person-centreed approach might be appropriate.

When looking for a personal therapist, we should consider our purpose: personal growth, personal problems, or personal training. We should consider the fit between our worldview and that of the therapist. We should also take into account the data suggesting that alliance accounts for more of the variance in outcome than technique (Hubble *et al.*, 1999), a finding apparently mirrored in the CBT literature (Trepka *et al.*, 2004). Therefore, perhaps we should be guided by the advice we would give our own patients, or when hiring a builder or plumber: get recommendations, find out the background and professional qualifications of the therapist, and make sure your therapist can do the job you want, and is someone with whom you feel comfortable and can trust.

The last section of this chapter features an in-depth report of a mental health professional's experience of receiving long-term CBT. We learn from the inside how and why the patient, Jess, experiences CBT as so valuable. In particular, she highlights both the importance of the therapeutic relationship—frequently illustrated with comments about empathy, genuineness, trust, curiosity, validation, and interest. And she also notes how effective CBT formulation and specific techniques can be. If as readers we can imbibe Jess' story, we too can gain quite a different and unique understanding about the process of therapy.

Jess: Physicians can't always heal themselves: a health professional's account of receiving CBT for multiple problems

I am a 38-year-old mental health professional. I was referred for CBT by my general practitioner (GP), having spent my adult life trying to overcome a number of difficulties on my own, and using knowledge gained from my professional training. These difficulties included anorexia and bulimia, panic attacks, low mood, obsessional thoughts, and perfectionist beliefs. At the core of these difficulties were low self-esteem, and being cut off from, and frightened of, emotions.

Somewhat ironically then, I went to the first CBT assessment appointment thinking I didn't have sufficient problems to 'deserve' help. I was *convinced* that the psychologist who saw me would conclude the same and 'reject' me straight away. I was shocked and horrified when I was accepted for therapy, concluding that I must have misled my therapist into thinking I was worthy of any help. This experience activated a whole set of beliefs and interpersonal difficulties that were to underlie, if not dominate, my experience of therapy. After that first assessment session I became unable to think about anything else other than 'having misled the therapist'. I couldn't eat, sleep, work, or engage with my family and friends.

This reaction to assessment and being offered therapy really surprised me. It has made me more aware of how the assessment process may activate core beliefs for people and that waiting for therapy, particularly having already been assessed, can be very difficult. Clients usually have to manage these difficulties without any interim therapeutic support. Fortunately, when it became clear how I had reacted to assessment, I was offered three scheduled telephone contacts to help me 'keep going' until therapy started. However, by the time therapy started (only a couple of months later) my mental health had deteriorated, and the first 18 months or so of CBT were extremely hard. Although I was 100% committed to therapy, engagement in it and forming a trusting therapeutic relationship were major problems that had to be addressed in order for me to make progress.

Engagement, early therapy, and the interpersonal relationship

At the outset I had a lot of thoughts that actively interfered with each therapy session. Firstly, dependency on anyone else was anathema. It took me some time to find a position of semi-dependence on my therapist which was needed to work effectively in therapy. Also, beliefs about my appearance ('I'm so repulsive') and my social skills ('I'm boring and thick') meant that I hated being seen by people and hated having to talk to people, both clearly problematic in a therapeutic relationship. I was, without doubt, the worst person imaginable; therefore everything I said in therapy was not to be trusted. I didn't deserve any therapy time and I certainly did not deserve to make any sort of recovery. Crucially, I fully expected abandonment, disgust, and criticism from the therapist.

Therefore, absolutely fundamental to my experience of therapy has been establishing a good therapeutic relationship. Without this, no manner of well-executed CBT techniques would have had any effect. To my surprise it took me almost two years to trust my therapist. It took a lot of misunderstandings and several therapeutic ruptures to reach a position where I genuinely realized that this person was reliable, dependable, and consistent. He was not going to suddenly disappear or abandon me. He was trying his best to help me, even though I found it very painful. He persisted with trying to help me even though I was certain about my beliefs.

I now think it's important, as a therapist, to have a reasonably robust sense of self and a relative ease with being alive. I learnt to feel safe in the room because my therapist conveyed a sense of solidity, that is, 'I'm OK, I can handle this, I am calm'. It also meant that we could work through therapy misunderstandings without fear that this would taint the rest of therapy. I reflect back on therapy I have given and wonder how different it would have been had I been both clearer about, and happier with, who I was.

Throughout therapy I have been extremely oversensitive to interpersonal cues and construed meanings from my therapist's behaviour. So, for example, if my therapist was one minute late, according to the waiting room clock, it meant he was really dreading seeing me. I would scrutinize his expression and tone of voice when he greeted me in the waiting room to try and ascertain his state of mind. I was highly sensitive to small changes in my therapist's mood and made catastrophic interpretations about these (e.g. therapist is a fraction less cheerful than usual, therefore he's depressed, therefore he'll go off sick from work and abandon me). Having my homework handed back to me 'meant' I was being rejected/it was too boring to keep. The only day my therapist was ill I was convinced he was going to die and I waited to be contacted with news of his death. It sounds irrational with hindsight but it was very real to me, and repeatedly intruded on the therapy process. Attendance to these sensitivities using a cognitive behavioural framework provided a very rich source for learning in therapy.

Some of my intratherapy behaviour would have been difficult for me to deal with, particularly as a novice therapist. For example, when any emotional subject matter was touched on, particularly relating to sadness, I would grin broadly and laugh inappropriately. Such incongruence of affect could easily disconcert or trigger judgements in the mind of the therapist. This was, however, my way of coping with uncomfortable feelings, given that I had no way of escaping them in the session, and served as a way of dismissing anything emotional. It was certainly a response learnt through my upbringing. My therapist was probably rather startled by this but he took the time to understand what it was about and linked it into our formulation. I also learnt from this that if, as therapist, one is feeling frustrated or bewildered by a client's unusual behaviour in a session, bear in mind that your client is employing the best coping strategy he/she can in that moment of time. The client may be acutely aware of his/her behaviour and be highly critical of himself/herself for it too.

I was struck by how gruelling and exhausting therapy was. I absolutely dreaded attending! Waiting in the waiting room with other people, all of whom I was sure were much more 'deserving' than me made me feel really ashamed. Sitting in the therapy room, feeling bombarded with feelings I could neither work out, nor escape, was really stressful. I always felt extremely tired and raw after therapy, particularly for the first 18 months or so. I quickly learnt that having any engagement immediately after therapy was a bad idea. I found that I needed a couple of hours to recover from each session and start to reflect, though it would usually take some days to truly be able to think a bit more objectively. My partner learnt to steer clear of me after therapy sessions as I was much more irritable, preoccupied, and withdrawn.

Having this experience made me realize that I have practiced with the belief that therapy should be a comfortable, almost enjoyable experience for the recipient. However, I have come to realize this is not how it has to be to be effective. For me, therapy was a physically painful experience, probably because of my specific difficulties with emotions. There were numerous times when, if it wasn't for my own professional background, and my ultimate trust in my therapist, I'd have cancelled or even dropped out of therapy. I am more sensitive to this with my own clients now and at the end of a difficult session, I try to troubleshoot any difficulties which may lead to future non-attendance.

CBT-specific reflections

Reflecting on specific CBT skills and techniques that I experienced, several are particularly memorable. Setting an agenda every session was always important. I have often felt uncomfortable using this exact term with my own clients, thinking it sounds too business-like and uncaring. However, therapy without an agenda would have been unhelpful and unproductive. I found that agenda-setting reduced my anxiety about sitting in the sessions as I wasn't on edge all session wondering what the therapist was going to bring up. It fostered a true sense of collaboration and transparency.

Socratic questioning is clearly a fundamental part of CBT. What was especially valuable about this for me was that my therapist was not making assumptions. He probably had some pretty good ideas of the answers to some of his questions but to appear genuinely curious allowed me to clarify some details and, particularly importantly, helped me to feel understood.

Having the therapist point out that, while I might tend to see the world in black and white terms, it didn't mean that *he* did, was really valuable. I can remember my therapist saying 'Yes, that could be true, but so could…'; 'That's possible but is it really likely or not?' I really didn't like this as I wanted '*certainty*' and not to talk in probabilities. I thought 'This middle ground is *so* unrealistic!' However, with repetition it became more tolerable as a concept. My therapist also highlighted that I *start off* from a position (a core belief) rather than *conclude it* on the basis of evidence. I was similarly very doubtful about this, but with time this too made sense.

In the session, I noticed that strong emotion, shame in particular, made it extremely difficult to think about my thoughts. Often, when talking about core issues, I couldn't think at all. I can best describe it as hearing the words, recognizing that they were in English, but being completely unable to translate them into anything that made any sense. At times like this I found diagrams helpful; having something written down on a whiteboard helped me focus and helped my understanding.

The educational component of therapy was one of the things that I valued the most. Lots of questions cropped up that I simply couldn't answer. For example, 'What sort of positive feelings are there?'; 'How do you distinguish between different types?' Here, judicious use of self-disclosure was extremely helpful. This wasn't about the therapist disclosing anything really personal, he simply modeled some normal thoughts, feelings, and behaviours. I'd have found a glib 'Well, what do you think?' very unhelpful as I just hadn't a clue and I lacked the knowledge to enable me to develop a view.

I really liked having homework! It helped me feel like I was doing everything I could between sessions to help myself. It also helped me feel less alone with the difficulties I was struggling with. There were often things I couldn't comprehend at all in therapy that a homework task would help me process between sessions.

As a therapist I sometimes think 'Well, we've talked about this already, and that hasn't worked, so I need to try a different approach', that is, there is something 'wrong' with the treatment strategies I'm using, or the original formulation. However, I found repetition of formulations, maintenance cycles, and alternative coping strategies really important. Often these things don't sink in first time around and need to be reiterated, rather than necessarily reinvented.

Difficulties that I had with CBT

Aside from the problems I had forming a trusting therapeutic relationship, I had several specific difficulties with CBT.

I am already quite a logical, scientific person. I come from a family in which 'be sensible and unemotional' were key messages. At first I felt that CBT was simply reinforcing these messages so I did not feel understood. I could, after all, be analytical and unemotional; but that was clearly insufficient on its own.

In a similar vein, I had gone too far with my version of self-CBT in that I went straight to analysing and changing my thoughts in a situation, giving no thought or weight to any feelings. I had used CBT to eradicate feelings from my life. I found it confusing that I was actually being encouraged to attend to feelings in therapy. I now understand that feelings are important too and shouldn't be completely ignored or reasoned away.

I didn't enjoy having my beliefs directly challenged; in fact I found this extremely uncomfortable. I think this is because I considered them to be 100% accurate and therefore not negotiable. They were 'facts' not 'thoughts'. They were also central to my identity and I didn't have any alternatives to believe. I also interpreted these challenges as meaning that 'my therapist thinks I'm stupid'. However, I can see that, in the long run, my discomfort may have been necessary. One of my beliefs was that I was 'the most terrible person in the world'. Now, with some distance from that belief, any approach other than questioning its validity doesn't really make sense. Sometimes though, an empathic, compassionate response helped much more than head-to-head challenging, particularly with regards to self-critical thoughts. I think it's really important to strike a balance between challenging beliefs and encouraging more rational responses, with validating a person's feelings and making sure they feel understood.

Advice for therapists

In one's attempt to be a good CBT therapist, I think it's crucial not to lose sight of the fundamental importance of a warm and strong therapeutic alliance.

For me therapy was helpful mainly because of this relationship. Specific cognitive behavioural techniques were less important, although conceptualizing problems using this model and being truly collaborative were essential. Also, don't underestimate the impact of giving a fundamentally human response to your client. I remember an occasion when I shared a belief about myself with my therapist. He simply looked me in the eye and said 'I don't think so'. That genuine response really surprised and affected me.

Try not to get bogged down by someone's complex history. Keep hopeful, it's contagious! I think my number of difficulties, on paper, could make me look like a real 'heart sink' patient. It is important to acknowledge, understand, and validate someone's history, but to remember that here-and-now change is absolutely possible, and probably needs to be the main focus. Also, sometimes the simplest techniques make the most impact; in my case the use of an activity diary.

Sometimes I think we assume that people who generate 'yes buts' in therapy 'don't want to change'; they are just unhelpfully coming up with difficulties, rather than gracefully accepting the sensible alternative suggested by the therapist! My 'yes buts' were frequent, but it was absolutely ok to express these. The therapist did not take them personally or respond to them in an irritated way, indeed he seemed genuinely interested in what the 'yes but' was. For me this was crucial—I could do the basic cognitive challenges but these 'yes buts' were really blocking me on a day-to-day basis outside of the therapy room.

Therapist enthusiasm and cheerfulness in response to my positive reports actually increased my anxiety ('now I'll be abandoned') and my feelings of guilt ('I'm bad so I don't deserve positive things'). For me it was much more rewarding to recognize that I was trying really hard and 'making some progress but not yet "better"'. This really enabled me to consolidate on any positive experiences I was having.

As a mental health professional I value kindness and have always felt uncomfortable being more challenging in style. However, this experience has reminded me that warmth and compassion are rarely enough on their own, particularly with complex difficulties. So now I spend a little less time being empathic, and a little more time being challenging. So far this change hasn't had any disastrous effects and seems to be helping people.

I think that in some spheres there is a tendency to be rather reductionist about CBT; that it's 'simply' about changing unhelpful patterns of thinking. Yet I experienced many of the intricacies of CBT, with a focus on meta-cognitive and interpersonal processes. My therapist clearly had CBT as his model but it's the process, the relationship and the learning through conversation that has made the most impact for me. For me professionally I have become aware that there is enough to think about in order to do CBT well, without worrying about being integrative and using other therapeutic models.

What I think I'll have learnt

Reflecting on what I've learnt from therapy is difficult at the moment; as my CBT is ongoing; but I have a sense that its effects will be quite profound. There are a lot of specific things that I have learnt, for example, about the nature of feelings. Regular reference back to a formulation has helped me develop a less critical understanding of my difficulties. I am much less anxious, my self-esteem is improving, and my daily life is more manageable.

I know there will also be a lot of things that I will take away from therapy that it is harder to quantify. Most of these have been learnt through the therapeutic relationship. I have told someone all the 'terrible' things about me and he has not acted as though I am the worst person alive. The mere fact that someone has been prepared to give me his time, considered me worthy of help and persisted, despite my intransigence, means a great deal.

I think therapy is also changing my personality. It seems to be helping me form a sense of identity, feel braver about having opinions, and be more prepared to take risks. As my difficulties started as a young adolescent, I feel that therapy has given me the space and encouragement to grow up.

Key points

- CBT therapists have been slow to recognize the value of CBT for themselves both for professional and personal development. There are now a range of self-experiential options available to CBT therapists for enhancing skills, identifying and changing beliefs and assumptions, addressing personal problems, and engaging in other personal development. Possibilities range from SP/SR to personal therapy.
- Our choice of method to use for ourselves should be determined by a range of factors such as: our aims (personal growth, personal problems, or personal training?), our context (with others? colleagues, friends, not known?), ensuring a sense of safety, and ensuring we have the time, resources, and motivation to reflect and engage with the work.
- With the ever greater demands of CBT therapists, we may find considerable survival benefit in applying our tools of the trade to ourselves.

Further reading

Bennett-Levy, J., Turner, F., Beaty, T., Smith, M., Paterson, B. and Farmer, S. (2001). The value of self-practice of cognitive therapy techniques and self-reflection in the training of cognitive therapists. *Behavioural and Cognitive Psychotherapy*, **29**, 203–220.

Butler, G. and Hope, T. (2008). *Manage your Mind.* Oxford: Oxford University Press.

Gilbert, P. and Leahy, R.L. (2007). *The Therapeutic Relationship in Cognitive Behavioural Psychotherapies.* London: Routledge.

Kottler, J. (1993). *On being a Therapist.* Englewood Cliffs, NJ: Jossey-Bass.

Yalom, Y.D. (2003). *The Gift of Therapy: Reflections on being a Therapist.* London: Piatkus.

References

BABCP (2000). *Minimum Training Standards for the Practice of CBT.* London: BABCP.

Beck, J.S. (1995). *Cognitive Therapy: Basics and Beyond.* New York: Guildford.

Beck, J.S. and Butler, A.C. (2005). Treating psychotherapists with cognitive therapy, in Geller, J.D., Norcross, J.C. and Orlinsky, D.E. (eds.), *The Psychotherapists' Own Psychotherapy.* New York: Oxford University Press, pp. 254–264.

Beck, A.T., Steer, R.A., Ball, R. and Ranieri, W. (1996). Comparison of Beck Depression Inventories—I and II in psychiatric outpatients. *Journal of Personality Assessment*, **67**, 588–597.

Bennett-Levy, J., Turner, F., Beaty, T., Smith, M., Paterson, B. and Farmer, S. (2001). The value of self-practice of cognitive therapy techniques and self-reflection in the training of cognitive therapists. *Behavioural and Cognitive Psychotherapy*, **29**, 203–220.

Bennett-Levy, J., Lee, N., Travers, K., Pohlman, S. and Hamernik, E. (2003). Cognitive therapy from the inside: enhancing therapist skills through practising what we preach. *Behavioural and Cognitive Psychotherapy*, **31**, 145–163.

Bennett-Levy, J. and Thwaites, R. (2007). Self and self-reflection in the therapeutic relationship: a conceptual map and practical strategies for the training, supervision and self-supervision of interpersonal skills, in Gilbert, P. and Leahy, R. (eds.), *The Therapeutic Relationship in the Cognitive Behavioural Therapies.* London: Routledge, pp. 255–281.

Bennett-Levy, J., Thwaites, R., Chaddock, A. and Davis, M. (2009). Reflective practice in cognitive behavioural therapy: the engine of lifelong learning, in Stedmon, J. and Dallos, R. (eds.), *Reflective Practice in Psychotherapy and Counselling.* Maidenhead: Open University Press.

Davis, M., Thwaites, R., Freeston, M., Bennett-Levy, J. and Chaddock, A. (2008). *SP/SR with Experienced CBT Therapists: A Measurable Impact on Beliefs and Therapeutic Skills.* BABCP Conference. Edinburgh.

EABCT (2000). *Minimum Training Standards.* Utrecht: EABCT.

Fussell, F.W. and Bonney, W.C. (1990). A comparative study of childhood experiences of psychotherapists and physicists: implications for clinical practice. *Psychotherapy: Theory, Research, Practice, Training*, **27**, 505–512.

Gilbert, P. and Leahy, R.L. (2007). *The Therapeutic Relationship in Cognitive Behavioural Psychotherapies.* London: Routledge.

Gilroy, P.J., Carroll, L. and Murra, J. (2002). A preliminary survey of counseling psychologists' personal experiences with depression and treatment. *Professional Psychology, Research and Practice*, **33**, 402–407.

Haarhoff, B. (2006). The importance of identifying and understanding therapist schema in cognitive therapy training and supervision. *New Zealand Journal of Psychology*, **35**, 126–131.

Haarhoff, B. and Kazantzis, N. (2007). How to supervise the use of homework in cognitive behavior therapy: the role of trainee therapist beliefs. *Cognitive and Behavioral Practice*, **14**, 325–332.

Hubble, M.A., Duncan, B.L. and Miller, S.D. (1999). *The Heart and Soul of Change: What Works in Therapy.* Washington, DC: American Psychological Association.

Laireiter, A-R. and Willutzki, U. (2003). Self-reflection and self-practice in training of cognitive behaviour therapy: an overview. *Clinical Psychology and Psychotherapy*, **10**, 19–30.

Lao-tzu, L. (1963). *Tao te ching.* London: Penguin Classics.

Macran, S. and Shapiro, D. (1998). The role of personal therapy for therapists: a review. *British Journal of Medical Psychology*, **71**, 13–25.

Moorey, S., Williams, R. and Cobb, J. (1990). The Institute of Psychiatry cognitive behaviour therapy course. *Psychiatric Bulletin*, **14**, 219–221.

Norcross, J. (2005). The psychotherapists own psychotherapy: educating and developing psychologists. *American Psychologist*, **60**, 840–850.

Orlinsky, D.E., Botermans, J.F., Rønnestad, M.H. and the SPR Collaborative Research Network (2001). Towards an empirically grounded model of psychotherapy training: four thousand therapists rate influences on their development. *Australian Psychologist*, **36**, 139–148.

Orlinsky, D.E., Rønnestad, M.H., Willutzski, U., Wiseman, H., Botermans, J.F. and the SPR Collaborative Research Network (2005). The prevalence and parameters of personal therapy in Europe and elsewhere, in Geller, J.D., Norcross, J.C. and Orlinsky, D.E. (eds.), *The Psychotherapist's Own Psychotherapy.* New York: Oxford University Press, pp. 254–264.

Padesky, C.A. (1996). Developing cognitive therapist competency: teaching and supervision models, in Salkovskis, P.M. (ed.), *Frontiers of Cognitive Therapy.* New York: Guilford, pp. 266–292.

Persons, J.B. (1989). *Cognitive Therapy in Practice: A Case Formulation Approach.* New York: W.W. Norton.

Sanders, D. (2006). *Will I Still Be Me? A Journey Through a Transplant.* Charlbury, Oxfordshire: Day Books.

Sanders, D. (2008). When therapist turns patient. *Journal of Healthcare Counselling and Psychotherapy*, **8**, 22–25.

Sanders, D. and Wills, F. (2006). *Cognitive Therapy: An Introduction.* London: Sage.

Schutte, N., Toppinen, S., Kalimo, R. and Schaufeli, W. (2000). The factorial validity of the Maslach Burnout Inventory-General Survey (MBI-GS) across occupational groups and nations. *Journal of Occupational and Organizational Psychology*, **73**, 53–66.

Trepka, C., Rees, A., Shapiro, D.A., Hardy, G.E. and Barkham, M. (2004). Therapist competence and outcome of cognitive therapy for depression. *Cognitive Therapy and Research*, **28**, 143–157.

Wilkins, P. (2006). Personal and professional development, in Feltham, C. and Horton, I. (eds.), *The Sage Handbook of Counselling and Psychotherapy*. Second edition. London: Sage, pp. 158–165.

Index